P9-BIC-962

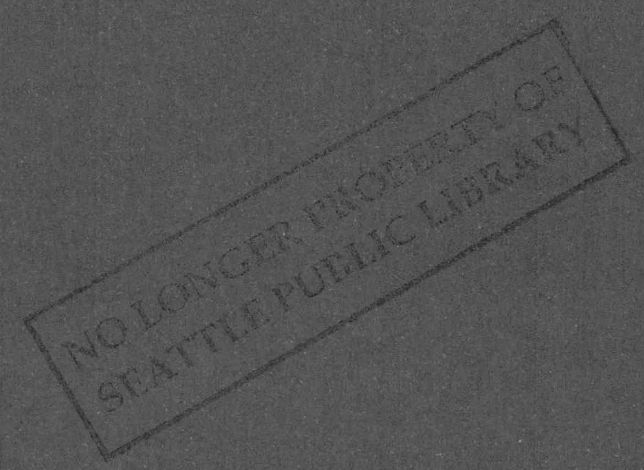
NO LONGER PROPERTY OF
SEATTLE PUBLIC LIBRARY

INTEGRATIVE NUTRITION

A Whole-Life Approach to Health and Happiness

INTEGRATIVE NUTRITION

A Whole-Life Approach to Health and Happiness

Joshua Rosenthal, MScEd

FOUNDER AND DIRECTOR, INSTITUTE FOR INTEGRATIVE NUTRITION

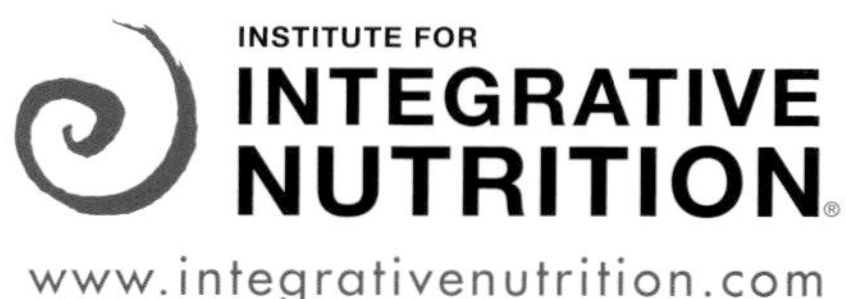

www.integrativenutrition.com

Integrative Nutrition: A Whole-Life Approach to Health and Happiness

ISBN: 978-1-941908-08-2 (hardcover)
ISBN: 978-1-941908-09-9 (e-book)

Library of Congress Control Number: 2017954818

Published by Integrative Nutrition, Inc., New York, NY
www.integrativenutrition.com

Notice: This book is not intended to replace recommendations or advice from physicians or other healthcare providers. Rather, it is intended to help you make informed decisions about your health and to cooperate with your healthcare provider in a joint quest for optimal wellness. If you suspect you have a medical problem, we urge you to seek medical attention from a competent healthcare provider.

Printed in China

10 9 8 7 6 5 4 3 2 1

Fourth Edition

This book is dedicated to the health and happiness of people throughout the world and to the future of nutrition, which will offer new possibilities for everyone.

Contents

Acknowledgments

I am grateful for the work I do every day and the opportunity to interact with so many intelligent, motivated people who share a vision to improve health and happiness in the world.

I would especially like to thank:

Those who supported in the creation of this book: Suzanne Boothby, Tim Tate, Joline Seavey, Shannon Howard, Bonnie Brinegar, and Amie Olson

The staff of Integrative Nutrition (IIN)—you all contribute to the mission of the school. Your vision, creativity, intelligence, love, and support consistently take the school to new levels

The guest speakers who continue to inspire my students and offer new perspectives on the health and nutrition puzzle

The students, graduates, and their clients who helped shape my view of things and have helped to spread health and happiness in the world

The love of my life, Alexandra Anzalone, for her daily love and support

My dear parents for their love and encouragement

My friends who add love, laughter, and support to my life

Anyone who has ever purchased my books, joined the school's community, and everyone I've met along the way.

This book could not have happened without you.

Other Titles by Joshua Rosenthal

The Integrative Nutrition Cookbook: Simple recipes for health and happiness

The Power of Primary Food: Nourishment Beyond the Plate

Crack the Code on Cravings: What Your Cravings Really Mean

Serendipity: How to Attract a Life You Love (Second Edition)

Integrative Nutrition Daily Journal

Nutrición Integrativa: Alimenta tu salud & felicidad

Foreword

A huge contributing factor to illness in the 21st century is stress. Stress is best defined as the perception of physical or psychological threat. While we are no longer threatened by predatory species, our bodies and minds have started perceiving everyday situations, such as traffic, career stress, and endless to-do lists as threatening.

To prevent illness, we must learn to reduce stress; and to reduce stress, we must consider what impacts a person's life, such as their relationships, career, and spirituality.

A complete approach considers them all, and health coaches are a modern application of that approach. They work with clients to find balance in every area of their lives, understanding that true nourishment is not just about the food on your plate, but what is happening in your everyday life.

As a physician and teacher, I have had the privilege of speaking at many universities, schools, and institutions. I have had the pleasure of speaking at Joshua Rosenthal's school, the Institute for Integrative Nutrition (IIN), which, for over 25 years, has been training Health Coaches around the world.

In this book, you will discover the power of the work that Joshua and his students are doing to transform healthcare from the inside out. You will learn about the unique concepts he teaches at the school, that Integrative Nutrition Health Coaches practice around the world, including the concept of bio-individuality—one man's food is another man's poison. Beyond that, you will learn how to take back control of your own health—not just your physical health, but your mental, emotional, and physical health as well.

Keep an open mind as you read this book, as it will undoubtedly transform your perspective of, and relationship, with your health.

Deepak Chopra, MD, FACP, *founder of the Chopra Foundation, cofounder of the Chopra Center for Wellbeing, and IIN Visiting Teacher*

How to Use This Book

Set an Intention

To help you prepare for the journey ahead, please take a moment now to clarify your personal goals around health and well-being. What are your main health concerns? What is it you wish to learn or accomplish by reading this book? Devoting a small amount of time now to understanding your optimal personal nutrition will result in a healthier, happier future later.

Experiment

In this book, you will find discussion of major dietary theories, but the food that is best for you is not going to be found in the pages of a nutrition book. No one diet is perfect for everyone. To best determine what is appropriate for your unique body and lifestyle, this book will guide you through experimenting with new foods and learning to listen to your body's responses.

Be Open to Discovery

A permanent shift in health may seem like a big challenge requiring a lot of dedication, but this approach is not about acquiring more self-discipline or willpower. It's about personally discovering what feeds you, what nourishes you, and, ultimately, what makes your life extraordinary.

Climb One Rung of the Ladder at a Time

With this book, you will unlearn old habits and absorb new information. Give yourself permission to go slowly. Big changes do not require big leaps. As far as your body is concerned, permanent change is more likely to happen gradually rather than through severe, austere diets. Proceed with care for yourself. Have fun.

Introduction

We all eat, all day every day, and we all know the saying, "We are what we eat." But for some reason, no one knows what to eat. Should we eat more grapes or drink more red wine? Are eggs a good source of protein or a source of bad cholesterol? Do dairy foods help us gain weight or lose weight?

Nutrition is a funny science. It's the only field where people can scientifically prove opposing theories and still be right. In science, we stick to facts. The earth rotates on an axis around the sun. The freezing point of water is 32 degrees Fahrenheit/0 degrees Celsius. But we have yet to discover the same definitive truths about nutrition. We are only beginning to understand the relationship between our diet and our health. Despite all the nutritional research that's been done and all the diet books that have been published, most Americans are increasingly confused about food.

I have been working in the field of nutrition for more than 30 years, and what I've learned is that there is probably no one right way of eating. I keep an open mind about new ideas that are published and respect others who are bravely working in this still-emerging field. My own background is in macrobiotics, an approach to healthy eating and balanced living developed in Japan that emphasizes the importance of whole foods and a plant-based diet. I've always been fascinated by food and health, and I spent years experimenting with different ways of eating, noticing their effects and looking for the best ones for me and for my clients. I studied with the top macrobiotics experts and appreciated the simplicity and balance of their system. I spent years counseling and teaching others to follow the principles of macrobiotics to improve their health.

As I went along, I began to realize that macrobiotics was getting some people well but not everyone. I started thinking there is more to health than simply eating healthy food. What was the missing ingredient? As I began to work with more and more clients, I found some interesting results. Some of my clients got better if they ate more raw foods, while others got better if they ate fewer raw foods. I had one client who didn't get better until she started eating some high-quality dairy products, even though macrobiotics advises against eating dairy. For other clients, it didn't matter what they ate. They got well by leaving a dysfunctional career or falling in love.

The more I observed human behavior, the more convinced I became that the key to health is understanding each person's individual needs, rather than following a set of predetermined rules. I saw plenty of evidence that having happy relationships, a fulfilling career, an exercise routine, and a spiritual practice are even more important to health than daily diet. From these ideas, I developed the concepts of Integrative Nutrition.

As I began evolving this new approach with clients, their results improved dramatically. I found many people were hungry for information about how to create a happy, healthy life and relieved to discover an approach that is flexible, fun, and free of dogma and discipline. Drawing on my background in education, I started my own school to help individuals discover the foods and lifestyle choices that work best for them and to empower them to change the world.

Integrative Nutrition (IIN) is a thriving school and community dedicated to helping evolve the future of nutrition so that all beings can live healthier, happier, and more fulfilling lives. For almost 20 years, people traveled far and wide to study at IIN in New York City. We now offer a life-changing online course, allowing students from all over the world to experience our unique program. As we spread our message to a global audience, the IIN community has grown exponentially. We are now 100,000 strong, with students and graduates in all 50 states and more than 155 countries.

We are the only school in the world integrating all of the various dietary theories—combining the knowledge of traditional philosophies, like Ayurveda, macrobiotics, and Chinese medicine, with modern concepts like the USDA food guides, the glycemic index, the Zone, and raw foods. We teach more than 100 different dietary theories and address the fundamental concepts, issues, and ethics of eating in a modern world.

We combine this information with simple steps for living a more balanced life full of laughter, joy, and abundance. My intention is for you to uncover this process for yourself and share it with others.

I have noticed that, as people improve their health, they become empowered to pursue the life of their dreams—the life they came here to live. If this book found its way to you, or you found your way to this book, I trust it means you are a highly intelligent, highly sensitive human being with an appreciation for the benefits of whole foods and holistic living. Let this book empower you to stand up, speak up, and act up for what you believe to be true. May your aliveness create a ripple effect in the world, and may all your hopes and dreams come true.

Chapter 1

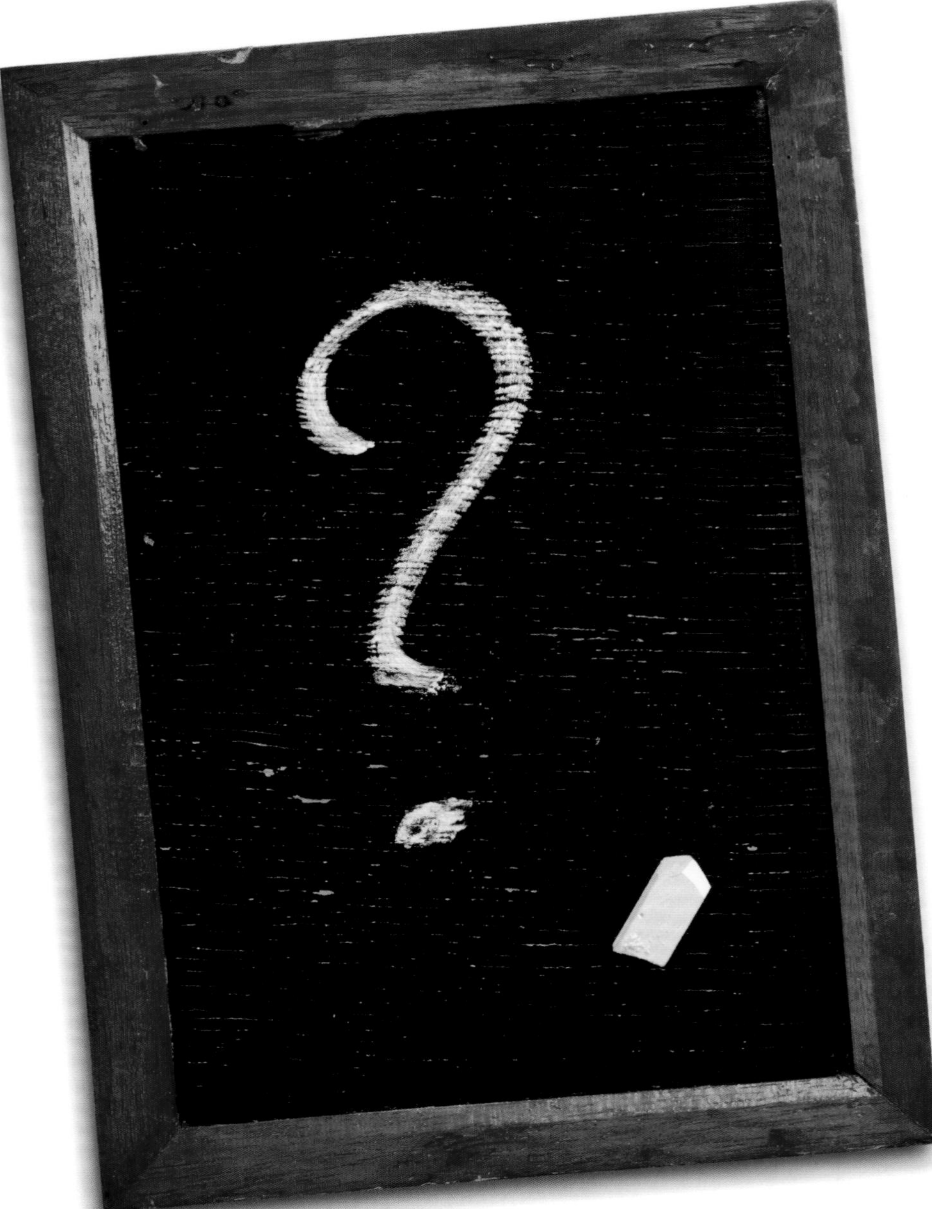

Question What You're Told

The important thing is not to stop questioning. Curiosity has its own reason for existing.

—Albert Einstein

The Global Health Crisis

It's no secret that we live amidst a healthcare crisis today. Rates of chronic lifestyle diseases continue to rise throughout the world. Healthcare is exceedingly expensive, particularly in the United States. Trillions of dollars are spent every year, while people become sicker than ever before. These high healthcare costs put a strain on individuals, governments, and companies alike.

How did we get here? On the most basic level, people today overexert their bodies. If life has a speed limit of working five days a week and resting two days, almost everyone exceeds it. We live with very little downtime, and then, on top of that, many people don't feed their body nutritious foods, don't sleep well, and don't move their bodies or spend much time in nature. We push, push, push our bodies, and then they break down.

What is most needed today is more education, support, and preventative measures to create lifelong healthy behaviors across the world. Instead, we have a system in which the cause of health problems isn't really addressed. Prescription medications and surgery remain the focus, while the lifestyle factors—diet, exercise, sleep, stress, and more—that actually contribute to disease have only recently entered the conversation.

Chronic diseases are the leading cause of death and disability in the U.S.[1] (and are growing throughout the world).[2]

"The worldwide increase of non-communicable diseases is a slow-motion disaster... But the unhealthy lifestyles that fuel these diseases are spreading with a stunning speed and sweep," said Margaret Chan, Director-General of the World Health Organization (WHO).[3]

I believe that just like a plant will lean toward the light, human beings will lean toward greater health. If we weren't influenced by millions of dollars of advertising and corporate agendas, we would instinctually eat well, take time to rest, and move our bodies naturally. We would take greater interest in and responsibility for our own self-care.

From my perspective, it all begins with the food we eat. People in many parts of the world have had little education about how to eat well and to live a healthy, happy life. We need change. The government isn't going to save us. Big companies aren't going to save us. It's people like you and me who can see the issues and want to be part of the solution who can make a difference.

When I started IIN, I was just one person who felt that if I could improve what people eat, I would play a role in making the world a better place. I started in New York City because it's a place that sets trends for the world. The United States has the security, freedom, and lifestyle desired by many people around the world. But Americans have become increasingly overweight, unhappy, and unhealthy. Every year, healthcare costs increase, while overall health decreases; people continue to eat poorly, don't get enough physical exercise, gain weight, and depend on medications and operations to maintain their health.

As our drinking and eating habits have spread throughout the world, so have our health concerns. People around the world are hungry for American products—movies, television shows, and cigarettes—and they love our food and drinks. American fast food restaurants and soda drinks can be found in every corner of the globe.

The results? We now have countries where more than 70% of the adult population is obese or overweight.[4] WHO estimates that, since 1980, worldwide prevalence of obesity has more than doubled. More than half (59%) of the population is now overweight or obese.[5] One-third of Mexicans are now clinically obese, while seven out of ten are considered overweight. They are rapidly catching up to America, where more than 70% of Americans 20 years of age or older are overweight or obese.[6]

After decades of food scarcity, the rates of obesity have more than doubled in China, and it now contends with the U.S. as the country with the largest population of overweight citizens. And it's not just city dwellers. In China, rates of overweight and obese children and adolescents are increasing rapidly in rural areas.[7] Overweight people now outnumber undernourished people in the world.[8] The WHO's estimates agree: Globally, there are about 1.9 billion overweight adults, and 600 million of them are obese; by contrast, about 800 million do not have enough to eat. Even Africa, a continent previously thought of as being synonymous with hunger and food scarcity, is seeing a drastic rise in obesity and diabetes.

I saw firsthand the spreading of American food and health concerns when I visited Japan in 2005, after having been there twelve years prior. On my first trip, I traveled throughout Japan with Michio and Aveline Kushi, founders of the macrobiotic movement. During this time, I was impressed with the health of the Japanese people and spoke with many of them about their traditional ways of eating. The people talked about the value of their diet, which was rich in organic whole grains, vegetables, sea vegetables, fish, and miso. They had perfect skin, clear eyes, slim bodies, and a strong sense of peace and tranquility. However, on my last trip, I was shocked by the extent to which people's health had declined. Fast food restaurants were everywhere. Many of the young Japanese people I saw were overweight, had acne, and were missing that healthy glow I remembered so fondly from years before.

Obesity rates are climbing. Worldwide, 422 million people have diabetes.[9] More than 14 million cases of cancer were detected globally in 2012, with rates expected to increase to 24 million by 2035.[10] Every day, 2,200 Americans die from cardiovascular disease, such as coronary heart disease, heart attacks, and stroke.[11] By 2030, almost 24 million people will die from heart disease, which is predicted to remain the single leading cause of death.[12] Why are we so unhealthy and overweight?

Originally, the medical establishment's aim was to promote healing, but it increasingly relies on a pro-business model instead of a pro-health model at the expense of patients. The goal has become to increase profit, decrease expenses, and let the chips fall where they may. This healthcare system is failing. In the U.S., Americans pay more for health insurance and have less time with doctors. Americans get more prescriptions and less guidance on how to create long-term health. U.S. health insurance today is really just prepaid medical expenses. Paying our monthly fees to insurance companies does not promise health; it just ensures that when you get sick you won't have to pay in full for your treatment.

The United States has the world's most expensive healthcare system. Yet, despite massive spending, Americans die earlier and experience higher rates of disease than people in other countries.[13] We suffer in increasing numbers from chronic health concerns, such as heart disease, obesity, diabetes, reproductive issues, and depression.

An exorbitant amount of money is spent on medications and operations, while virtually nothing is spent on prevention, education, and holistic health. The system is essentially saying, "Live it up. Do what you want, and when you get sick, we'll give you a magic pill that will make it all go away. If that pill doesn't work, we'll give you a different one, or a combination of a few, and if that doesn't work, we'll perform a quick operation, remove the problem, and you'll be as good as new." What kind of system is this? Instead of asking citizens to pay for more pills and doctor's bills, wouldn't it be better to spend money on answering the question: *What would it take to have a country full of healthy, happy people?*

But it is not just Americans suffering. Healthcare costs are straining governments and individuals around the world. About 150 million people a year are pushed into poverty by their medical bills.[14] Aging populations, the growing burden of chronic diseases, and more expensive treatments are the main challenges governments face in funding healthcare.

In Australia, the health system is too complicated for patients to navigate, according to the Organization for Economic Co-operation and Development (OECD), whose mission is to promote policies that will improve the economic and social well-being of people around the world.

> "...With an aging population and the anticipated rise in chronic disease, Australia needs to strengthen primary health care to better coordinate the care of patients," reads the 2015 OECD Health Care Quality Review of Australia. "Poor coordination of care increases the risk of medical errors that are unacceptable to patients and costly for the health system."[15]

2013
Health Care Spending

TOTAL HEALTH CARE SPENDING PER CAPITA[c]	
AUSTRALIA	$4,115[a]
CANADA	$4,569
DENMARK	$4,847
FRANCE	$4,361
GERMANY	$4,920
JAPAN	$3,713
NETHERLANDS	$5,131[b]
NEW ZEALAND	$3,855
NORWAY	$6,170
SWEDEN	$5,153
SWITZERLAND	$6,325[b]
UNITED KINGDOM	$3,364
UNITED STATES[c]	$9,086
OECD MEDIAN	$3,661

[a] 2012.

[b] Current spending only: excludes spending on capital formation of health care providers.

[c] Adjusted for differences in the cost of living.

SOURCE: OECD Health Data 2015.

In 2000, the World Health Organization completed the first ever assessment and comparison of the world's healthcare systems. Examining various data, including patient satisfaction, overall national health, medical responsiveness, and distribution of services amongst the population, they rated the healthcare systems of 191 countries. The United States ranked 37th, despite the fact that we spend the highest proportion (over 16%) of our gross domestic product on healthcare. The United States spends more than $8,500 per capita on medical care, compared with the average of more than $3,000 spent by other industrialized countries and twice as much as European countries, like the United Kingdom, Sweden, and France.[16] Our expenditure is significantly higher, yet we are the only industrialized nation that fails to offer universal healthcare to all of our citizens. In fact, uninsured Americans reached an all-time high in 2010 at almost 50 million people.[17] Many of these Americans forgo treatment because of prohibitive costs. Bankruptcy from lack of coverage and the excessive subsequent medical bills is commonplace. Job-based insurance premiums continue to rise, resulting in higher co-pays, deductibles, and out-of-pocket expenses, according to the 2012 Employer Health Benefits Survey by the Kaiser Family Foundation and the Health Research & Educational Trust. Even after much-needed reform, insurance coverage in the U.S. continues to be a complicated system, with premiums increasing in most states each year.

In addition, American patients report the greatest number of medical errors, including getting the wrong medication or dosage, incorrect test results, a mistake in treatment, or late notification about abnormal test results. It's the third leading cause of death in the U.S. today, ranking right below heart disease and cancer.[18] After carefully examining numerous indicators of performance, the Commonwealth Fund, a nonpartisan health policy think tank, gave the United States healthcare system a score of 64 out of a possible 100.[19] If we were in school, this grade would be equivalent to a big, fat D.

If you were shopping in a store that had high-priced and low-quality products along with poor customer service, chances are you would not go back to that store. Why do we continue to tolerate this archaic, ineffective form of healthcare? Before blood pressure units and stethoscopes, doctors in Asia went from village to village caring for their patients. Using their ancient, traditional, and so-called primitive skills of diagnosis, they would ask a few questions, look into a patient's eyes, check the tongue, take a pulse, and then make recommendations. The next year, when the doctor returned, he was paid only if the patient was still healthy. If the patient had been sick, the doctor was not paid. Now that's a healthy healthcare system!

My passionate prayer is that people in the U.S. will become increasingly vocal about the exceptionally high cost of healthcare and demand answers from government officials at the local, state, and federal levels. As Americans recognize the fundamental relationship between poor nutrition, expensive healthcare, and the lamentable state of the public's health, my hope is that we can begin to set new trends for the world. What we eat makes a huge difference, yet very few doctors, corporations, or politicians stand up for this truth.

The USDA

Good nutrition is straightforward and simple, but in America, pressure from the food industry makes it almost impossible for any public official to state the plain truth. Public nutrition policy is dictated by the political process, which is now heavily impacted by a corporate agenda to maximize profits.

The primary agency responsible for American food policy is the U.S. Department of Agriculture (USDA), which was created in 1862 as a regulatory agency to ensure an adequate and safe food supply for the American public. The agency also took on the role of providing dietary advice to the public. From the start, the government had conflicting priorities. How can you protect public health on one hand and protect the interests of the food industry on the other? This opposition alone has led to decades of confusing and economically charged dietary advice.

As far back as 1917, when the USDA released its first dietary recommendations and launched the food-group format, it ignored research that Americans were eating too much, especially too much fat and sugar, because food manufacturers wanted to encourage the public to eat more.[20] It wasn't until the 1970s, when senators like George McGovern started to speak about the connection between overeating—especially fats, sugar, salt, and cholesterol—and chronic disease, that the USDA began advising people to restrict these foods in their diets with the *Dietary Goals* of 1977. With this new advice came strong objections from the meat, dairy, and sugar industries.

The food industry's greatest allies are in Congress. It's the job of these politicians to protect the interests of their states, which includes not only the citizens but also the corporations and industries that operate there. So a senator from Texas will support the cattle industry. A senator from Wisconsin is going to fight for dairy by not allowing any wording into government guidelines that will negatively affect the dairy industry. Politicians, together with skilled, well-paid lobbyists, control legislation and nutritional information put out by the government. In 1977, when senators from meat-producing states such as Texas, Nebraska, and Kansas saw the new dietary guidelines, they worked quickly, with the help of lobbyists for the National Cattlemen's Beef Association, among others, to amend the national dietary recommendations, removing any mention of decreasing the amount of meat in one's diet for optimal health.

This back and forth between the USDA, politicians, and corporations continues to shape the public's awareness about what to eat. In 1991, the USDA and the Department of Health and Human Services (HHS) created the first ever Food Guide Pyramid in an attempt to provide accurate guidelines about what to eat for optimal nutrition. Immediately, the meat and dairy industries blocked publication because they claimed it stigmatized their products. Marion Nestle, professor and former chair of the Department of Nutrition at New York University, chronicled the saga in her pioneering book *Food Politics: How the Food Industry Influences Nutrition and Health*. The meat and dairy industries were upset because the Food Guide Pyramid placed their products in a category labeled "eat less." The USDA then withdrew the guide. It took more than a year to create a pyramid that was acceptable to the two industries. And that, my friends, is how our "politically correct" Food Guide Pyramid was created.

Let's take a moment to examine the pyramid that shaped American attitudes about health, diet, and nutrition for more than 20 years. The USDA designed the pyramid in hierarchical form to indicate the importance and recommended quantity of each food group. The broad foundation is carbohydrates, including bread, cereal, rice, and pasta. Next up is a slightly narrower band of fruits and vegetables, then a smaller layer of protein-rich foods, including meat and dairy. The very top has a small section of fats, oils and sweets.

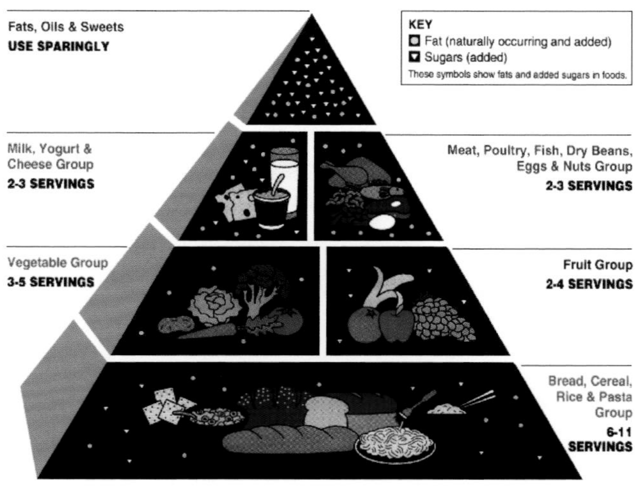

Source: U.S. Department of Agriculture/U.S. Department of Health and Human Services

Do you find anything odd about this picture? Anything you might question or disagree with? Almost everyone I meet has numerous issues with this pyramid. Even the experts who put it together must have known something was wrong here. Let's face it: The 1991 USDA Food Guide Pyramid is a political document, not a scientific one. It encourages people to eat a lot of everything. This advice certainly helps the food industry and the senators protecting their financial interests.

The insurance companies, politicians, and bureaucrats all advocated this Food Guide Pyramid from 1991 to 2005. The guidelines influenced government nutrition programs, food labeling, and food promotion. Nutrition professionals used this as their foundation for working with clients, as did the makers of school lunch programs. These recommendations were the foundation of America's outlook on health, diet, and nutrition for a time period that had a substantial increase in obesity and diet-related health concerns.

In 2001, the Physicians Committee for Responsible Medicine (PCRM) won a lawsuit on the topic of the USDA's ties to the food industry. PCRM objected to the over-promotion of meat and dairy products by the government because of the prevalence of diet-related diseases such as heart disease, diabetes, and hypertension. PCRM showed that the majority of the committee that reviews and updates the federal dietary guidelines had strong financial ties to the meat, dairy, or egg industries.

"Having advisors tied to the meat or dairy industries is as inappropriate as letting tobacco companies decide our standards for air quality," said Dr. Neal Barnard, president of PCRM.

The verdict found that the USDA had violated federal law by withholding documents that revealed a strong bias by the committee. PCRM's victory was a huge embarrassment to the USDA, especially because the government ruled against itself, which very rarely happens. Four years after the PCRM verdict, the Dietary Guidelines Advisory Committee reviewed and updated the dietary guidelines again. This time, they had the task of responding to recent statistics showing skyrocketing rates of obesity across the nation. The 2005 Dietary Guidelines were described as "the most health-oriented ever."

The report recommended that Americans eat more vegetables and whole grain products, cut down on certain fats, such as butter, margarine, and lard, and consume less sugar. The report strongly recommended that people "engage in regular physical activity and reduce sedentary activities to promote health, psychological well-being, and a healthy body weight." In other words: Get up, America, and start exercising.

Despite the improvements, the 2005 Dietary Guidelines still had many limitations. First, the guidelines were supposed to be about diet, and emphasizing weight loss through exercise shifts the responsibility for dietary change to the individual and away from the food industry's multibillion-dollar budget for marketing and promoting unhealthy foods. In addition, the guidelines didn't speak a language easily understood by the people who most needed the advice. Imagine if the guidelines said, "Stop eating Oreos, Jiffy peanut butter, and Hostess cupcakes. Stop eating McDonald's, Burger King, and Taco Bell." Now that's something we would understand!

MyPyramid

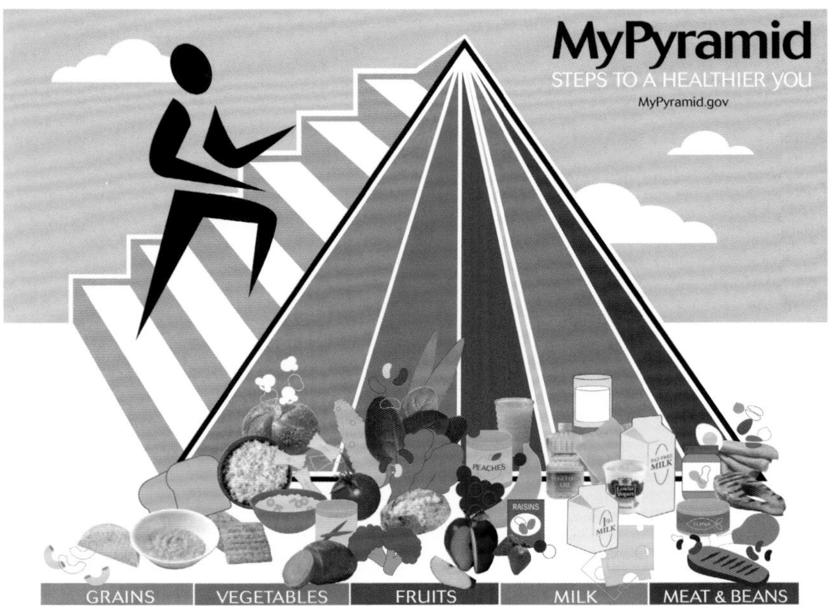

Source: U.S. Department of Agriculture/U.S. Department of Health and Human Services

Following the release of the Dietary Guidelines in April 2005, the USDA redesigned the food pyramid, which had stood more or less unchanged since its first appearance in 1992, and renamed it "MyPyramid." MyPyramid showed some improvements from the previous pyramid. It drew attention to both leafy green vegetables and whole grains, two groups the old pyramid was missing. It also addressed the concept of healthy fats, with advice to get most of your fat from fish, nuts, and vegetable oils. For the first time, beans, seeds, and nuts were recognized as legitimate sources of protein, and the pyramid even recommended to "vary your protein routine" and "choose more fish, beans, peas, nuts, and seeds." The milk section included a comment for people who "don't or can't consume milk," marking the first time the USDA has acknowledged that not everyone can digest dairy. Even with these advances, MyPyramid was still far from an easily understood and accurate representation of which foods are necessary for health. The vegetable section was about the same size as the milk section, which seemed to imply you should consume the same amount of milk and vegetables.

MyPyramid promoted the idea that we can eat as much as we want, as long as we exercise every day. "Calories in, calories out" is a concept that benefits both the food and the exercise industries. The pyramid was constructed for people who exercise 30 to 60 minutes a day. A better plan would have been to create a pyramid for people who do not exercise at all, since most Americans are not active.

2010 Dietary Guidelines

The USDA released the 2010 Dietary Guidelines for Americans in January 2011. Like the 2005 report, the 2010 guidelines point out that Americans don't eat enough vegetables or whole grains and, instead, eat too much fat and sugar. Unfortunately, the guidelines continued to miss the mark and use vague terminology. "SoFAS" is used to describe solid fats and added sugars. To even a well-educated person, the word *sofa* is generally used to describe a small couch.

It's the use of these misleading words that led the Physician's Committee for Responsible Medicine (PCRM) to file yet another lawsuit against the federal government, on February 15, 2011. PCRM states that using biochemical terms instead of naming actual foods like "meat and cheese" keeps Americans eating these unhealthy foods. "What Americans really should be told is we need to eat less red meat, less cheese, less ice cream, and less refined grains," Dr. Walter Willett said in a National Public Radio interview. Why is it so hard for the government to call out the main culprits?

Although the potential for conflict of interest still exists among committee members, these guidelines seem to be significantly more transparent than in years past. The guidelines committee recommended more action by requesting that the USDA and HHS convene separate committees to develop strategies for implementing these recommendations. They even admitted, "The actions needed to implement key recommendations likely differ by goal."

MyPlate

In response to the updated dietary guidelines of 2010, the USDA replaced MyPyramid with MyPlate. The goal was to simplify nutritional information to make it more useful to the average family. I commend the plate, as most people can understand that image.

Unlike the pyramids of the past, which attempted to convey how much you should eat based on the colors and relative sizes of sections on the pyramid, MyPlate focuses on the portion sizes at each meal through simple divisions of a plate. It makes it visually obvious that half of your plate should be filled with fruits and vegetables. The MyPlate icon also features selected messages, like "avoid oversized portions" and "enjoy your food, but eat less." However, as with the pyramid, you must visit the MyPlate website for specific instructions on what to eat. While MyPlate is a huge step toward instilling healthy changes in Americans, it still has many shortcomings, such as dairy's continuing to be an essential part of the meal and the lack of a clear definition for grains.

The Integrative Nutrition® Plate solves many of these issues. Adapted from the USDA MyPlate, this version also emphasizes the importance of vegetables, fruits, and protein, but I swapped dairy with water and added fats and oils, which are essential to the diet. To complete the full picture of health, the plate is surrounded with lifestyle factors—primary foods—that create optimal health. The four main types of primary foods are: relationships, physical activity, career, and spirituality. I encourage people to look at these aspects of life as a form of nourishment—a way to feed themselves at a much deeper level than food. The food you eat plays a critical role in your health and happiness, and discovering the right foods for you is very important. But primary foods truly nourish you and make your life extraordinary. We will explore these areas in depth later in the book.

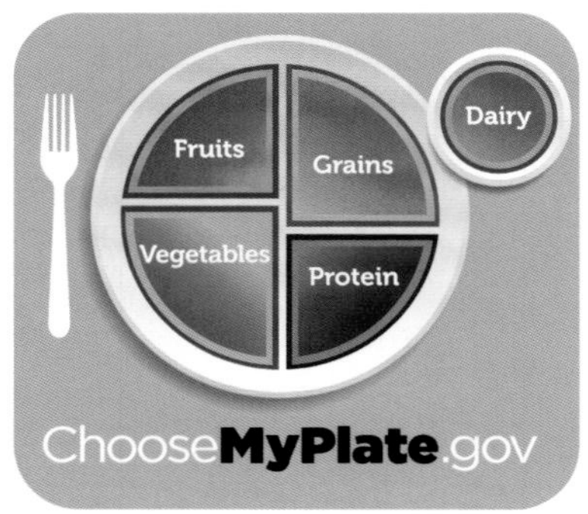

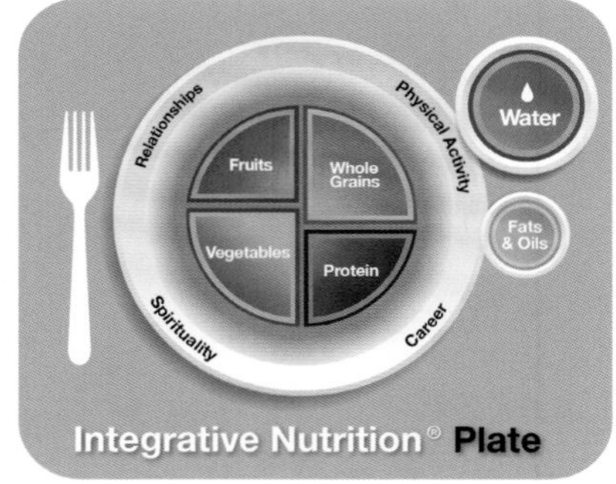

® Source: U.S. Department of Agriculture/U.S. Department of Health and Human Services

Food Corporations

Food corporations are more or less free to deceive the public about the nature of their products, often using the guidelines—like the Food Guide Pyramid, MyPyramid, and now MyPlate—as vehicles for their own agendas. The U.S. government even contributes to many food-marketing campaigns. Just think of popular campaigns like "Got Milk?" "Beef. It's What's for Dinner," and "Pork. The Other White Meat." These campaigns, aimed at increasing Americans' consumption of dairy, beef, and pork products, are part of the federal government's commodity promotion programs, called "checkoff" programs. Checkoff programs demonstrate the dual role of the federal government to educate the public about nutrition and health while still promoting its food. The question is, where are all of the ads for vegetables or whole grains?

When MyPyramid was released in 2005, General Mills announced that about 100 million boxes of its Big G cereal brands would carry MyPyramid on them, citing the cereal box as one of the most-read items in the home.[21]

The company also announced that they would reformulate their products to include whole grains, which was in line with the recommendation of the 2005 pyramid to eat more whole grains, thereby implying that their cereals, including Lucky Charms, Trix, and Golden Grahams, are healthy. Now that's savvy marketing. Even today, many of these same brands are coming out with gluten-free versions that are touted as "healthy," while these products are still highly processed and full of sugar.

Also in 2005, Frito-Lay, the potato chip manufacturer, devised its own food pyramid, showing packets of chips with happy, smiling faces filling the bottom section, implying that chips provide the carbohydrate foundation needed for good health. This is nonsense. The carbohydrates in chips are covered in fat, drenched in artificial flavoring, and so highly refined that they immediately break down into simple sugars in the body.

It seems like every food corporation is trying to create a healthy image and pass off its products as being good for you. While the Food and Drug Administration (FDA) now has standards for labels, many companies continue to make claims about their products on the front of their packages. Food corporations use their millions or billions of dollars to trick the public into thinking their products are healthy simply because one of the ingredients is derived from a whole grain.

Of course, if people consumed junk foods only occasionally, we would not have a global health crisis. But food and beverage corporations are big business. In 2012, Nestlé had more than $92 billion in sales, PepsiCo more than $62 billion in sales, and Kellogg more than $13 billion. The list goes on and on.[22] The fast food and restaurant industries also generate billions in annual sales. And even though sales are down at McDonald's, they still managed to rake in over $25 billion in 2012, and they open new franchises all the time.[23] These corporations put a big hunk of this money back into advertising.

You might be wondering how food corporations can get away with these tactics. Let me explain. The food industry spends a tremendous amount of money on lobbyists in Washington. In fact, in 2016, $30 million was spent on specific food and beverage lobbying. These big bucks pay off, giving these corporations major unfair advantages when it comes to food policy and regulations. In 2015, Big Food (along with farm and biotechnology companies) spent more than $101 million on lobbying to help prevent labeling of food containing genetically engineered ingredients. Big Soda has spent about $67 million since 2009 to help squash soda taxes and warning labels in states throughout the U.S. and about $14 million annually at the federal level.[24]

Soda companies have aggressively worked to deceive the public. In 2013 Coca-Cola released a new commercial touting their efforts to fight obesity, saying, "All calories count, no matter where they come from, including Coca-Cola and everything else with calories." The American Beverage Association says its members have cut 88% of the calories shipped to schools since 2004 by offering fewer sugary drinks and emphasizing water, low-fat milk, and juice in schools. But these are the same soda companies that made sure to solidify relationships with young customers through exclusive "pouring rights" contracts in public schools starting in the early '90s. In exchange for exclusive selling rights in school districts, Big Soda companies supplied schools all of the beverages sold at snack bars, in vending machines, and at sporting events, offering the struggling schools massive payments.[25]

Along with the drinks, the companies also filled the school with advertisements. But in response to growing pressure from parent groups and public health advocates, the ABA eventually announced voluntary restrictions on soft drink sales in elementary and middle schools, instead ramping up sales of bottled water and juices.[26]

Big Soda continues to market heavily overseas, trying to maintain that their products can be included as part of a healthy diet. In the U.K., Coca-Cola launched a Work It Out Calculator on their website, showing that you can still enjoy your soda; you just need to keep active. How about everyone keeps moving and ditches the soda? Back in 2012, Pepsi launched a high-fiber, fat-burning soda in Japan called Pepsi Special. The drink contained a fiber-rich starch, dextrin, that can be derived from arrowroot, potato, or wheat. Japan's soda market is valued at almost $48 billion, but it's still a wonder why people would ever think getting fiber from empty, sugary calories could make them healthy.[27]

Not all food news is bad, however. Thanks to more awareness around health, we are seeing changes. Organic food sales in the U.S. have reached all-time highs. Soda sales have fizzled in recent years, with soda consumption dropping to a 30-year low in the U.S. Additionally, major cities like Boulder,

Colorado; Philadelphia, Pennsylvania; and San Francisco, California, have passed measures that discourage soda drinking by taxing sugar-sweetened beverages, joining places like Mexico, France, Hungary, Ireland, and the United Kingdom. And so far, studies have found that the taxes help reduce purchases. Consumer demand for more natural and nutritious ingredients has many Big Food companies, like Hershey, Nestlé, and McDonald's, shifting to "cleaner labels" or reducing sugar in their products. They are replacing artificial colors and flavors with more natural ingredients and switching to animal products raised more humanely and without antibiotics.

Government Policies

Ever notice that unhealthy foods are cheaper than healthy foods? You may think nothing of it, but in the U.S., government policies and practices help lower the prices of unhealthy foods. Since the 1920s, American farmers have received government subsidies to help maximize production, reduce the cost of raw materials, stabilize crop prices, and keep the cost of food down for the American public, allowing farmers to stay in business. This originally well-intentioned government money has led to the overproduction of corn and soybeans and, consequently, lower prices for these crops and for foods containing them as ingredients. This may seem harmless. Corn and soybeans are healthy, right? In their natural states, these foods are not bad, but the overproduction of these crops has led to their increased use as cheap, unhealthy ingredients in processed foods on the grocery store aisles. High fructose corn syrup, an artificial ingredient found in most sodas and junk foods, is an inexpensive use of corn. Low corn prices have led to artificially low meat prices, because corn has become the number one feed for cattle—a major shift from a traditional grazing diet. The overproduction of soybeans and corn provides an inexpensive way to add flavor to packaged junk food, fast food, corn-fed beef and pork, and soft drinks. For consumers, these less nutritious foods are cheaper and particularly tempting to people living on a budget. These subsidies contribute to the obesity epidemic by making it cheaper to produce and purchase unhealthy packaged foods.[28]

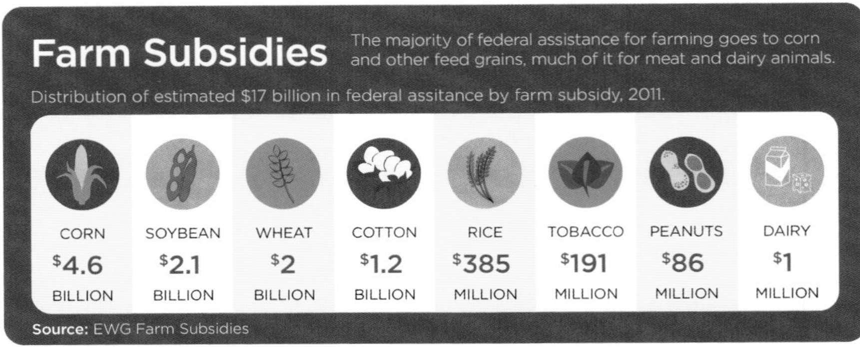

As a result of the subsidies, growing a variety of fruits, vegetables, and other grains is less lucrative for farmers. Less than 10% of USDA subsidies are spent on fruits and vegetables. We should be asking why vegetables, fruits, and whole grains aren't heavily subsidized so they can be cheaper and more accessible to everyone. Obviously, this change in policy would go a long way toward helping Americans follow their own government's nutritional guidelines. This disparity in government funding points out an awkward truth about the USDA: What it urges people to eat does not match what it pays farmers to grow.

Decades of food policy designed to benefit agribusiness and megafarms plays a big role in American public health. Every five years, Congress must look at the national policies for agriculture, nutrition, conservation, and forestry policy under a bundle of legislation commonly known as the "Farm Bill."[29, 30] This legislation has the power to influence everything from the cost and availability of food to the protection of farmland throughout the country. The foods subsidized by the farm bill have an enormous impact on how the country eats. It's important to follow this legislation and continue to make our voices heard to expand the Farmers Market and Local Food Promotion Program and to encourage the purchase of fruits and vegetables in the Supplemental Nutrition Assistance Program, which serves the nation's low-income communities.

Another influential factor is political campaign contributions. Dependence on financial contributions from powerful lobbies prevents government agencies from stating the simple truths about nutrition. Politicians say the money they receive from corporate donors does not influence the policies they promote, but why would companies give money if this were true? Corporations are not known for their spontaneous generosity. Politicians need a lot of money to get elected, and food and drug companies are some of their biggest backers. McDonald's, Pepsi, General Mills, Kraft, Nestlé, and Hershey depend on their friends in Washington, who make the food laws and guidelines. The top contributors to the former chairman of the Agricultural Committee, Frank D. Lucas (R-OK), were American Crystal Sugar, Dairy Farmers of America, National Beer Wholesalers Association, and National Cattlemen's Beef Association.[31] Of course, they want some return on their investment.

The Growing Drug Problem

Something has gone terribly wrong in the pharmaceutical industry today. Medications in America are increasingly expensive. Every month, a new magic pill emerges, and we are bombarded with commercials for drugs that cite side effects that sound worse than the original ailment. Does this sound familiar? "Warning: may cause nausea, headaches, constipation, dizziness, drowsiness, or, in extreme cases, death."

Americans spent $425 billion on prescription drugs in 2015.[32] This boom is fueled in part by expensive new drugs for cancer and other diseases hitting the market, along with price hikes for older drugs. Drug advertisements, which usually feature attractive people, sometimes celebrities, smiling in the outdoors, also help send the message that what people need to be healthy is more prescription drugs. Name the health concern; a drug is out there for it. Drugs help us control cholesterol, lower blood pressure, regulate the menstrual cycle, prevent osteoporosis, and end acid reflux. I frequently say that Americans are not prescription drug deficient. We are nutritionally deficient.

In addition to inundating the market with drugs and creating advanced marketing strategies, the pharmaceutical industry makes a killing charging exorbitantly high prices for their products. In *The Truth About Drug Companies: How They Deceive Us and What to Do About It*, Dr. Marcia Angell argues that drug companies must find a better, less expensive way of doing business. She says profits for pharmaceutical manufacturers really took off in 1980, when new legislation allowed university medical researchers and big drug companies to form an alliance. Before that time, taxpayers funded drug research, and findings were available to any pharmaceutical company that wanted to use them. With the new law, universities could patent their discoveries and grant exclusive licenses to drug companies. Suddenly, unbiased research disappeared. Then, Congress passed another series of laws extending monopoly rights for brand-name drugs to 14 years, another big win for the pharmaceutical industry. Under this law, pharmaceutical companies could market their drugs without competition for 14 years, charging whatever they liked. Only after the 14-year period could companies sell generic copies of the drug. This law allowed government-granted monopolies in the form of patents and FDA-approved exclusive marketing rights. As profits increased from these new policies, so did the political clout of drug companies.

Drug companies have one of the largest lobbying groups in Washington and give generously to political campaigns. By 1990, the industry had unprecedented control over its own fortunes. If it didn't like something that its regulatory body, the FDA, decreed, it could force change on the policy through direct pressure on friends in Congress.

The FDA has the task of approving and regulating not only prescription drugs but also food, supplements, and other products that can be harmful to health. Their mission statement says:

> The FDA is responsible for protecting the public health by assuring the safety, efficacy, and security of human and veterinary drugs, biological products, medical devices, our nation's food supply, cosmetics, and products that emit radiation. The FDA is also responsible for advancing the public health by helping to speed innovations that make medicines and foods more effective, safer, and more affordable and helping the public get the accurate, science-based information they need to use medicines and foods to improve their health.

In 2008, poisoning became the leading cause of injury death in the U.S., and nearly 9 out of 10 poisoning deaths were caused by drugs.[33] This same year, these deaths exceeded the number of motor vehicle traffic deaths. Celebrities like Michael Jackson, Heath Ledger, Prince, and Whitney Houston all died from overdoses and complications related to FDA-approved pharmaceutical drugs, specifically prescription painkillers. These kinds of overdoses have tripled in the last decade and now have a larger toll than deaths from cocaine and heroin combined, according to a report from the Centers for Disease Control and Prevention (CDC).[34] Opioid medications are among the most commonly dispensed class of drugs.

Hello, where is the FDA? They appear to be overly focused on helping drug companies maximize profits rather than protecting consumer interests. Almost no one in the government is asking the right questions. People don't need more drugs. Maybe they need to understand disease prevention, the importance of exercise, and how to eat a nutritious, balanced diet.

The reason I share this information is not to blame the FDA or drug companies. I want the public to wake up to the fact that our system is broken. I want people to understand that, even though a pill is out there claiming to help with a particular condition, there may be another way—a path that involves nutritious food, physical activity, and a fulfilling life.

I want to tell you a little bit about my father. He is a fit, healthy, clever, and humorous man who lives in Canada, and until he was 82 years old, he was on no medication. My American friends and colleagues are surprised by this fact, but it is actually normal in other parts of the world for people not to take medication.

Scientists have even started studying certain regions around the world where people commonly live past the age of 100 with little disease and no need for medication. These areas are called Blue Zones and are found in the mountain villages of Sardinia, Italy; the islands of Okinawa, Japan; the beach area of Nicoya Peninsula, Costa Rica; and a community of Seventh-day Adventists living in Loma Linda, California. What the people in these areas have in common is a healthy lifestyle, including staying active, engaging in social activities with people of all ages, putting family first, eating mostly plant-based diets, and not smoking, which is a far cry from lifestyles found in the Western world. I'll talk more about the Blue Zones later in the book.

The Turning Point

If we want to be healthy, we need to eat nutritious foods. It really isn't difficult. Unfortunately, billions of dollars are spent every day trying to seduce us not to do it. The food industry, drug companies, politicians, civil servants, and even the medical profession all have strong vested interests in making money and not in protecting our health. In one way or another, almost all of the sources of information we would expect to support our quest for overall health are contaminated for reasons of financial gain. If we face the facts, being sick and overweight keeps corporate profits healthy.

But the world is beginning to wake up to the reality that healthy food creates healthy people. We see it in the papers and on television commercials, and we hear all sorts of people talking about it. Corporations are responding. The success of stores such as Whole Foods and Trader Joe's and the incorporation of organic sections at Walmart and Costco illustrate that consumers are concerned about their health and the quality of their food. When individuals like you and I stand up for improving our own health, things do change. If we buy our food from health food stores and farmers' markets and don't spend our money on unhealthy foods, corporations get the message loud and clear. Don't become a silent victim within the system. Think globally. Act locally. Get involved with your local government, your school system, your office, your church or temple, and your family. With our dollars, our voices, and our forks, we have the power to create change. If we all stand up and speak up for what we know to be true, we can dramatically improve the world's health and happiness. Margaret Mead said, "Never doubt that a small group of thoughtful, committed citizens can change the world; indeed, it's the only thing that ever has."

Exercises

1. Supermarket Field Trip

Go to your local supermarket with a friend or family member, and walk around, looking into people's shopping carts. This should give you a good understanding of what people in your community are eating today.

- Take out a piece of paper, and write down the most common food items you see in people's carts.
- What is missing from the carts?
- Imagine, how would you feel if you were eating these foods?
- What attracts you to the foods people have chosen (packaging, colors, etc.)?

2. Get Involved

Contact your government and find out where your local officials stand on food and health issues. Here are some web resources to get you started:

- U.S.: House of Representatives: www.house.gov;
U.S. Senate: www.senate.gov
- U.S.: Project Vote Smart provides non-partisan information on each elected official and candidate for office: www.votesmart.org
- Australia: www.australia.gov.au
- Brazil: www.brasil.gov.br
- Canada: www.canada.ca
- India: www.india.gov.in
- Japan: www.japan.go.jp
- Mexico: en.presidencia.gob.mx
- U.K.: www.gov.uk
- United Arab Emirates: www.government.ae/en

Chapter 2

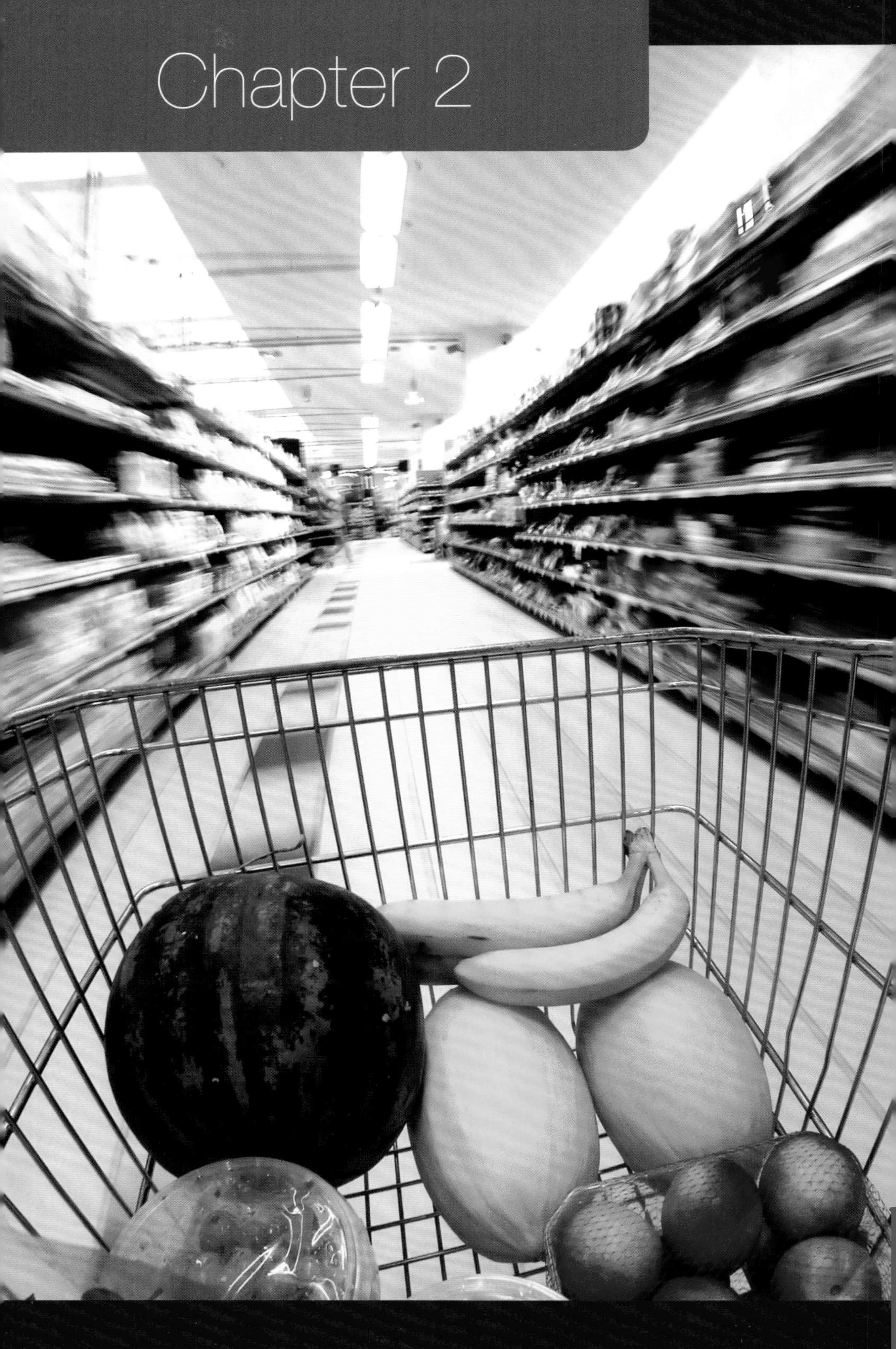

What Is Integrative Nutrition?

> This approach is not about acquiring more self-discipline or willpower. It's about personally discovering what nourishes you, what feeds you, and ultimately what makes your life extraordinary.
>
> —Joshua Rosenthal

We live in a world of conventional and modern nutrition. Let me explain. Conventional nutrition is the kind of information we get from food pyramids and government agencies. It's similar to conventional healthcare. People who dwell on calories, carbs, fats, proteins, restrictions, and lists of good and bad foods are relying on conventional nutrition. Advice such as "always choose lean cuts of meat," "switch to low-fat dairy," or "eat more whole grains" comes from conventional nutrition.

Then we have modern nutrition, where we are hit with a new discovery each day, proclaiming the health benefits of a certain food or the fastest way to gain more energy this week. This approach is prescriptive, touting a one-size-fits-all mentality, like eating low carb, slow carb, raw food, high fat, or avoiding all animal products. Modern nutrition bombards us, from the brightly colored covers of diet books to the trends we see captured on social media feeds with opinions and images of what to eat. Avocado toast, anyone?

The message of both conventional and modern nutrition is: Eat healthy. But we've lost a connection to what *healthy* really means. Are energy bars good for breakfast or as an afternoon snack? Can I enjoy oatmeal if I'm gluten free? Is a grass-fed burger on a lettuce wrap good for me, or should I avoid meat altogether? We have so many questions about what to eat, and many people feel like they are constantly getting it wrong, even those of us who study nutrition.

"If people stay confused about what a healthy diet is, you can keep selling the next and the next and the next diet book. Our culture has been making a ton of money out of sowing confusion, while the food industry has been exploiting the messages of experts and turning them into nonsense," said David Katz, founding director of Yale University's Yale-Griffin Prevention Research Center.

It wasn't too long ago that humans existed without this media blitz or diet gurus telling them what to eat. Instead, they relied on intuition. People simply knew what to eat and how to prepare it. They didn't go to the gym to exercise; they just exercised. They didn't have a complicated career; they just worked. They didn't have such a cerebral interpretation of basic human needs. People naturally lived in harmony with the seasons and with their surroundings. They ate what was local, traditional, and available and what gave them proper nutrients for their lives.

The worlds of conventional and modern nutrition are incredibly complex. Nutrition is the only science in which two parties can comprehensively prove two different theories that are diametrically opposed to one another. Scientists unanimously agree that the speed of light is 670 million miles per hour, gravity is an attractive force between all matter, and water is made of two parts hydrogen and one part oxygen. How is it possible, then, that one expert can prove dairy is a necessary component of a healthy diet while another expert can prove dairy is extremely detrimental to health? That one expert can claim meat is essential to a healthy human body while another expert says meat is an unnecessary and unhealthy part of the human diet?

The publishing industry has largely shaped our beliefs about food and health. Eager to earn money from the next bestseller, they are the ones who "discover" and promote nutritional truths, not the medical industry. Think about it. Did you ever try to *Eat This, Not That!*? What about *The Baby Food Diet* or *The FastDiet*? The *Dukan Diet* was a phenomenon in Europe. In Japan, an actor created *The Long Breath Diet*, which involved daily breathing exercises to shed unwanted pounds. I'm sure you can think of at least a few that you have tried or were intrigued by. Popular diet books are not always scrutinized for truth and scientific evidence about healthy eating; they simply aim to be bestsellers. They grab attention by shocking, entertaining, and providing quick-fix solutions. But the dietary theories in these books are not usually sustainable for long periods of time, and some may even be unhealthy in the long term. Once they stop working, the reader will try another diet book, and so on, and so on, consistently supporting the publishing industry. Back in 2001, the Atkins Diet craze hit the market with a splash. Sales of *Dr. Atkins' New Diet Revolution* exceeded 10 million copies, even though the book provided no medical evidence that the diet worked. In fact, it went against the conventional nutritional advice to eat more vegetables and get more exercise.

My point is not to bash these diets. The Atkins Diet was the beginning of public awareness about the glycemic index of certain foods and the unfavorable effects of refined carbohydrates. Each new diet may expose one more piece of the nutrition puzzle, but they also end up sensationalizing or blowing that one piece out of proportion and missing the larger picture. Nutrition is still an emerging field in many ways, and we are only just beginning to understand all its facets.

Experts agree that we all need variety in our diets. But many disagree about other issues, such as how much water to drink throughout the day, or whether organic vegetables have more nutrient value than nonorganic. Their theories are all missing a huge part of what nutrition is really about: the individual. Most nutrition books tell you what to eat without any reference to age, constitution, gender, culture, size, or lifestyle. Most don't clarify their diets for people who are well or people who are dealing with disease. We need to point out that each person has very specific needs for his or her own health and that everyone can benefit from being open-minded about exploring different ways of eating.

To avoid this perplexed, media-driven nonsense, I take a different approach to nutrition, simply called Integrative Nutrition. One of the main concepts is recognizing your bio-individuality. No way of eating works for everybody. The food that is perfect for your unique body, age, and lifestyle may make another person gain weight and feel lethargic. Similarly, no perfect way of eating will work for you all the time. You may notice you eat different foods on days when you are working eight hours than on a relaxing day spent reading. Foods you ate as a child may not agree with you as an adult. What you crave in the winter may be completely different from what you crave in the summer.

Another huge concept in Integrative Nutrition has to do with primary food. As mentioned in Chapter 1, all that we consider nutrition today is really just a secondary source of energy or nourishment. The foods you eat are secondary to all of the other parts of life that feed you—your relationships, career, spirituality, and exercise routine. I call these elements of life primary foods. Integrative Nutrition also bridges the gap between nutrition and personal growth and development. These two entities are absolutely linked; you can't look at one without the other. People really want to be better. They crave growth. But very few experts in the realm of personal growth and development address the importance of nutrition. Likewise, conventional and modern nutrition will simply give you a list of foods to eat and not to eat, but their advice will not work until you start to identify what in your life is keeping you from making healthy choices. Look at it this way: A person stuck in an unhealthy relationship can eat all the broccoli in the world, but it won't change their relationship. This unhealthy relationship will cause their health and well-being to suffer. Similarly, if your career is opposed to your spiritual values, you will have a hard time making big breakthroughs with a health concern. The energy spent at a draining job will ultimately outweigh the benefits of eating healthy food.

Being healthy is really not that complicated. The body knows what to eat. It's the brain that makes mistakes. Maybe you've heard about a diet that sounded great in theory, but after a week of eating that way, you started to feel weak or bloated. You don't have to read nutrition books to know what to eat. Instead, you can foster a deep relationship with your body in which it naturally tells you what it needs to function at its highest potential. This integrative approach will help you cultivate the ability to eat intuitively, trusting your body—not some book, chef, or research study—to guide you to the foods that best support you and allow your body and mind to operate at their fullest potential. As you learn to trust your gut more about what to eat, you learn that it's also worthy of your trust about everything else in life.

Bio-Individuality

In 1956, Roger Williams published *Biochemical Individuality*, asserting that individuality permeates each part of the human body. This book explained how personal differences in anatomy, metabolism, composition of bodily fluids, and cell structure influence your overall health. Each person, Williams wrote, has genetically determined and highly individualistic nutrition requirements. This theory influenced some independent-thinking minds in the nutrition world but is still largely ignored by mainstream medicine.

Watching fad diets sweep through the U.S., from high-carb diets in the '70s, to low fat in the '80s, to high protein and high fat in the 21st century, I wondered how each of these nutrition experts could claim their diets worked for everyone. We are too individualistic to eat the exact same food. Ever notice that men eat very differently from women? Children, teens, and adults all have very different preferences. Office workers eat differently from those who do physical labor. People eat according to their age, whether they are 25, 55, or 85.

Scientific research is starting to catch on to this concept. In a 2008 study, scientists found that men and women really do eat differently. The population survey of the Foodborne Disease Active Surveillance Network (FoodNet) looked at the eating habits of more than 14,000 American adults and found that, generally, men are more likely to report eating meat and poultry, and women are more likely to report eating fruits and vegetables.[1] I've noticed over the years that, many times, women try to get their male partners to eat more like a woman, with more salads and vegetables. Years later, they wonder, where's my man? Now I know that both men and women enjoy a variety of foods, but isn't it interesting to tune in to these subtle differences?

A November 2015 study published in *Cell* found that universal dietary recommendations simply don't work. Israeli researchers wanted to understand which foods cause people's blood sugar levels to spike, so they measured responses of 800 people over the course of a week, gathering data from more than 46,000 meals. They found that—surprise, surprise—each person had different responses to similar foods. In fact, many people in the study had low glucose responses to ice cream—a sugary food that should certainly increase glucose levels. This research knocks out traditional ideas of good and bad foods and the idea that any one diet can work for everyone. Again, it depends on your individual makeup.

Working in the field for so many years, bio-individuality is something I've always known to be true. In my heart I could feel that no one way of eating could possibly be helpful for everyone, yet medicine and science are constantly in search of the magic bullet—the one perfect way of eating that will solve all of humanity's problems related to diet. But the tides are shifting. One of the top health trends in 2017? Personalization.

One of the major factors shaping bio-individuality is ancestry. If your ancestors were Japanese, you will most likely thrive on a Japanese-type diet, high in rice, sea vegetables, and fish. If your ancestors were from India, your digestive system will probably love basmati rice, cooked beans, and curry. If many generations of your ancestors from Scandinavia were accustomed to eating dairy on a daily basis, it's natural that your body will be able to assimilate dairy-based foods. This theory also applies to foods that you have difficulty digesting. For example, many traditional African communities had an abundance of beans, grains, animal protein, sweet potatoes, and green vegetables. Dairy was not easily accessible or easy to store in hot regions and, therefore, not a part of the traditional diet. So it makes sense that a lot of people of African descent are lactose intolerant.

My mother, who is now in her late eighties, grew up in Hungary, where dairy was an important part of the daily diet. She drank warm, raw milk straight from the cow. When I first became involved with nutrition and health, I rejected dairy. I came to see that no other species naturally consumes dairy after infancy and that cow's milk is the perfect food to help a baby calf grow into a big, heavy cow but had no place in the adult human diet. I was eating brown rice and veggies, following my macrobiotic diet by the book. For years, I felt really good being off dairy. I stopped getting colds in the winter and stopped having mucus. Then I went on my first trip to India and visited several Ayurvedic doctors, who all agreed I needed more dairy in my diet. They said I was lacking the calming, soothing, feminine energy that dairy holds. I remembered how strong my mom was and how much dairy she drank growing up. So I gradually let go of my rigid attitude and began to experiment with milk, cheese, and yogurt. Some people cannot tolerate any dairy; they get mucus, digestive trouble, and allergies. Because my ancestors consumed dairy on a regular basis, it makes sense that I benefit from moderate amounts of high-quality dairy products in my diet.

Inside your body are bacteria that play a huge role in unlocking your bio-individuality. Right now, governments and independent foundations around the world are funding millions of dollars of research to understand it more fully. I'm talking about the microbiome, a DNA record made up of trillions of bacteria that live in your gut, your skin, and throughout your body. These microorganisms play a major role in maintaining immune function and digestion, but they are also unique to each person. The health of your microbiome can have an effect on your ability to gain energy from the foods you eat, for example. These tiny microbes may be used to both prevent and treat diseases in the future, ranging from autoimmune disorders to cancer.

Another aspect of bio-individuality is metabolism, or the rate at which you convert food into energy. Knowing your personal metabolic rate is useful when gauging the quantity of food your digestive system can process. Depending on your metabolic rate, your body may quickly convert calories to energy, or it may store the extra calories. You may recall that, as a teenager, you could wolf down a burger, fries, milkshake, and ice cream all in one meal, without any indigestion or tightening of your jeans. That's because young people are still growing, have fast metabolic rates, and burn calories more quickly than adults.

Keep in mind that even your metabolic rate and sensitivity can shift as you age or as stress levels or nutrient levels change in your diet or lifestyle. If this all seems too confusing and complicated, don't worry. Just observe how your own body responds to the food you give it. People are different, and getting to know your own body is an essential first step in discovering how to stay healthy.

Metabolic theory demonstrates that no one diet is right for all of us. You may know people who can eat processed carbohydrates, such as bread and pasta, and stay very thin, while you gain weight on such a diet. It's not because carbohydrates are "evil" or your body isn't as healthy; it just shows that all people metabolize these foods differently. You might do better on a high-protein diet with lots of fresh vegetables and some whole grains. Knowing which foods you metabolize best will help you choose foods that make you feel good and support your individual body.

Our personal tastes and preferences, natural shapes and sizes, gut bacterial profile, metabolic rates, and genetic backgrounds influence which foods will and won't nourish us. So, when the experts say "tomatoes are good for you" or "red meat is unhealthy," it's too much of a generalization. One person's food is another person's poison, and that's why fad diets don't work in the long run. They are not based on the reality that we all have different dietary needs.

Sometimes it takes millions of dollars in funding and years of research for scientists to prove what we already know. I am certain that science will soon discover that dietary needs are based on bio-individuality.

Primary Food

OK, so let's get back to this idea that the food on your plate is only providing nourishment and that other aspects of life also feed you.

Please think back to a time when you were passionately in love. Everything was exciting. Colors were vibrant. Intimacy was magical. Your lover's touch and feelings of exhilaration sustained you. You were floating on air, gazing into each other's eyes. You forgot about food and were high on life.

Recall a time when you were deeply involved in an exciting project. You truly believed in what you were doing and felt confident and stimulated. Time fell away. Hours passed. You developed single-pointed focus. Mealtime and sleep time were irrelevant.

Remember when, as a child, you were playing outside, having fun? Suddenly, your mother announced dinner was ready, but you were not hungry at all. The passion of play took all your attention.

Sometimes we are fed not by food but by the energy in our lives. These moments and feelings demonstrate that everything is food. We take in thousands of experiences of life that can fulfill us physically, mentally, emotionally, and spiritually. We hunger for play, fun, touch, romance, intimacy, love, achievement, success, art, music, self-expression, leadership, excitement, adventure, and spirituality. All of these elements are essential forms of nourishment. The extent to which we are able to incorporate them determines how enjoyable and worthwhile our lives feel.

Conventional and modern nutrition—with its focus on carbs or proteins, fresh produce or fast food—is really just one source of nourishment, which I call secondary food. If we are not starving, other dimensions of the human experience are generally much more important to us than what we put in our mouths. Secondary foods don't come close to giving us the joy, meaning, and fulfillment primary food provides. When we use secondary food as a way to alleviate or suppress our hunger for primary food, the body and mind suffer. Weight gain is just one of the consequences. Diet-related disorders, such as heart disease, cancer, obesity, high blood pressure, and diabetes, are national epidemics, and one of the main reasons is because we are stuffing ourselves with secondary foods when we are really starving for primary food.

Chronic depression is also widespread in our society. Globally, an estimated 300 million people suffer from depression, according to the World Health Organization.[2] Eleven percent of people over the age of 12 take antidepressants,[3] and their use is on the rise throughout the world. Many also experience frustration, anger, disappointment, sadness, and isolation. These conditions and emotions are all cries for primary food, but instead of giving ourselves what we really need, we often turn to secondary food for comfort and solace. The problem is that this substitution does not work. If you are not getting the primary food you need, eating all the food in the world won't satisfy your hunger.

The Laboratory of Your Body

Fortunately, you already have free, 24-hour access to the world's most sophisticated laboratory for testing how food affects your body and your health. Where is this lab? You're living in it. Your body is a sophisticated bio-computer. By learning to listen to your body and developing an understanding of what foods it needs and when it needs them, you will discover what is best for you.

If you doubt this connection to your body, begin by acknowledging that your body is highly intelligent. Your heart never misses a beat, and your lungs are always breathing in and out. Even if you break up with a romantic partner, even if you receive traumatic news, your heart's four little chambers go right on pumping, and your lungs continue to expand and contract. You can trust your body. It has evolved helpful instincts to keep you alive and well.

Just as a tree will always lean toward light, humans and animals know instinctively how and where to get food that is best for them. Animals don't read nutrition books. Their bodies tell them which plants to eat and which to avoid, or, if they're predators, which animals to kill when they're hungry. They heal themselves when they are sick, usually by resting a lot and eating very little until the sickness passes.

We have the same instincts, but many of us ignore the messages our bodies are constantly sending. Dark circles under the eyes signal exhaustion; your body is telling you to slow down and get some rest. Constipation and bloating are signs that something you are eating, or the way you are eating it, is not appropriate. We disregard these messages until they become unbearable, and that's when we go to the doctor for medications and operations.

Additional signs that the food you're eating may not agree with your personal constitution include poor energy levels, lack of focus, irregular bowel movements, disturbed sleep, aches and pains, weight fluctuations, frequent colds or getting sick in general, intense cravings, or mucus buildup in the body. Does this sound like most people on a standard Western diet? It's important to remember that our bodies are designed to be healthy, not sick. If you are dealing with some of these issues, consider getting back to basics. Switch up your diet, get some rest, drink plenty of water, and see if your symptoms clear up.

A somewhat extreme example of the body speaking out loud and clear comes from a 2016 news story about a young boy who was admitted to the hospital in Michigan with strange symptoms: bleeding gums, a full-body rash, and leg pain when he walked. The doctors did what they do best and ran a full range of tests from CT scans and MRIs to blood tests. After four days at the hospital, they still couldn't figure out what was causing his issues, other than a slight case of anemia. Eventually, one of the doctors, a radiologist, asked about his diet. His mother said he is a picky eater. And after more questions, the medical team discovered that his diet consisted of chocolate milk and graham crackers—and that's it. A simple blood test confirmed that he had scurvy because he had zero vitamin C in his diet. The doctors didn't even think to scan for this disease, which is characterized by skin rashes, joint pain, and bleeding gums, because it's so unfathomable that a young child would not get the proper nutrients to prevent it.

Of course, he was a young boy, and his parents were just doing the best that they could. He made a full recovery within four months by adding fresh foods to his diet. But I hope you get my point. The food we eat has an impact on our bodies. Notice the feedback you are receiving.

Give yourself time to explore the laboratory of your body, and you will be surprised by its responsiveness, sophistication, and intelligence. At the end of the day, you can never really make a mistake with food. Everything you do is an experiment.

Food-Mood Connection

Scientific research and personal experience both demonstrate that what we eat affects how we think and how we act. Still, most people don't acknowledge the connection between their food and their mood. Stop and think for a moment about how you feel throughout the day. Do you sometimes feel fuzzy and tired after lunch? Angry and irritable between meals? Energized by a great meal?

Food undoubtedly changes your mood. The most extreme examples are coffee and alcohol, which change your state of mind within minutes. The standard American diet, high in processed carbohydrates and poor-quality animal meat, while lacking in vegetables and water, leaves many people in a bad mood. It's hard to feel inspired and happy when you're living on processed junk foods. Julia Ross, author of *The Mood Cure* and a pioneer in the field of nutritional psychology, refers to this relationship as the law of malnutrition. The current epidemic of bad moods is definitely linked to an epidemic of deteriorating food quality and quantity: Junk moods come from junk foods, she writes. Soda, chocolates, ice cream, potato chips, and fries are all easily accessible foods that people turn to when they want to be lifted out of a bad mood, but the irony is that these foods are a big part of the problem. Salt can mess with your mood, making you feel tense. Sugar can give you a high and make you feel energized. When your blood sugar goes up, you get that woo-hoo good feeling. But as soon as it goes down, that feeling quickly disappears.

Think about the idea of comfort food. If you have a bowl of soup, you somehow feel all warm inside. It's soothing. The opposite of comfort food is focus food, which helps you work harder. Many people refer to protein, such as eggs, nuts, or meat, as brain food. Ever notice how you crave more comfort food after work or more sharpening food to focus during a busy day at the office? We even crave more aphrodisiac food, such as chili peppers and spice, avocado, and chocolate, when we are out on a date. What we are really doing with all of this food is a form of self-medicating, or seeking balance. We already understand the food-mood connection; we just don't have a language to discuss these habits with each other.

From a scientific perspective, the food-mood relationship is maintained by neurotransmitters—chemical messengers that relay thoughts and actions throughout the brain and in the gut. Some neurotransmitters, such as serotonin, can make us feel relaxed. Others, such as dopamine, have a stimulating effect. The food we eat breaks down in the digestive tract, enters the bloodstream, and creates changes in the behavior of these neurotransmitters, thus impacting our mood. Eating carbohydrates releases serotonin in the brain, which makes people feel more relaxed. Eating too many carbs or overly-processed carbs, like sugar and flour, releases even more serotonin, causing drowsiness. You've probably experienced that sleepy feeling after eating too much pasta or heavy carbohydrates. Eating protein produces dopamine and norepinephrine in the brain, which makes people feel more alert and full of energy when protein is eaten in the appropriate portions. On the other hand, overeating protein can lead to tension and irritability.

To take this one step further, some people with mood disorders are told, "It's all in your head," when the truth is that most serotonin (about 90%) is found in the gut. The bacteria in our gut send signals to the brain, altering our hormonal system, which in turn affects our mood. Research has shown that people with depression have an abundance of harmful bacteria and low levels of beneficial bacteria. So simply changing your diet to increase beneficial bacteria and decrease the harmful ones can have a huge impact on how you feel, especially for those dealing with depression. Perhaps we can listen more to those gut feelings about what to eat and the intelligence from what many scientists now call our "second brain."

Another experience of the food-mood connection comes from eating too much. Think of a big holiday dinner and how tired you become after indulging. Overeating often leads to drowsiness. To handle the excess food, blood flow is directed to the stomach and away from the brain. The result is a feeling of lethargy.

It's surprising how deeply food affects us. In relationships, we often get irritated and blame our partner when actually it's our own mood swings that are causing the rift. Our moods go up and down like a yo-yo, and as soon as we come into a nutritional state of balance, suddenly our partner turns out to be a wonderful person.

Each person's food-mood sensitivity varies. Only you can determine the right amount of proteins, carbs, and fats to keep yourself in balance. Once the correlation enters your consciousness, you will be more careful with your food choices. I simply encourage you to notice, explore, experiment, and determine what works for you. I'm sure you've met people who are vibrantly healthy, despite the fact that they eat donuts and drink coffee for breakfast on a regular basis. You probably think to yourself, "If I ate that way, I'd be a mess." And you're probably right. There's nothing wrong with you or with the coffee and donut person, other than the fact that your food-mood sensitivity is different.

One of the best ways to discover how different foods affect your mood is to simply record what you eat and how you feel afterward. Try the exercises at the end of this chapter, both the **Breakfast Experiment** and the **Food-Mood Journal**, to explore how your body and mind respond to different foods.

Energy of Food

As you increase your awareness about the foods you consume, consider that each food has its own unique energy, beyond vitamins, minerals, fats, and carbohydrates. When we eat, we assimilate not only the nutrients but also the energy of the food. Food has distinct qualities and energetic properties, depending on where, when, and how it grows, as well as how it is prepared. By understanding the energy of food, we can choose meals that will create the energy we are seeking in our lives. Virtually no one in the field of health and nutrition speaks about the concept of food having energy, but if you stop and think about it, it intuitively makes sense. Vegetables have a more vibrant energy than proteins. Animal meat from tortured animals has a different energy than meat from animals that lived a peaceful existence. Food energetics is all about how the foods you choose to eat affect your body.

If you practice yoga or have been to India, you may have heard the word *prana*, a Sanskrit word simply translated as "energy." This word is just one way to describe the vital life force energy that exists around us and inside of us. Energy comes from the universe, from air, and from food. Yogis believe that certain foods, such as fresh produce, have a greater amount of energy than foods that are heavily processed or that have been reused a day or two later. It makes sense: When you eat foods with more energy, you will have more energy.

Steve Gagné, author of *Energetics of Food: Encounters with Your Most Intimate Relationships*, says that all food has an essential character. He analyzes where foods come from to help identify their essence. Plants sprout from a seed; some animals are hatched from eggs, while others are birthed by their mothers and nurtured through infancy. Regarding plant food, consider where, when, and in what direction it grows. Greens, such as kale, collards, and bok choy, reach up toward the sun, soaking up the chlorophyll. Eating foods that are rich in chlorophyll provides the blood with oxygen. For this reason, greens are powerful mood enhancers, lifting the spirit. Squash and gourds grow level with the ground and help balance moods and energy levels. Root vegetables, such as carrots, parsnips, beets, and burdock, grow into the ground and absorb the nutrients from the soil in which they grow. Therefore, they have a strong downward energy and are great for grounding us when we feel overstimulated.

In contrast to these vegetables, reflect for a moment on the character of a donut. It starts with dough, made of wheat and sugar. Then it's deep fried, probably in a less-than-desirable oil. Often it's filled with jam, cream, or custard, or topped with a sweet glaze of icing. What kind of energy do you imagine you get from this donut? How would that differ from the energy you get from eating organic roasted root vegetables? As you cultivate awareness around the energy of your food and how it is passed on to you, you will begin to make greater strides in recognizing your own mind-body connection.

Another important point about the energy of food is how nutrients in our food work together, a concept known as food synergy. Whole foods contain an array of components, such as phytonutrients and vitamins, which offer health benefits when consumed together. So, while taking a vitamin C supplement can be helpful at times, if we can find foods like citrus, strawberries, and red pepper, even better. For years, research has found that, when single antioxidants are studied in clinical trials, they do not hold up to the amazing preventive benefits of the whole foods themselves. No individual compound can replace what's found naturally in fruits and vegetables. So eating a wide range of these foods is what helps keep us healthy. It's simple, really.

Taking food energetics to the next level, I have a theory I call Cross-Species Transference, which asserts that character traits can be passed from animals to humans. Essentially, you become more like the species you eat. Modern nutrition experts claim that a protein is a protein is a protein. The current dietary guidelines say that meat, poultry, fish, beans, eggs, and nuts are basically the same. I have to disagree. Energetically, it makes an enormous difference if you are getting protein from any of the following sources: dal or minestrone soup; soy milk or cow's milk; beef, chicken, or fish; and organic or nonorganic protein.

This theory may seem esoteric and difficult to prove, but I became convinced during my years of working with clients that I could spot the influence of specific animal foods on individuals. When I would meet people with pronounced, beak-like noses and tense, nervous dispositions, I would ask, "Have you eaten a lot of chicken?" Nine times out of 10, they would answer "yes." Think about Frank Purdue in all those commercials for his chicken conglomerate. He looked like a chicken. When I'd bump into someone strong and muscular, with a red face, and ask if they ate a lot of beef, they would invariably answer "yes."

Our bodies absorb the energetic qualities of our foods, especially when we eat meat. Once you open your eyes to this information, it's amazing to discover how much it impacts us daily. What impresses me is how sensitive and adaptable the human body can be. We can change our moods, our bodies, and our mind-sets by making small changes in our daily diet. I hope understanding the flexible nature of your own biological organism will encourage you to explore and experiment with different foods. Your body will respond to the changes you make, and you will feel the difference. Just give it a try.

Back to Basics

I really try to keep it as simple as possible when it comes to my health. I know it's hard to sort through all of the theories out there, but when it comes down to it, the average person needs to have less meat, milk, sugar, and processed junk food, and more vegetables, fruit, water, exercise, and sleep. People think they need to understand all of the nuances of complex science, but, in my experience, all of this information is not what wins the day. It's really about the basics of exploring your habits, being open to new strategies for health, and sticking to a simple, whole-foods diet most of the time.

I do want to talk for a moment about our relationship between food and weight. Our society idolizes people who are thin. But with an overabundance of snack foods, junk foods, and fast foods, combined with a lack of daily exercise, many people struggle with their weight. The World Health Organization says that most of the world lives in countries where health issues related to being overweight and obese kill more people than those related to being underweight. More than 1.9 billion adults 18 years or older are overweight, and more than 600 million of these people are obese.

People turn to conventional and modern nutrition's approach of counting calories and trying to get fit. When they have trouble following their own diet regimen, they look for help in the more than $60 billion diet and weight loss industry, which includes everything from commercial chains like Weight Watchers and Jenny Craig to diet pills, artificial sweeteners, diet books and magazines, meal replacement shakes, and belly-stapling surgeries.[4]

Year after year, many Americans realize that these fad diets don't work. In fact, about 90% of all dieters regain some or all of the weight originally lost. Diet and exercise theories like the 40-day, 20-day, or even 8-minutes-a-day to a thinner you are aimed at quick results and book sales.

Many people who have lost weight and maintained their health have looked past the diet books and fads and found what works best for their own bodies. I encourage people who want to lose weight to experiment with different methods and see what works.

We also live in a culture where we get a lot of negative messages about our bodies, and many people, especially women, feel the need to fix, improve, or change their bodies in some way. Healthy bodies come in all sizes. The emphasis should be on proper nutritional intake and overall health, not trying to get as skinny as possible. When we love and respect our bodies, we are much more apt to take care of them and make healthier choices to prevent chronic health issues.

In the current nutrition discussion, most people really miss the idea of keeping your health simple and getting back to the basic food and lifestyle choices that help the vast majority of people live well. In that vein, please review these wellness tips as a reminder of how you can always get back to basics.

Wellness Tips (That Work for Almost Everyone)

Be a food detective. Read food labels, and don't eat anything you can't pronounce. Stick to simple, whole foods that will nourish your body.

Drink more water. By replacing soda, coffee, or energy drinks with water, you can cut a significant number of stimulants from your daily routine. Many people report more energy by simply replacing these drinks with water throughout the day.

Make your own meals. Restaurant food generally has more salt, more fat, and more unknown ingredients than food cooked at home. When you make your own meals, you can control the quality of your food, your portion sizes, and the environment you eat in. If you have to eat out, try eating somewhere with an emphasis on slow food or farm-to-table practices. Remember: The food you eat has energy, and how you eat it will impact how you feel.

Reduce your stress levels. Many people eat more when they feel stress; the stuffed feeling makes them feel comfortable and helps them relax. Try other ways of relaxing, like a hot bath or a walk around the block. Also try slowing down, breathing, and enjoying each meal. Say a prayer beforehand, or take a moment to be grateful for the food you are eating.

Get enough sleep each night. Growing evidence supports that missing out on sleep can increase your appetite, which many times makes you reach for processed snack foods. Most people need about 7 to 9 hours of sleep each night.

Keep moving. Start with small changes, like getting off one stop earlier on a train and walking the rest of the way or parking in the back of a parking lot. Take the stairs whenever possible. Instead of meeting a friend for coffee, meet for a walk or a bike ride, or take a dance class together.

Explore cravings. Cravings are not something you need to squash; they are messages from your body. Tune in and listen to learn more about what your cravings might mean.

Be mindful. A little attention to your health can go a long way. You can try a food journal or use an app on your phone, but explore ways to connect with what you are eating and how different foods affect your mood and overall health.

Exercises

1. The Breakfast Experiment[5]

As a way of tuning into your body and learning how to listen to its messages, explore eating a different breakfast every day for a week. Jot down what you eat and how you feel, both right after the meal and then again two hours later.

Day 1: scrambled eggs

Day 2: scrambled tofu

Day 3: oatmeal

Day 4: boxed breakfast cereal

Day 5: muffin and coffee

Day 6: fresh fruit smoothie

Day 7: fresh green juice and a handful of nuts

Day 1 Breakfast:

Right after eating I felt:

Two hours after eating I felt:

Day 2 Breakfast:

Right after eating I felt:

Two hours after eating I felt:

Day 3 Breakfast:

Right after eating I felt:

Two hours after eating I felt:

Day 4 Breakfast:

Right after eating I felt:

Two hours after eating I felt:

Day 5 Breakfast:

Right after eating I felt:

Two hours after eating I felt:

Day 6 Breakfast:

Right after eating I felt:

Two hours after eating I felt:

Day 7 Breakfast:

Right after eating I felt:

Two hours after eating I felt:

Once you get the knack of this experiment, you can expand it to include your whole daily intake, exploring how different foods and liquids affect you. For example, for one week, make a point of drinking more water during the day, eating more leafy greens, or experimenting with different protein sources. Notice how your body feels and how each change of diet affects your mood.

2. Food-Mood Journal

Write down what you eat at each meal or snack and how you feel afterwards. Be sure to record how you feel immediately after and then again a few hours later. You may feel great right after eating candy or drinking coffee, but two hours later it's often a different story. You may write, "I had tea first thing this morning, and I felt good. I had coffee at 11 a.m. and still felt okay, but the second cup of coffee after lunch put me over the top." Or you may notice, "I had too much animal meat today and felt lethargic." Or, perhaps, "Every time I eat bread, my stomach hurts." Or, "Yesterday, I had a nice spinach and lentil soup, but I wanted something more. I had a small piece of chocolate for dessert and felt satisfied." Soon you will know what energizes you and what drains you. Certain foods will give you gas; certain foods will prevent you from sleeping well, and other foods will enhance your ability to concentrate at work.

3. Friend Food Inventory

List the three healthiest people you know and the three unhealthiest people you know. Write down what they eat. See how the foods correlate with their level of vibrancy.

Chapter 3

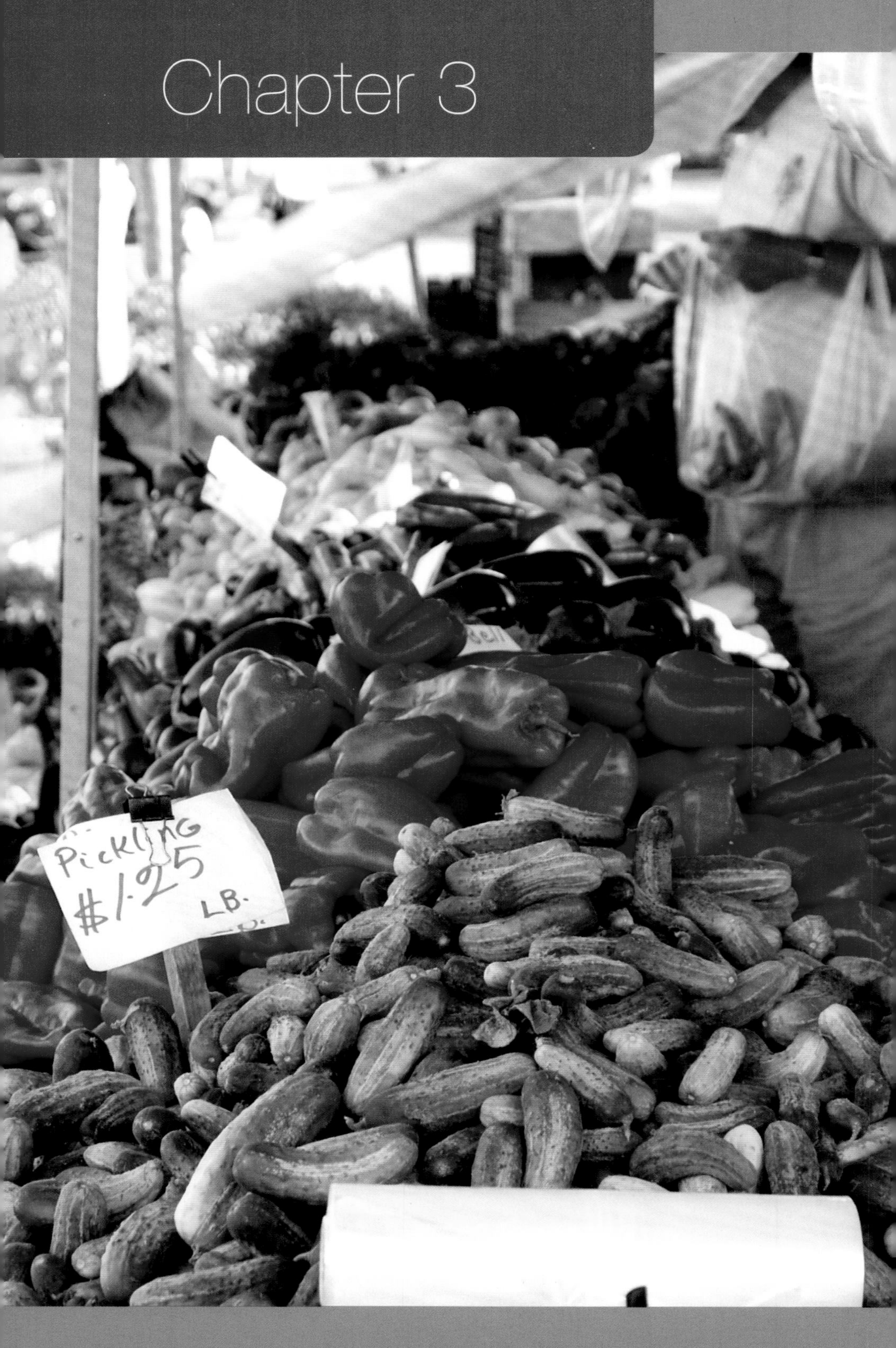

The Ethics of Eating

> The energies of nature and the infinite universe are absorbed through the foods we eat and are transmuted into our thoughts and actions.
>
> —Michio Kushi

Now that you know the fundamentals of postmodern nutrition, let's go a little deeper. Part of the modern experience of eating has to do with the quality of the food we eat and the quality of our eating experience. In just a few generations, humans have completely transformed what, when, and how we eat. Supermarket food contains chemicals, additives, and sweeteners wrapped in boxes with bright colors and catchy slogans. Labels on packages have become sneakier, with phrases like "lightly sweetened" or "made with whole grains" as savvier shoppers look for healthier options. We eat this stuff, along with fried fast foods, in our cars, in front of our TVs, or at our desks, giving little thought to where our food comes from and how our food choices impact the world around us. We eat with all of our senses, but many of us never stop to enjoy the look, smell, sound, texture, or even taste of our food. Most people don't really chew their food. They spend time at doctors' offices complaining of upset stomachs, constipation, and a range of other digestive disorders without thinking about these larger issues.

The Integrative Nutrition approach to this problem is quite simple: Eat and *enjoy* high-quality food. Take a look at what you're eating, when you're eating it, and how you eat it. You may be surprised to find that, by making a few adjustments, you can dramatically improve the quality of your life. Better food equals better health. It's really that simple.

What We Eat

The Food Our Ancestors Ate

Throughout history, people have eaten food essentially as nature produced it. People ate whole and unprocessed vegetables, fruit, grains, beans, chicken, fish, and other animal foods. Small amounts of sugar and honey or some wine and beer in the diet were balanced by regular physical labor, from sunrise to sunset, for every member of the family. They had no cars, planes, trains, or bicycles for transportation. Life was active.

Our ancestors would not recognize the food in today's supermarket. In the last 100 years or so, large-scale food processing has become the norm. Breads and other baked goods that were once made of whole-grain flour are now made from processed, white, bleached flour that is far less nutritious. American consumers have developed a taste for processed foods, like pastries, cookies, crackers, chips, and other foods that are far removed from their origins. I think most people would agree that Doritos don't grow on trees.

Many people don't realize that processing food strips it of many nutrients. Think of the difference between white bread and wheat bread. Both come from wheat. But wheat bread uses the entire grain, while white bread is made by removing the bran and the germ (parts of the grain) during the milling process. Manufacturers remove these parts to create lighter, fluffier bread and to extend its shelf life. The germ, specifically, contains natural oils that could make bread go rancid. Wonder Bread can sit on the shelf for about 21 days before it loses its moisture and gets hard, while bakeries typically sell their fresh-baked bread within 24 hours. With gluten sensitivities on the rise, some experts have speculated that the processing may have something to do with it. Research from the Whole Grains Council has found that wheat foods are higher in gluten these days, which may account for increased health issues.

In addition to leaving out or removing essential nutrients, processing foods generally involves adding sweeteners, colors, flavors, and preservatives. Manufacturers now add sugar to everything from ketchup to toothpaste. Supermarket shelves are filled with highly processed foods, including soft drinks, packaged snacks, frozen dinners, boxed desserts, and condiments. Nearly all of these items contain artificial ingredients, rather than fresh food.

Sometimes manufacturers try to reintroduce nutrients into foods by a process called enrichment. But a laboratory can't possibly reintroduce all of the vitamins, minerals, carotenoids, and fiber that the original plant source contained. A single tomato contains more than 10,000 phytochemicals. Scientists have identified thousands of phytochemicals that can help boost immune function, prevent DNA damage, and protect cells from the damaging effects of toxic substances that can result in cancer and heart disease.[1] When you see the word "enriched" on bread labels, such as "enriched white flour" or "enriched wheat flour," it means they took out the good stuff in the processing and tried to put some of it back at the end. A similar process occurs with fortified cereals, which typically feature highly processed grains and sweeteners doused with a few vitamins. A simple way to think about enriched foods is to imagine you have $100 in your wallet. If someone stole the $100 but then decided to put back $20, would you feel enriched? I think most people would feel like they're still missing $80.

The fact that we have to inject nutrients back into our food demonstrates how strange our eating habits have become. Not that long ago, we ate what was fresh and available. Now we eat foods that are cheap, fast, and convenient with little thought about whether they give our bodies the nutrients we need to get us through our day. I wonder what our ancestors would think. My guess is that, if they could see us buying food from drive-thru windows and from automated vending machines, they would think we were from another planet. If they tasted all of the chemicals, preservatives, and added fats and sugars, the flavor of our modern foods would be so intense they would probably spit them out.

What we buy in the grocery store may look like food, and it may taste like food, but it's not the food our great-grandmothers ate. I encourage you to eat foods in their whole, natural states as much as possible. But let's distinguish the difference between processing and refining. When you peel a carrot at home, that's a form of food processing. So not all processing is necessarily a bad thing. But there's another kind of processing where foods get highly refined, meaning a core part of the food gets removed, like the germ from a grain, or they become unrecognizable from their original form. Before you put products in your cart at the store, or before you place your order at a restaurant, think about the process your food went through to get to you. If you're at a Mexican restaurant, the corn tortillas are probably made from processed corn flour and a mix of preservatives. If you're buying Twinkies from the store, think about how they were created—using highly processed flour and sugar—and stuffed with a white filling made from cream, which comes from cow's milk and contains added sugar. Many different machines are involved in both the production and the packaging of processed foods like this one.

Many people are disconnected from real, whole foods and have lost touch with the reality that our food comes from the earth. We don't even know how most of the fruit and vegetables we buy are grown. Simple eating celebrates the richness of whole foods. Think of the juiciness of a ripe piece of fruit, the crunchiness of a whole carrot, or the creaminess of mashing an avocado. I encourage you to find simple pleasures in the foods you eat. An easy strategy is to stick with foods that have five or fewer ingredients and foods with labels that include ingredients you recognize, rather than chemicals and preservatives.

Organics

One of the most profound ways to experience the energetic nature of food is to notice the properties of organic food. Have you noticed that eating organic food can make you feel more vital and that the taste is cleaner and more flavorful? It's not surprising that organic products continue to be one of the fastest-growing categories of food. Worldwide, 2.3 million producers farm organically, and the countries with the most producers are India, Uganda, and Mexico. The global market for organic sales reached $80 billion in 2014, according to Organic Monitor. The U.S., Germany, France, and China have the largest markets for organic. In the U.S., almost 5% of all food sold was organic in 2015.[2]

Originally, all foods were "organic"—grown without synthetic pesticides, herbicides, chemical fertilizers, or hormones. Large-scale farming with chemicals began during World War II, around the same time that food processing exploded. Large-scale farming works against the natural cycles of the earth, relying on chemicals to produce big returns. This process has depleted much of the world's soil of its minerals and nutrients. The resulting vegetable and animal foods are not only deficient in nutrients but also full of pollutants and agrochemicals.

The modern denaturing of foods through massive refining and chemical treatment degrades their original life force, making it difficult to foster equilibrium and health for the people eating them. Pesticides, which are present in most commercial produce, must be processed by our immune systems and have been shown to cause cancer as well as liver, kidney, and blood diseases. In addition, as pesticides build up in our tissues, our immune systems weaken, allowing other carcinogens and pathogens to affect our health. They even pass through breast milk!

In contrast, organic farming works with the land. Crops are rotated from year to year to allow the soil to replenish its nutrients between growing cycles. Animals graze in different areas each season to let grasses recover and replenish between seasons. Farmers feed the soil with broken-down plant waste (compost), rather than using artificial fertilizing methods. Some farms even cultivate good pests to help rid the area of bad pests and plant seeds in coordination with the cycles of the moon. All of these practices are long-term, sustainable methods of farming that work with the natural environment, instead of adding chemicals to it.

Fresh, organic produce contains more vitamins, minerals, enzymes, and other micronutrients than intensively farmed produce. According to research published in the *Journal of Agricultural and Food Chemistry*, organic fruits and veggies have 50% to 60% higher levels of cancer-fighting antioxidants than nonorganic fruits and veggies.[3] Similarly, research published in the *British Journal of Nutrition* found that both organic dairy and meat contain about 50% more omega-3s than conventionally raised counterparts, thanks to the animals foraging on their natural diet—grasses full of omega-3s. Though organic food is usually more expensive, you can rest assured that you're limiting your exposure to chemicals, GMOs, hormones, and antibiotics. If you're on a budget, consider money-saving tips, like growing more of your own organic produce, buying in bulk whenever you can, and reducing waste by being mindful about how you store your food. Don't forget to shop deals at your co-op or grocery store; foods in season tend to cost less.

Some people avoid organic produce because it sometimes looks less colorful and less perfectly shaped than conventionally grown produce. But have you ever bought a big, red, juicy tomato from the store, only to find that when you bite into it at home, it has no flavor? Have you ever picked a small, funny-shaped tomato right off the vine and found it incredibly sweet? It hasn't spent weeks on a truck or been exposed to harsh chemicals, so its natural taste is preserved. Organic fruits and vegetables may not always look as bright or "perfect" as some conventionally grown foods (which are sometimes dyed to look more appealing), but they certainly taste fresh off the vine. Another thing people notice when first buying organic produce is that the fruits seem smaller. Our society tends to believe that bigger is better, but try to reverse this saying when you look at organic produce. It is actually grown to its natural size, resulting in a more flavorful, and often sweeter, taste than its larger, non-organic counterpart.

Another reason to eat organic is to avoid genetically modified organisms (GMOs), also known as genetically engineered foods. A GMO is any organism in which the genetic material has been altered or shuffled around in a way that does not occur naturally. This technology allows individual genes to be transferred from one organism to another. This science is used to cultivate genetically modified (GM) plants, which are then used to grow GM food crops. GMOs on the market have been given genetic traits to provide protection from pests and diseases, to provide resistance to pesticides, or to improve the quality of the crop. The most prevalent GM crops were created to resist harsh chemicals; these crops have DNA traits from bacteria, fungi, or other plants that create this resistance. Farmers who use GM crops can spray their fields to kill everything growing in the area except the food crop. Imagine what is being killed in our bodies when we eat these foods.

The most common genetically engineered crops in the United States, which is the largest grower of GM crops in the world, are canola, corn, soy, and cotton. Genetically engineered soy, corn, and canola are used in many processed foods. In fact, experts estimate that about 70% of the foods in grocery stores in the U.S. and Canada contain genetically engineered ingredients.

During the past decade, food safety experts have identified several potential problems with genetically engineered food crops, according to reports from the Union of Concerned Scientists. These problems include the possibility of introducing new toxins or allergens into previously safe foods, increasing toxins to dangerous levels in foods that typically produce harmless amounts, and diminishing foods' nutritional values. Many scientists have raised environmental concerns about these crops, as GM crops tend to dominate wild plants and conventional crops, potentially disrupting natural ecosystems.

About 64 countries throughout the world require labeling of genetically modified foods—including Australia, Brazil, Russia, Saudi Arabia, and the United Kingdom. In 2016, U.S. legislation passed after a long fight to label GMO foods. While the bill that passed established a national standard for labeling, it also gives a lot of flexibility to big food companies about how they choose to label. They can put labels directly on food packages or make consumers do more research by directing them to scan a code, call an 800 number, or visit a website.

Proponents of labeling argue that it allows consumers to know which foods on supermarket shelves contain genetically engineered ingredients and prohibit these products from getting labeled as "natural." Big food companies, like Monsanto, Dupont, PepsiCo, Coca-Cola, Kraft, General Mills, and Kellogg, have spent millions of dollars fighting labeling.[4] But change is afoot, and big food companies are slowly changing their tune. In 2016, ConAgra, Kellogg, Mars, General Mills, and Campbell's pledged to label their products that contain GMOs, even before legislation passed.

If you live in a place where these foods are not labeled, and you want to avoid them, become a food detective. Look for "organic" or for products labeled by the Non-GMO Project, a collaboration of manufacturers, retailers, farmers, and consumers who have developed the first independent third-party Non-GMO Product Verification Program.[5]

Most and Least Contaminated Produce

Each year analysts at Environmental Working Group (EWG) create lists of fruits and vegetables that have been found to have the most and least amounts of pesticide residue. Their work is based on laboratory tests done by the USDA Pesticide Testing Program and the Food and Drug Administration. EWG is a not-for-profit environmental research organization dedicated to improving public health and protecting the environment. In general, more delicate foods, such as leafy greens and fruits with soft peels like apples and peaches, tend to have higher amounts of residue. Heartier foods, like avocadoes, pineapples, and onions, tend to have less. Use these lists to help you make food choices, and if you can't buy all organic, consider these lists to help you prioritize what to buy organic. Check out their website at https://www.ewg.org/foodnews/.

Environmental Effects of Food Choices

Our personal food choices have an impact not only on our bodies, but also on our environment. Each meal is made up of food that requires a significant amount of energy and resources to reach your plate. The journey of our food is a much longer process than many of us realize. Some people refer to this journey as food miles, which is the distance food travels from field to plate, and the higher the mileage, the larger the impact on the environment. Food travels farther these days partly because of large corporate grocery stores, which have centralized methods for distributing food. In some cases, a crop of cherries may travel across the country to be packaged and then sent back close to where the cherries were originally grown. In other cases, stores fly in food from all over the world to ensure they have fresh produce, whatever the season. This practice causes us to have organic bananas from Peru, organic kiwis from New Zealand, and organic avocados from Mexico, at any time of year. Locally produced, seasonal foods cut energy use and, therefore, leave a smaller impact on the environment.

The decision about whether to eat meat is also a big one, and it can have a significant impact on the environment. In John Robbins's book *Diet for a New America*, he points to many areas that are impacted by factory-farmed beef consumption. Cattle require huge amounts of water every day. Giving up one pound of beef a year could save more water than if you stopped showering for six months, according to his book. Corn-fed cattle also impact the environment, because each bushel of corn they eat has been treated with about 1.2 gallons of oil-based fertilizers. Each cow consumes about 25 pounds of corn each day, which translates into a lot of fossil fuel energy. Cattle also need land for grazing. About 70% of the lands in Western national forests are used for grazing, according to the book. And although the U.S. is the world's largest producer of beef, worldwide demand for beef has caused massive deforestation in other parts of the world. An international team of scientists estimates that close to 15 billion trees get cut down each year, and in large part this deforestation is for agriculture. Since 1978, more than 750,000 square kilometers (289,000 square miles) of the Amazon rainforest has been destroyed throughout Brazil, Peru, Colombia, Bolivia, and Venezuela.[6]

The leading cause of deforestation in the Amazon is cattle ranching. The growth in cattle production—80% of which was in the Amazon—was largely export driven. While deforestation has slowed since 2008, it continues. Environmental groups are working with scientists to help achieve zero net deforestation by 2020, according to the Living Planet Report.[7]

But you don't have to eat a strict vegan diet to eat in an environmentally friendly manner. Get to know where your meat comes from by making friends with your local farmers and ranchers, or look online to find better sources than what's available at your local store. Look for quality meat that is grass-fed, humanely raised, and local, whenever possible. Experiment with adding into your diet wild game meats, like rabbit, venison, bison, or duck, which do not contribute to deforestation. Think about reducing the amount of meat in your diet and, therefore, lessening your overall environmental footprint.

When We Eat

Seasonal Foods

One Christmas when I was visiting India, I went to the market to buy fruit. It was still frigid in Massachusetts, where I lived at the time, and I hadn't had good, fresh fruit in several months. I filled bags with grapes, pomegranates, mangoes, and limes, and, after feeling the ache in my arms on the walk home, realized I had overdone it. As I came to the gate of my apartment building, I offered some of the fruit to the guard outside the apartment where I was staying.

"No, thank you, sir," he said, smiling politely. I knew he was a poor man and fruit was a relative luxury for him, so I was confused.

"Do you eat fruit?" I asked him with curiosity.

"Yes, sir, thank you, sir. You are very generous, sir. But I don't eat fruit in the wintertime because the weather gets cold at night."

Although he'd probably never read a diet book, the guard instinctively knew that fruit is a cooling food. He knew not to eat food that reduced his body temperature during a cold time of year because it would lead to sickness. Returning to my apartment, I realized it probably wasn't such a great idea for me to be eating all of this fruit either. I had some anyway, but it was an "aha" moment. I learned more from this man than from all of the diet experts' books. Our ancestors ate seasonally because they had no choice. Fresh greens grew in spring, fruit ripened in summer, root vegetables kept them going in the fall, and people relied on animal food to get them through the winter. But when California and Florida were settled and highway transportation and refrigerated trucks were invented, pretty soon Americans could eat more or less anything they wanted, anytime they wanted. But there are costs to this kind of convenience. When we have ice cream in the middle of January and hot barbecued foods on the 4th of July, it's likely to confuse the body. Eating locally grown food in accordance with the seasons will help you live in harmony with yourself, your body, and the earth.

In the wintertime, it's natural for many people to crave animal protien, more substantial vegetables (like potatoes and squash), and warming grains because that's when the body needs to feel more solid and insulated from the cold. Look at how animals get ready for the winter. Squirrels gather nuts and fatten up to prepare for the cold season. Humans also need more fat in the winter. Allow yourself to eat heavier meals at this time, and be sure to have plenty of oils, protein, and nuts. If you want to remain on a vegetarian diet through these cold months, it may be an interesting experiment to grill your vegetables, giving them more heat and density, and to avoid raw vegetables and salads. Thick soups, such as pumpkin, pea, or potato, will help keep your body feeling sturdy.

Because produce is available year-round, choosing what's in season can be confusing. Generally, look for ripe, fresh produce in abundance, and check with your local farmers to get location-specific assistance for each season. Focus on eating warming foods during cool seasons and cooling foods during the warm seasons. Notice what works best for your body.

Daily Eating Habits

Pay attention to the times of the day when you eat. Most of us eat habitually at regular, clocked times: before work, during the lunch break, and in the evening. We may take a couple of coffee or snack breaks during the day or make a late-night visit to the fridge. Few of us pause to check whether we are really hungry when we eat. We use food as entertainment and comfort, whether we are socializing or alone, passing time or feeling bored.

When we eat determines how well our bodies assimilate food. Ayurvedic philosophy advocates for people to eat their biggest meal in the middle of the day, because it's the best time for our bodies to take in and digest a large meal. If you look at many cultures in Europe, this practice is very common. People close shop, go home, and eat a large meal with their families and friends. In our country it's harder to find this time during the day, but you can find creative ways to have your largest meal at lunch hour. You may find that this works best for your body, or you might find you feel best when you have a large meal at breakfast or at dinner instead. Some people eat a large breakfast and lunch and then have a small snack for dinner; others do best with five small meals throughout the day. Experiment with the size and timing of your meals; only you can determine what is best for your body. Each meal is an experiment. Take the time to listen to your body and notice what it needs.

Many health experts emphasize that we should not eat after 7 p.m. or 8 p.m. I agree that it's a good idea to avoid eating three hours before bed, because when we sleep, digestion slows, and, rather than using this time to repair, our bodies are using energy to digest, which is why you may wake up and still feel tired. Strange dreams and restless sleep can result from late-night eating and affect the next day's energy. New research has suggested that we gain more weight from food we eat at night. I know I don't sleep well on a full stomach, a strong indication that it's not working well for my system. But, again, it's something for you to explore, using your own body as your laboratory.

How We Eat

Drive-thru Eating

People dine in odd ways and places: standing up, driving a car, on the subway, discussing business deals, watching television, reading a book, and playing video games. Eating is no longer viewed as an activity in and of itself, worthy of exclusive quality time. What most people don't realize is that, while we eat food, we are also assimilating energetically whatever else is going on around us. The body is in an open and receiving mode while we eat, and we take in more than just the vitamins and nutrients in our meal. We also absorb what is happening in the environment around us. If we eat in an ugly, noisy, neon-lit room, the energy of that space is going to penetrate us. If we eat quietly in a beautiful park or by the ocean, we will also absorb the positive qualities of those surroundings. When eating with other people, we often absorb their moods, their laughter, their complaints, and their busy minds.

Many people suffer from a range of digestive disorders, from acid reflux to irritable bowel syndrome and more. These conditions are connected not just to what we eat, but to how we eat it. Our bodies have sensors that connect our guts to our brains and our five senses. When these sensors are triggered, they get our digestive juices flowing, helping us properly process our food. They tell us when we have had enough to eat so we don't overload our systems. When we eat too fast, on the run, or under stress, these sensors don't have enough time to go off. Our bodies are unable to rev up and prepare for digestion. By the time our brains get the message that we are getting full, we've already scarfed down a huge meal and moved on to our next activity. As a result, our bodies barely recognize that we have eaten, even though there is plenty of food in our stomachs. I'm sure you've had this experience. For example, many of us eat while driving and then wonder why we feel hungry a few hours later and crave or eat more food. This overeating can overwhelm the body and eventually lead to chronic conditions.

Because the nature of our bodies is to "rest and digest," the body likes to be relaxed, inactive, and in a peaceful environment when assimilating food. The body doesn't want to be in a tense "fight, flight, or freeze" mode, alert for danger and unexpected events. In this state, the eyes tighten, the heart beats faster, and blood goes from the center of the body to our extremities to prepare the body to fight or flee. Stress contributes to poor digestion because the body is ready to run, not digest. Proper assimilation of the nutrients in food is essential to health, and if we want this assimilation to take place, we need to be calmer when we sit down to meals.

People used to enjoy food by eating dinner together. This traditional daily ritual had a binding effect on the family as an organic unit. As the saying goes, "A family that eats together stays together." Sharing meals made the family more cohesive and, in turn, kept them interwoven within a much bigger collective fabric, a whole mind-set about the kind of society we all wanted. This mind-set is rapidly changing. Now kids eat prepackaged microwave dinners because both parents are working and have no time to prepare home-cooked meals. If Dad eats a burger for dinner, Mom has a large salad, and the kids eat pizza on the run, it's natural that the family will have difficulty relating to one another later in the evening. Each member of the family will have different energy, thoughts, and feelings depending on his or her individual meal.

Whether you are a single person or part of a family unit, experiment with ways to eat in a calmer, quieter, more loving way. Cultivate a "slow food" mentality, offering balance to our fast food world by cooking more at home and eating slowly and mindfully. Healthy eating means eating with all of our senses. We need to see our food, smell it, and spend time enjoying it. Maybe you can organize your family to eat a home-cooked meal together once a week. Notice the difference this makes in your energy and connection. Try simple rituals to make mealtime special, like eating off of your good plates, lighting a candle, or saying a blessing before your meal. If you tend to eat at your desk at work, try to change this habit. Simply going into a different room to eat, or better yet, eating outside, may make a big difference. Be creative, and discover what you can do to bring your body into a more relaxed state during your meals. It could make a big difference to your overall health.

The Importance of Chewing

Many of us inhale our food. We use our fork as a shovel, putting the next bite in before we've finished the previous one. It's part of our fast-paced culture. Aside from missing the enjoyment of a long, relaxing meal, eating quickly can be detrimental to our health. Digestion actually begins with the chewing process. If you think about your stomach working to break down every little bit of food you put into your mouth, it makes sense that the more you break it down in the chewing process, the easier the digestion process will be. In addition, the action of chewing and the resulting production of saliva send a message to the stomach, intestines, and entire gastrointestinal system that the digestion process has begun. These organs can then prepare for their digestion tasks and keep the body in balance.

Chewing also makes food more enjoyable. The sweet flavor of whole foods is released only after they have been chewed thoroughly. Complex carbohydrates start breaking down in the mouth by an enzyme in saliva known as amylase. It is only by chewing the carbs thoroughly and mixing them with amylase that we can taste all of their sweetness. This sweet flavor becomes a reward for chewing. Do you see the brilliance of the natural food system involved in this process? Leveraging our inherent craving for sweetness, our body works with nature to ensure we get the nutrients we need.

I do not have a recommended amount of time people should take to chew each bite, although some of my students experiment with chewing each bite 20 to 50 times. In general, I recommend putting down your fork or utensils in between each bite to help you focus on the food in your mouth. Once you are done chewing, then you can take your next bite. It can be difficult to focus on chewing when eating with others, so try eating on your own and focusing on fully chewing each bite. Turn off the TV, resist the urge to text, and really focus on your eating experience. You'll see that it takes you longer to eat your meal but that you get full faster. Another useful tip to help people slow down is to try eating with chopsticks. They can only pick up a limited amount of food at a time, and it can be a fun eating adventure.

The Changing Health Food Scene

Since the original publication of this book, the food scene has changed quite a bit. Health food markets and healthy restaurants used to be few and far between. They mostly catered to the fringes of society—people who were looking for vegetarian or macrobiotic food or people who liked sprout wraps and kitchari. Now, we have juice bars everywhere, farm-to-table restaurants abound, and many healthy, fresh foods are available, even at regular grocery stores.

Food is a really big deal today. When I was a kid, I took a sandwich to school. Dinner was typically a piece of meat and veggies. Life was simple. Today, we are all much more sophisticated. But there's still an enormous emphasis on eating for flavor and taste, not for health. So, while I applaud more fresh food available to all, we still need to be mindful when it comes to "foodie" items, like artisanal kale and blueberry ice cream. It's still ice cream! And while the rise of fast casual restaurants throughout the world means higher-quality on-the-go options (including organic), don't forget that these chain restaurants are simply better dressed cousins to the fast food world. They are still selling chips, fries, and milkshakes, which are not typically foods you would make at home. Similarly, it's refreshing to see food companies responding to trends by reducing or even eliminating unhealthy ingredients in their processed foods. In 2015 Kraft announced that it would replace food dyes in its signature boxed mac and cheese product with annatto seed and paprika extract. It's a first in my lifetime to see mainstream companies making these shifts. Yet, we still have a long road ahead.

Ultimately, my advice in this changing landscape is to continue listening to what feels right for your body. Keep it simple, and stick to good ol' fashioned real food as much as possible. Enjoy the benefits of more healthy food when you are out and about, and stay attentive at every meal.

Exercises

1. Your Local Farmers' Market

Find a farmers' market in your area. Walk around the market, and notice all of the fresh vegetables. Talk to the farmers about where they come from and ask about the journey the vegetables took to get there. If they are local and organic, they are most likely in season. Filling your bag with local produce is a way to ensure that you are cooking and eating in season. Share some of your favorite finds with your friends and family. Consider trying something new each time you visit.

2. Mindful Eating

At your next meal, count how many times you chew each mouthful of food. See if you can chew 100 times per bite. Or try 50. Become more aware of each bite, and practice chewing slowly and with intention. Notice how you feel at the end of your meal. Share your experience with your friends and family, and encourage them to chew as well.

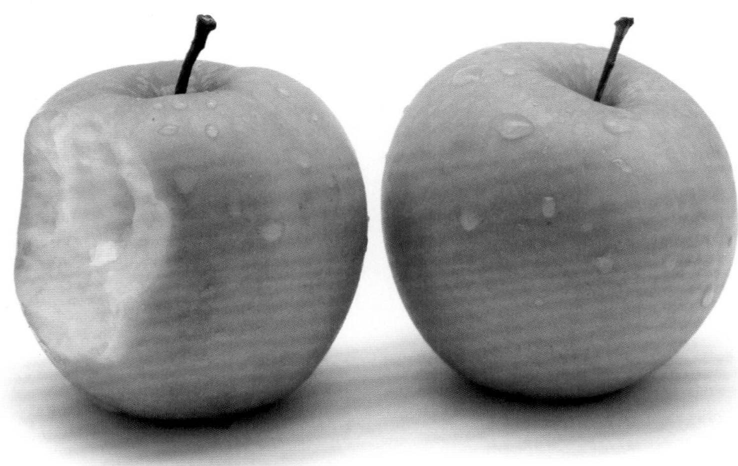

Chapter 4

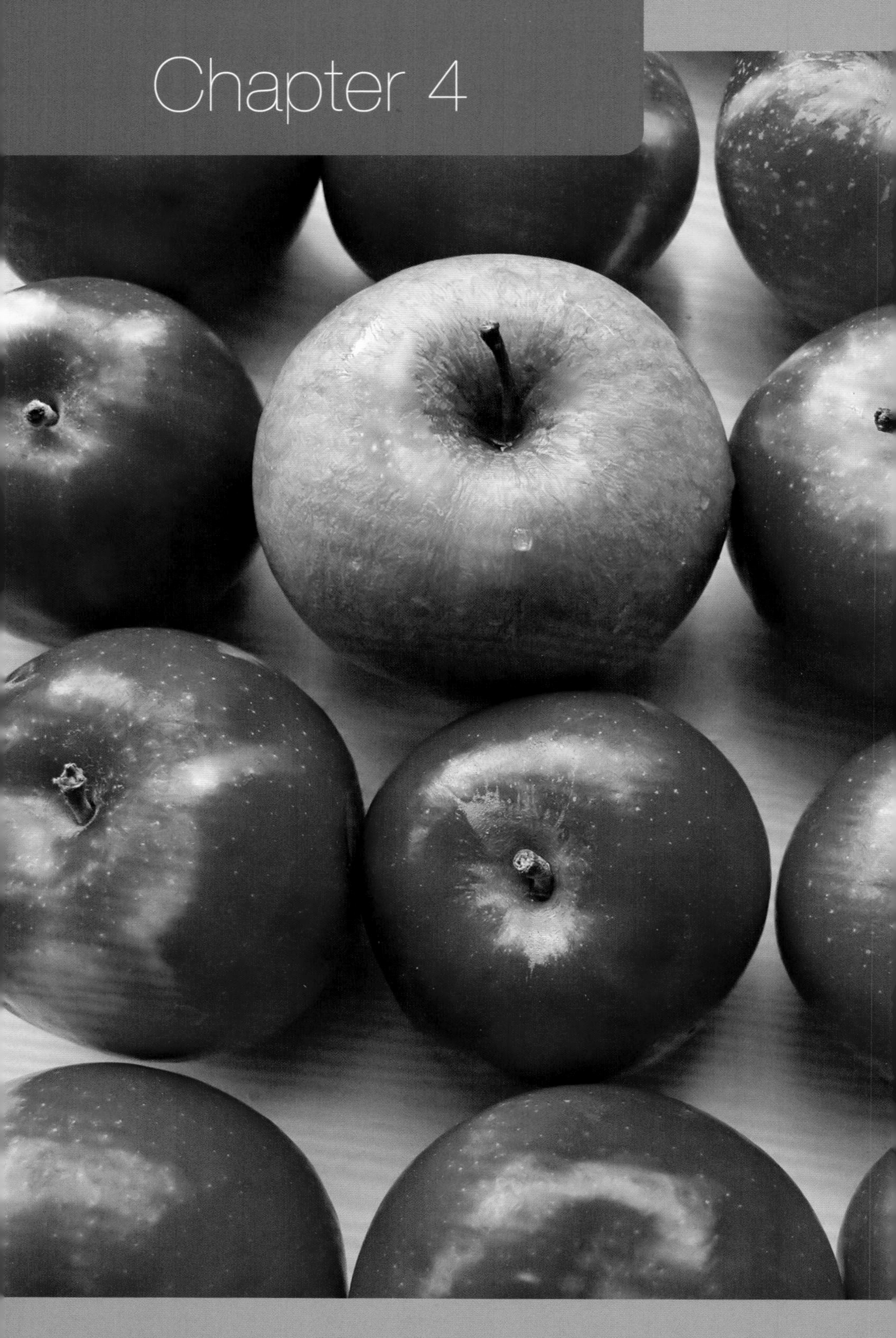

Dietary Theory

> When it comes to diet, one size definitely doesn't fit all.
> —Christiane Northrup, MD

I have always been interested in food. As a child, I was excited to go shopping with my mother. I was enthralled by the enormous supermarket filled with shopping carts and aisles upon aisles of food. I wondered how my mother knew which foods to choose and which to leave on the shelf. At home, I would help put the food away in cupboards or in the fridge, and my mom would systematically take it out again throughout the week for meals. The whole process—how food transformed from packages on shelves to warm, delicious meals on a plate—fascinated me.

As I grew up, my passion for food continued. In my 20s, while getting my master's in education with a specialization in counseling, I noticed that there was no overlap between the sciences of psychology and nutrition, but I knew a connection existed. At that time, I encountered someone on a vegetarian diet. With that friendship, I became much more conscious of my eating habits, which led to a further understanding of the food-mood connection. I realized that, to best support my clients emotionally, I would have to incorporate dialogue about food. The clients who upgraded the quality of their food became more clear, optimistic, and healthy. In turn, I became clear that emotional counseling had to be preceded by counseling on food and diet.

At the age of 25, my interest in natural foods led me to macrobiotics. I read every book on the topic that I could find (about 50 at the time), went to macrobiotics conferences, studied at the macrobiotics center in Toronto, and eventually studied extensively with Michio and Aveline Kushi, two of the chief students of George Ohsawa, the man who created macrobiotics as it is known today. Then, when I was director of the macrobiotics center in

Toronto, I increased my frequency of visits to the Kushi Institute, learning as much as I possibly could. Considering that my nutrition philosophy evolved out of this Japanese-based theory, I'd like to share a few stories to illustrate why macrobiotics initially attracted me.

Michio invited me to go with him to Japan, where I met people whose families had grown traditional macrobiotic foods for centuries, such as umeboshi plums and high-quality brown rice. I met miso masters and even someone who made sake from brown rice. On this trip, I gained a deep understanding of Michio, Aveline, and traditional macrobiotics. Upon our return, I enrolled in their intensive 10-day Macrobiotic Educator Course, which boasts such esteemed alumni as Paul Pitchford, Dr. Dean Ornish, and Dr. Christiane Northrup, to become an official, expert macrobiotic teacher. We studied medicinal cooking, visual diagnosis, and shiatsu massage, and we learned how to perform consultations to gain an in-depth understanding of macrobiotic theory and practice. Students would take turns cooking and eat three meals a day together. Michio and Aveline were known for their finely tuned taste buds and skills in judging how food was prepared by its taste alone. At mealtimes, they would intuitively know who at the table had prepared each dish and what his or her thoughts and feelings had been as they cooked. They could tell a lot about a person by just tasting his or her food.

Macrobiotics follows the premise that every action on the food affects the quality and nutritional value of the meal. Every single slice, chop, and shake, the speed of the stirring, the mood the cook is in, as well as the cleanliness and order of the kitchen, is consumed with the food. One day my friend Vince decided to challenge the precision of Michio and Aveline's intuition, as well as test the legitimacy of this theory. He cooked the meal in a messy kitchen and went wild running around the kitchen singing, shouting, and dancing. He also manipulated the food much more than was necessary, but all along maintained the integrity of the ingredients for a proper macrobiotic meal.

As Michio tasted the food, he commented, with studied Japanese politeness, "This is good, but very strange." At the end of the meal, he turned to my colleague and said calmly, "Maybe you need a doctor."

Another time, I was preparing a meal for 10 people as part of my certification exam, when, thirty minutes before mealtime, someone announced that Michio had returned from a visit to Japan and would be joining us for dinner. He had an entourage of 10 students with him. Since I had no time to prepare extra carrot-burdock sauté or roasted root vegetables, I decided to quickly add more soba noodles to the soba dish and more water to the miso soup and cross my fingers that it would all still taste okay. When Michio and Aveline arrived, they inspected the food, admired its appearance, and offered a prayer. Everyone sat down and began to eat. Utter silence filled the room as Michio and Aveline tasted the food.

After a few bites, Michio looked up and said, simply, "Noodles are good. But why did you add water to the soup at the end of its cooking?" He looked at me steadily, waiting for an answer. With his wise eyes on me, I suddenly felt like I was the only person in the room.

"Uh, no I didn't," I stammered.

Michio continued watching me, but I could see a smile playing on the corners of his lips. Everyone else at the table had looked up from their plates and was watching me too.

"Okay, I did, I did," I admitted, blushing. "I didn't know how to make the meal feed everyone." He just smiled in a non-egotistical way without needing to say another word.

During the time I spent training at the Kushi Institute, I was repeatedly awed by the depth of Michio's awareness of the subtle aspects of cooking and consuming food. He inspired me to commit my life to the development of this kind of understanding and, eventually, to help my students develop this understanding as well. Studying with him, I learned how to use my body as a walking, talking laboratory to conduct a vast array of experiments in my search for optimum health.

For a while, macrobiotics supplied all of the answers for me. Like many dietary theories, it promised longevity, peace of mind, and extreme wellness to those who followed its complex rules. But I also encountered some issues that wouldn't go away. Many macrobiotic teachers smoke cigarettes, drink alcohol, and indulge in quite a few donuts on a regular basis. These habits always seemed odd to me, since the macrobiotic diet is so rigid in its prohibition of tomatoes, potatoes, oranges, and garlic, as well as other restrictions, yet the teachers were regularly consuming much more harmful foods. Over time, noticing these contradictions was helpful for me; they freed me from becoming a "true believer" about any theory of nutrition. My growing awareness of the limitations of macrobiotics spurred my quest to gather a broader base of knowledge and information about food and health.

Moving to Kripalu Center for Yoga & Health, the largest residential yoga center in the United States, was another formative step in the evolution of my thinking on nutrition. Part of Kripalu's philosophy is to expose students to many different types of yoga, from Iyengar to Anusara to Kundalini. Watching the skillful teachers move seamlessly between yogic styles, I began to see the beauty and wisdom of assimilating different learning styles from a variety of traditions, instead of having to decide on one alone. By applying the same principle to nutrition, I realized I could relieve a lot of needless suffering and release people from the notion of one "perfect diet." I decided to create a new kind of nutrition school, one that would cover the best of every diet system and support people in their own quest for nutritional knowledge.

Most nutrition professionals believe their theory is the right one and everyone else's theory is wrong. They see the emergence of new information as competition and attempt to dismiss all other diet plans as "fad diets." My approach is just the opposite. I am thrilled when new dietary theories emerge because it shows that people are continuing to uncover what will help us all live happier, healthier lives. When a new theory appears, I read about it, research it, try to understand where its creators are coming from, and then add their wisdom to my teaching.

I like to discuss various dietary theories, covering the pros and cons of each, because the interesting thing is that they all work to some degree. When people decide to go on a diet, they have already become conscious of their eating habits that could be improved and realize it's time for a change. Whatever diet they choose is going to work because they are often shifting from a chaotic, disordered way of eating to an ordered way of eating. They are going to stop eating overly processed junk food and get better. The general rule is that any attention to diet is better than none. Diet theorists miss this fact because they want to attribute success to their unique approach.

All diet programs contain elements of truth. When I talk about various diets to my students, including programs ranging from raw foods to Paleo, some students always swear that a particular diet really helped them. The extent to which people can benefit from specific diets is amazing. This fact reminds me to appreciate how we as a species are so diverse and unique. I believe that, when a diet is successful, a placebo effect may be responsible for at least some of the benefits. Many studies illustrate the power of the placebo effect. A group of patients all suffering from the same ailment take sugar pills and are told they contain a breakthrough medicine that will help cure them. With no active ingredients in the pills, a significant percentage of the patients will recover, simply because they believe they are being treated. It's the same with diets. Many of them work because of this mind-over-matter factor.

Most people will lose weight on any given diet program for a limited period of time and then revert to a less disciplined way of eating. Why? Because most diet books instruct people to eat a limited spectrum of recommended foods. People follow the program with the best of intentions, slowly narrowing their list of acceptable foods, squeezing their eyes shut while scurrying past a Dunkin' Donuts or Starbucks, determined not to stray from the chosen path. Sooner or later, though, the cravings become too intense, their determination fades, and they fall off the wagon. These people are not weak, ignorant, or lacking in willpower; many of these diets are simply not sustainable long-term. Their cravings occur because humans are omnivorous creatures with roving appetites. We all have unique bodies, cravings, and lifestyles, and a list of "acceptable" foods is not always going to align with our individual needs or satisfy our cravings. It's not how you eat some of the time but how you eat most of the time that really matters. We need balance in our daily eating habits. So, just as all diets work, they all also don't work.

I've learned this fact as much from my personal experience as from that of my students. Late one evening, after I had been more or less vegetarian for a few years, my craving for meat grew so strong I found my car pulling into a fast food drive-thru window. I saw myself ordering a burger with extra, extra vegetables and parking on a deserted street to wolf down the forbidden food. I had never experienced such exhilaration. The thrill of giving my body exactly what it needed, even though it went directly against my beliefs at the time, was undeniable. It felt so good and so bad at the same time! For years, I kept these clandestine moments of what I thought were weakness to myself, hiding them from my friends, family, and colleagues. They only stopped when I was able to come to a deeper, clearer understanding of balanced eating. This understanding came from listening to my own body and applying dietary theory.

The Diet Puzzle

If you are reading this book, I'm sure you've done a fair amount of research and experimentation with diets already in your life. The mere mention of the word *diet* can evoke many emotions. You may have been taught from a very young age that dieting was the way to solve "the problem with your body." Going on a diet was seen as either a quick fix or a pie-in-the-sky way to revolutionize your body. To shed a few pounds, you simply needed to cut out fries or stop eating sweets. If you needed to gain weight, you would do the opposite. But there's a bigger picture. It's not just calories in and calories out. If calorie counting were the answer, obesity and body image disorders wouldn't be such common issues.

The first step in healing is to get clear about your relationship with diets. What's your diet history? Have you bounced from one trendy plan to the next? Do you have an entire bookshelf (or two) of snazzy diet books? Before making any judgment, take a moment now to ask yourself: How has following these diets served you? Then take another moment, and just think about how they have potentially held you back. There's no need to beat yourself up about whatever you discover. The important piece is to become more conscious and begin the work of rewriting your story so you can achieve a more desirable outcome—a life you love!

One of the main issues I see with dieting is that it puts the responsibility and expertise outside of you. Instead of allowing yourself to be intuitive and aware of what you are thinking, feeling, or craving at any given moment, you place all of your focus on external rules or a specific regimen. It makes the diet the expert, rather than yourself.

In reality, your body already knows exactly what it needs. Your brain has its own sense of how much you should weigh—a "set point" that usually fluctuates within a few pounds. Chemical signals tell you to gain or lose weight, depending on your food consumption, environment, and countless other factors. When you put yourself on strict regimens, you produce less serotonin, an essential chemical for happiness and metabolic function. From that perspective alone, we know that diets can leave you feeling frustrated and guilty.

Another important piece of this puzzle is the seemingly endless diet-binge cycle. What about willpower? Unfortunately, we all know it's limited and exhaustible. When you deprive yourself for too long, you're bound to devour a jar of peanut butter at 11 p.m. or do whatever it takes to find balance. If you find yourself in a dieting cycle, I encourage you to break it by eating whatever you feel like, within moderation. The only catch is that you have to tune in to your body and acknowledge when it's full, when it needs some greens or protein, or when it needs a little sweetness.

Health is really much more about trusting yourself and getting in touch with both your physical and emotional needs. When you learn how to communicate effectively with your body, no food situation will make you feel out of control—not even the biggest tray of cookies.

The truth is that you're unlikely to lose weight permanently until you go off diets completely. When you fuel yourself intuitively and mindfully, your metabolism remains steady, and you reach and maintain your ideal weight.

So why talk about dietary theory at all? Many themes in the dietary world do contain wisdom. As I've mentioned, it all comes back to this idea of bio-individuality. What works for you will not work for anyone else, which is exactly why you see some people thrive when eating a certain way, while others feel terrible on the exact same diet. So it's not just applying the wisdom point blank, but figuring out how the knowledge can work for you.

The real thing we are all searching for is to live a healthy life without all of the worry. The secret is to explore secondary food and combine that with a balance of primary foods to nourish yourself each and every day. You can start by experimenting with different eating styles and see what feels good to you. Notice how you feel when you eat in different ways. The goal isn't to land on one perfect "diet"; the goal is to figure out which pieces of these different approaches make you feel your best. What food and lifestyle choices really work for you?

The rest of this chapter has descriptions of many of the dietary themes that I have found the most useful, interesting, and applicable throughout the years. I will look at traditional-style diets—or systems of eating—that have been around for extended periods of time. Traditional diets include Ayurveda, Chinese medicine, macrobiotics, and even the Mediterranean diet. Then I'll look at some modern, popular themes, too. The point is to inspire you with many different ways of eating so that you can tune in to what makes you feel good. But first, my favorite "diet."

Joshua's 90-10 Diet

I've noticed that when many people try to eat totally clean and pure diets, they can only do so for a limited period of time. Sometimes it's a day, a week, a month, or even a year. But at a certain point, no matter how strong your determination might be, certain foods that you are avoiding become increasingly appealing.

This realization inspired me to create my own dietary theory. Since so many other diets work on recommended proportions, I decided to express my diet in the same way, as the "90-10 diet." I'm not very much into rules, so this diet has only one rule. And even that rule is flexible. The rule is that 90% of the time you eat what is healthy for you, and 10% of the time you eat whatever you feel like eating.

A lot of people try to stay 100% on their chosen diet program, which is bound to cause stress and likely to result in failure. Why turn dietary "mistakes" into sins? Having fear and guilt around food is not healthy. Cravings are an opportunity to listen to the body and fine-tune eating habits. Instead of creeping guiltily to the fridge at 2 a.m. for a pint of ice cream, publicly enjoy an ice cream with friends at a pleasurable social occasion; or get a delicious ice cream cone, and eat it outside on a nice day. By giving yourself a 10% range of flexibility, you can indulge yourself without guilt and maintain a healthy diet.

The other great part about this "diet" is that it allows you to have fun. Balance means letting loose once in a while so you can simply enjoy yourself and feed your soul. The 90-10 theory is a helpful reminder that if you eat wholesome foods and take good care of yourself most of the time, then your body can handle a cookie or a glass of wine from time to time. The point of wellness is not to adhere to anything so strictly that you miss out on all of the joy in life. It allows room for you to have a piece of cake on your birthday or try new and exciting foods on vacation. And I want to be clear that 90-10 is not a yo-yo approach. It's not about eating something forbidden and bouncing back to good foods. It's about getting real that sometimes you will deviate from your typical foods and that's okay.

If you're anything like me, this rule may surprise some friends in your circle. They may think you're so healthy and that you would never eat certain "banned" foods. Isn't it fun to be flexible and make up your own rules? Part of the reward of being wellness-oriented is that you get to relax and indulge on occasion, too.

Traditional-Style Diets

Macrobiotics

Central Philosophy: Translated literally, macrobiotics means "great life." The philosophy is based on eating only natural foods and balancing yin and yang in the body. The idea is to live within the natural order of life.

The modern macrobiotic movement began in the early 1900s with George Ohsawa, a Japanese dietary innovator, who combined theories of Eastern philosophy with food and medicine. Macrobiotics is a modified version of the ancient concept of yin-yang, which points to an underlying order in the universe based on a dynamic, ever-changing balance between two apparently opposite yet complementary principles. Yang embodies the masculine qualities of hard, strong, active, tight, and contractive. Yin embodies the feminine qualities of soft, yielding, passive, receptive, loose, and expansive. The dance between these two universal energies includes not only men and women, but sweet and salty, day and night, winter and summer, and dark and light. The list goes on and on. Regarding food, the yin-yang theory of balance asserts that we should avoid foods that are too yin, or too yang, to avoid imbalance, which eventually leads to illness.

It wasn't the dietary aspect of macrobiotics that interested me initially, but the simple, ancient wisdom of the yin-yang philosophy, the dance of opposites. How could Western theorists overlook such a simple and self-evident system of universal dynamics? On further study, I learned that Ohsawa's key to good health is to maintain yin-yang balance by following a traditional, grain-based diet. He taught that there is only one basic cause of human disease: imbalance.

Macrobiotics is based on the age-old concept that grains are the principle food in the diet, sacred in virtually every traditional society. Ohsawa reintroduced this idea to the West, helping to establish brown rice and soy products as staple foods in Europe and America. Macrobiotics originated in an enclosed Japanese island culture with limited food resources, where people were obliged to eat the same foods—rice, local vegetables, fish, and seaweed—over and over again. They did not have dairy or much animal meat. To keep their meals appetizing and healthy, they developed different ways to cook the same foods, often based on the season of year.

When I first encountered macrobiotics in the 1970s, eating seasonal, locally grown, organic produce and traditional foods made me feel vibrant and energized. I was also intrigued by some of the lifestyle suggestions, including singing a happy song every day. The recommendation to sing really surprised me. A singing diet? Unbelievable! But when I did it, I noticed I felt better, happier, and more relaxed. This opened my mind to the concept of being nourished on different levels, not only physically, but also mentally, emotionally, and spiritually.

Other macrobiotic suggestions include keeping your home simple, neat, and clean, wearing more cotton clothes and fewer synthetic fibers, keeping a sense of humor, allowing time for prayer and meditation, avoiding excessive jewelry or chemical perfumes, and growing green plants in the home. Another recommendation is to be on good terms with all people, creating more balance in your personal life.

For several years I followed a vegan macrobiotic diet—eating no dairy, meat, honey, or eggs. I did eat fish about once a month. I became very healthy and strong, and anytime I went for a checkup all my blood tests were normal. Gradually, however, I began to notice the downside of this way of eating. Although macrobiotic theory advises people to eat the traditional diet of their ancestors, most macrobiotic teachers, books, and sections in natural food stores strongly emphasize Japanese foods. This issue wasn't too problematic when I started my nutrition school in Toronto, but when I moved to New York I was dealing with a much more diverse clientele—students who went home to feed Puerto Rican, African American, and Jewish families. Imposing a Japanese diet on these people wouldn't have been sustainable or aligned with their needs. Moreover, for New York's singles and working moms, preparing complex macrobiotic recipes added unnecessary stress to their already crowded daily lives.

The drawbacks of macrobiotics are largely due to the reliance on salt in the traditional Japanese diet. The diet rarely incorporates herbs and spices; and sugar is never recommended, so salt is the main flavoring for everything. Miso soup, for example, is very salty, as are soy sauce and umeboshi plums. Unfortunately, as a result of this overabundance of salt in the diet, stomach cancer is a significant problem among the Japanese. Every medical student and health practitioner knows that too much salt can lead to hypertension, accompanied by rising blood pressure. If a patient has high blood pressure, a macrobiotic diet is probably not appropriate for them.

One of the most difficult-to-follow aspects of the macrobiotic diet is the suggestion to drink only when thirsty. The body doesn't normally feel the urge to drink until it is already dehydrated, a kind of neurological time lag. Our body needs water, but our brain doesn't get the message in time. I spent years on a macrobiotic diet, and I never thought I was thirsty because my body was accustomed to a very low level of water. Too much salt and not enough water are both independently problematic for the body, but to combine the two is a recipe for disaster.

Even though your head can convince your body to obey a diet for a while, your body will reach a certain point and reassert itself, sometimes with tragic results. It's amazing how people get carried away with their beliefs, becoming almost militaristic in their eating habits, which can be ostracizing and unsustainable for most. Macrobiotics certainly has its share of fanatics. To such people I want to say, "It's just a diet. It doesn't matter that much. You are not going to heaven for eating so many vegetables, and you will not go to hell for drinking too much water."

Ayurveda

Central philosophy: Ayurveda is an ancient healing system from India that emphasizes eating in accordance with your individual body type and the seasons. The system promotes health and disease prevention through balancing the doshas, or mind-body types.

The ancient Indian healing system of Ayurveda, which translates as "the science of life" in Sanskrit, was developed at least 3,000 years ago. In recent times, Ayurvedic medicine and its accompanying herbal remedies have become increasingly popular in the United States and Europe. Ayurveda recognizes that all life—human, plant, and animal—must live in harmony with nature in order to survive. Creating optimal health and balance begins by adopting the concept of "food as medicine."

In Ayurveda, proper diet is determined by the three harvesting seasons: Late fall, spring, and summer. The late fall harvest is rich in nuts and grains—all warming and insulating to combat the cold, dry extremes of the coming winter. Meat is not typically recommended in an Ayurvedic diet, but it is more accepted during cold times of year. In the wet, rainy, and congested spring, the naturally occurring harvest is rich in low-fat and astringent roots, sprouts, grapefruits, and berries. These foods help to decrease the seasonal tendency to make mucus and fight against allergies, colds, and weight gain. In the summer months, the naturally occurring harvest is rich in cooling fruits and vegetables, and eating these foods moderates the accumulated heat of the season. Cultures that still rely on food from local farmers practice these universal principles of Ayurveda by naturally changing their diets with the rhythm of the seasons.

In Ayurvedic theory, the five elements of nature are space, air, fire, water, and earth. These elements materialize and combine to create the three basic fundamental principles in nature, called doshas. Space and air combine to form the principle called Vata. Fire and water combine to form the principle called Pitta. And earth and water combine to form Kapha. These principles are used to categorize mind-body types, also called doshas. Thus, Ayurveda has three seasons, three primary harvests, and three doshas.

Vata

The qualities of Vata as seen in nature are cold, dry, rough, and constantly moving. Winter is the season in which Vata predominates. During this time of year, it is cold, our skin gets dry, precipitation becomes cold and dry in the form of snow, and the wind blows without restriction, as the trees are without leaves. The Vata body type is thin-boned, tall, and skinny, or short, slim, and petite.

Vatas have sharp minds and a tendency to worry; they are light sleepers and have nervous dispositions. These people usually have a fast metabolism, experience difficulty gaining weight, and are characteristically weak in their intestines, suffering from poor absorption of nutrients. As the squirrel needs nuts in the winter and as the natural harvest is rich in warm, heavy foods, so the wintry Vata requires highly nutritious food, with an abundance of cooked vegetables and whole grains to promote healthy assimilation and bowel function.

Vatas benefit from eating small amounts of animal food but must be careful not to overdo it. Fish and low-fat meats are usually best. Vatas need regular exercise to release nervous tension. They do best with more meditative, gentle, and calming practices such as yoga.

Pitta

During the summer months, the environment accumulates heat. The property of fire or heat is called Pitta.

The Pitta body type embodies the qualities of fire. This body type is physically oriented, with more muscle and a fiery temperament. Pitta people usually have yellow- or reddish-colored skin that is sensitive to rashes. They often sweat profusely and are easily irritated. Their bodies and temperaments both tend to be hot. For the most part, they have a very strong and athletic constitution.

Pittas tend to be leaders and are well organized, intelligent, and charismatic. They are usually emotional, competitive, and passionate, and in need of a good eight hours' sleep per night to rest and cool off. They have enormous appetites for food and life experience and can become gluttons if not careful. Pittas benefit from seeking balance in eating, avoiding hot spices and too much animal food, and emphasizing sweet vegetables like squash and pumpkin and whole grains like barley and oats. Most importantly, Pittas must avoid excess and include regular exercise in their daily schedules.

Kapha

Spring, which is the Kapha season, is a very wet and heavy time of year. It is allergy season, the rainy season, full of heavy mud and potential congestion. Influenced by the qualities of springtime, those with Kapha body types are big-boned, full-bodied, and physically strong, and they tend toward weight gain. Their solid skeletons protect them from osteoporosis. Skin color is pale and cool, and eyes are large and often dark. They are frequently easygoing, slow, methodical types, with balanced, peaceful temperaments. Kapha types radiate competence, even when they are quiet or shy.

Kaphas have slow metabolisms and strong intestines, and the ease with which they assimilate nutrients means that they don't have to eat much to stay in good health. In fact, they should avoid overeating because their main health concern is danger of obesity. The heart is their weakest organ. Kaphas should eat lots of vegetables and light foods, including a wide range of grains. Their primary animal food should be eggs. All spices are good for Kaphas, but they need to restrict intake of oil as much as possible. Regular, non-strenuous physical exercise, like taking a stroll in the park, suits them best.

If this system intrigues you, I encourage you to study it further. In India, Ayurvedic doctors usually do not tell a patient his or her body type. Instead, they look at a patient's susceptibility to imbalance. With this information, they can employ preventative techniques to avoid disease and maintain good health. For some, this system might be too complex to follow, and if that's the case then just remember the basics. Our greatest lesson from Ayurveda is to learn from nature, eat in harmony with the seasons, and live a life of balance.

5 Element Theory

Central Philosophy: An ancient Chinese belief system that says we are surrounded by five energy fields: wood, fire, earth, metal, and water. Keeping all of the elements in balance promotes harmony in our surroundings and in ourselves.

Based on ancient Chinese philosophy, the 5 Element Theory relates all energy and substances to the elements—fire, earth, metal (or air), water, and wood. Each element is associated with a direction of the compass and a season of the year, with late summer as the fifth season. In the creation cycle, one element gives birth to the next and nourishes it through the flow of energy. Wood creates fire, which creates earth, which creates metal, which creates water, which creates wood. In the destruction cycle, wood injures earth, fire destroys metal, earth controls water, metal attacks wood, and water injures fire. Wood is associated with the morning and the spring season. It is associated with the liver and the gallbladder and the emotions of impatience and anger. Wood vegetables are artichokes, broccoli, carrots, string beans, zucchini, sprouts, parsley, and leafy greens. The effect of wood on the body is purification.

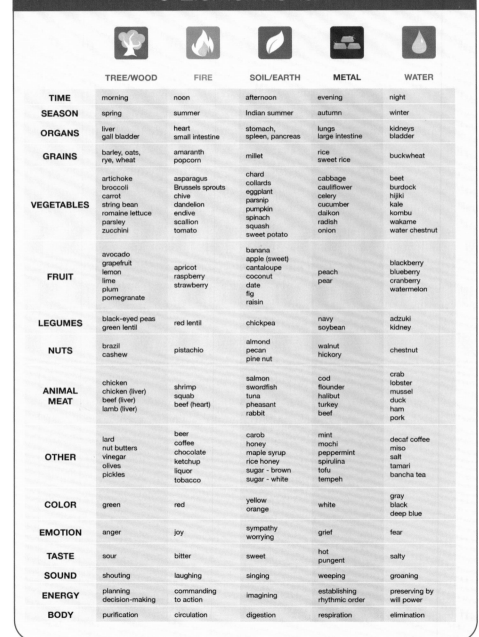

5 Element Chart

	TREE/WOOD	FIRE	SOIL/EARTH	METAL	WATER
TIME	morning	noon	afternoon	evening	night
SEASON	spring	summer	Indian summer	autumn	winter
ORGANS	liver gall bladder	heart small intestine	stomach, spleen, pancreas	lungs large intestine	kidneys bladder
GRAINS	barley, oats, rye, wheat	amaranth popcorn	millet	rice sweet rice	buckwheat
VEGETABLES	artichoke broccoli carrot string bean romaine lettuce parsley zucchini	asparagus Brussels sprouts chive dandelion endive scallion tomato	chard collards eggplant parsnip pumpkin spinach squash sweet potato	cabbage cauliflower celery cucumber daikon radish onion	beet burdock hijiki kale kombu wakame water chestnut
FRUIT	avocado grapefruit lemon lime plum pomegranate	apricot raspberry strawberry	banana apple (sweet) cantaloupe coconut date fig raisin	peach pear	blackberry blueberry cranberry watermelon
LEGUMES	black-eyed peas green lentil	red lentil	chickpea	navy soybean	adzuki kidney
NUTS	brazil cashew	pistachio	almond pecan pine nut	walnut hickory	chestnut
ANIMAL MEAT	chicken chicken (liver) beef (liver) lamb (liver)	shrimp squab beef (heart)	salmon swordfish tuna pheasant rabbit	cod flounder halibut turkey beef	crab lobster mussel duck ham pork
OTHER	lard nut butters vinegar olives pickles	beer coffee chocolate ketchup liquor tobacco	carob honey maple syrup rice honey sugar - brown sugar - white	mint mochi peppermint spirulina tofu tempeh	decaf coffee miso salt tamari bancha tea
COLOR	green	red	yellow orange	white	gray black deep blue
EMOTION	anger	joy	sympathy worrying	grief	fear
TASTE	sour	bitter	sweet	hot pungent	salty
SOUND	shouting	laughing	singing	weeping	groaning
ENERGY	planning decision-making	commanding to action	imagining	establishing rhythmic order	preserving by will power
BODY	purification	circulation	digestion	respiration	elimination

Fire is associated with twelve noon and the summer season. The related organs are the heart and small intestine. The related emotion is joy. Fire vegetables are asparagus, Brussels sprouts, chives, dandelion, scallions, and tomatoes. Coffee and tobacco are also fiery. Fire creates circulation in the body.

Earth is associated with the afternoon and the late summer season. The stomach and pancreas are the active organs, and sympathy and worry are the correlated emotions. Chard, collards, parsnips, spinach, squash, and sweet potato are the earth vegetables. The taste of earth is sweet, and other earth substances are carob, honey, maple syrup, and sugar. The related bodily function of earth is digestion.

Metal is associated with the evening and the autumn season. The lungs are the active organs. The emotion is grief. Cabbage, cauliflower, celery, cucumber, daikon, and radish are the metal vegetables. Peppermint, spirulina, tofu, and tempeh also belong to the metal family. Respiration is the related bodily function.

Water is associated with night and the winter season. The active organs are the kidneys and the bladder. The emotion is fear. Beets, burdock, sea vegetables, and kale are water vegetables. Miso, salt, and tamari are also water foods. Elimination is the bodily function.

By eating foods associated with each of the elements, you can promote balance in the body. Knowing which foods, seasons, emotions, and bodily functions are associated with which element can make you a master of balance. Say, for example, it's the middle of winter, and you are feeling constipated and tight. It's the water time of year, so increasing sea vegetables with water energy and drinking more water could help. Or say you are craving coffee and cigarettes, which both belong to the fire element. You could deconstruct those cravings and ask yourself, "Where else can I add fire, passion, and joy into my life?" You might also increase the fire vegetables, like green leafy vegetables, in your diet. Chances are your craving for coffee and cigarettes would subside.

According to 5 Element Theory, the way you cook changes the energy of your food. Stir-frying and deep frying give food a wood energy. Grilling and barbecuing add fire energy. Boiling imbues food, with water energy. Baking creates a metal energy, and steaming brings about an earth energy. If you are interested in exploring this theory further, use the chart with the elements and components of each element clearly listed. In your food journal, you can record what you eat from each element every day for breakfast, lunch, and dinner. This will help you see your natural tendencies and find balance. If you notice that you are eating mostly earth foods, it may help to increase wood foods because wood holds down the earth.

Traditional Diet

Central Philosophy: Traditional diets are just what they sound like, following the ancient traditions of our ancestors with food in its most pure, unprocessed form. These unrefined, natural foods are revered for their nutrient density and should be prepared just as your great-great-great-grandmother did.

Many foods have a long history of supporting good health. For centuries, humans existed without the need to read books about their diet. They ate from the land and grazed on what was around them, and the traditional diet looks to reclaim these ways.

Nina Planck, author of *Real Food* and *Real Food for Mother and Baby*, explains that "traditional" means that a food has been farmed or raised and processed pretty much the way it used to be. Foods like grass-fed beef and wild salmon are two to three million years old. By contrast, modern foods like corn syrup were developed in the 1970s. In her books, she explains how ancient foods like beef and butter have been falsely accused of causing health problems, while industrial foods like corn syrup and soybean oil have created a triple epidemic of obesity, diabetes, and heart disease. She writes that real food is never an imitation of something else.

The real food movement can be traced back to the early 1900s, when Dr. Weston Price, a dentist who believed nutrition is the foundation for well-being, studied the diets of many ancient societies and decided that by eating nourishing, traditional foods and farm produce, we could achieve optimal health. He traveled the world studying indigenous people's dental and physical health. He found that the farther away people lived from civilization, the healthier they were. They ate from local food sources. They had fewer cavities, and some cultures never experienced any cancer or heart disease.

Sally Fallon Morell brought Price's work to a larger audience in her book *Nourishing Traditions: The Cookbook That Challenges Politically Correct Nutrition and the Diet Dictocrats*. I really appreciate that her work ignores the current fads and politics around food and, instead, looks to our heritage to determine which foods are ideal for human consumption. Perhaps one of the most controversial parts of traditional diets is that raw dairy products are considered an important part of a healthy diet. Followers argue that, for the past 9,000 years, humans have relied on milk to meet their needs for protein and fat and that the problem is not milk, but the modern methods used to make dairy cows produce milk. Selective breeding and genetically engineered hormones, along with pasteurization, which makes the proteins in milk difficult to absorb, interfere with the benefits from milk. However, raw milk isn't advisable for everyone, particularly those who have a weakened immune system or are pregnant.

The traditional diet includes a variety of animal foods. Fallon Morrell cites studies of primitive cultures that relied on animal meat and had healthy bones and claims that certain health problems, such as bone loss and tuberculosis, developed when agriculture was introduced and people began depending on grains and beans for sustenance. Fallon Morrell says animal food is the only source of complete protein with all 22 amino acids necessary for the human body to thrive. She acknowledges that abstaining from commercial meats is a good practice and that avoiding meat for a certain period of time can be cleansing and healing, but she cautions against strict vegetarianism.

Fallon Morrell stresses the benefits of the natural fats in meat, eggs, and dairy, and encourages people to avoid the no-fat or low-fat alternatives to these products. In addition to high-quality animal meat, she recommends eating other quality fats, such as virgin olive oil, unrefined flax oil, coconut oil, and palm oil. Carbohydrates from organic whole grains are another essential element of her diet. She also recommends high-quality water, meat stocks, vegetable broths, unrefined sea salt, raw vinegar, fresh herbs, and naturally fermented soy sauce. Since this diet is very rich in protein and fat, it may not agree with everyone.

Mediterranean Diet

Central Philosophy: By adopting the eating style of the people who live in the Mediterranean region of the world, particularly Southern European countries like Greece, Italy, France, Portugal, and Spain, people can enjoy longer lifespans and less risk of developing chronic disease.

The Mediterranean diet is less a diet and more a lifestyle. People who live in the southern coastal regions of Europe and the Middle East dine leisurely, engage in regular physical activity, spend time with family, and, of course, eat a heart-healthy diet with lots of vegetables, healthy fats, and beans. The region emphasizes fresh, regional cuisine, simply prepared with very little fried or heavily processed foods.

Interestingly, a Minnesota physiologist named Ancel Keys was the first scientist to talk about the health value of a Mediterranean-style diet. He was also one of the first people to talk about the role of saturated fats in contributing to heart disease. His work began in the 1940s, but he became known for his landmark epidemiological research that he called the Seven Countries Study starting in the late '50s. He studied 12,000 healthy middle-aged men living in Europe, Japan, and the U.S. and revealed that the Mediterranean diet was protective against heart disease even though about 35% of the calories come from fat. Yet, most of those fats are monounsaturated fats from plant sources. Even more interestingly, Keys lived to be 100 years old.

In the last decade or so, scientists have continued to study this region extensively, mostly looking at how residents enjoy such good health. In 2011, researchers examined 50 studies linking the Mediterranean diet to reduced risk of developing metabolic syndrome, which leads to heart disease, diabetes, and stroke. But even more striking was the first major clinical trial to measure the diet's impact on heart risks. The study ended early, after only about five years, because the results were so staggering: About 30% of heart attacks, strokes, and deaths from heart disease could be prevented in high-risk people, simply by switching to the diet. The results were published in a 2013 *New England Journal of Medicine* article, marking the first time a diet was shown to be a powerful means to reduce disease risk in a clinical setting. In the study, a low-fat diet went head to head with the Mediterranean diet, which allows for healthy fats and a more balanced way of eating. Not only did the Mediterranean diet have better results, but the study participants were able to stick with it and feel satisfied. Other studies have shown that the diet can help maintain a healthy body weight and lower risk for diabetes.

I like this diet's traditional roots, and I agree that a balance of good food and lifestyle factors can help you live longer and enjoy your life. Of course, many people wonder whether this diet can really be recreated around the world and if it makes sense to advise, say, people in China to eat more like people in Italy. Again, I think people benefit more from adopting the traditional diet of their own region.

Modern Themes

High-Carbohydrate Diets

Central Philosophy: High-carbohydrate diets are a modern take on traditional diets that relied on whole grains, beans, and vegetables.

I pinpoint the publication of *Diet for a Small Planet* by Frances Moore Lappé in 1972 as the beginning of a trend toward high-carbohydrate diets in America. This book eventually sold more than three million copies worldwide. Lappé postulated that human practices, not natural disasters, cause worldwide hunger. Food scarcity results when grain, rich in nutrients and able to support vast populations, is fed to livestock to produce meat, which yields only a fraction of those nutrients to many fewer people. Lappé theorized that traditional cultures stay healthy by mixing vegetable proteins together, such as the pairing of beans and grains. Her book's publication coincided with an American hippie subculture that was turning its back on fast food and embracing natural foods, macrobiotics, Indian-style vegetarianism, and a grain-based diet as part of a general "back to the land" movement.

Then came Nathan Pritikin, a medical doctor who studied indigenous cultures around the world and noted they did not have the types of chronic disease suffered by people in developed countries. He attributed their health to a low-fat diet with lots of carbohydrates. Based on these insights, he created the Pritikin Longevity Center in 1976. In 1980, he co-authored a best-selling book, *The Pritikin Program for Diet and Exercise*, in which he advocated a low-fat, low-protein diet, with most nutrients coming from complex carbohydrates. Recommended foods included fresh and cooked fruits and vegetables, whole grains, breads, pasta, and small amounts of lean meat, fish, and poultry. He also encouraged a daily regimen of aerobic exercise.

In 1977, George McGovern, former director of the "Food for Peace" program under President Kennedy, headed the U.S. Senate Select Committee on Nutrition and Human Needs. After years of discussion, scientific review, and debate, the committee encouraged the movement toward vegetable and grain-based diets in America—unwelcome news for the meat and dairy industries. Six years later, in 1983, Dr. John McDougall attracted public attention by designing a vegan diet of high-carbohydrate, low-protein foods. In 1993, Dr. Dean Ornish published the best-selling *Eat More, Weigh Less*, shattering the commonly held notion that losing weight requires starvation. To actually eat more and still shed pounds was a truly revolutionary idea. Ornish embraced macrobiotics but had the foresight to realize that the Japanese foods, like seaweed and miso, and yin-yang philosophy were too foreign for most Americans. He incorporated the system's basic dietary principles into his new diet and used more familiar American foods and concepts.

In 1988, the U.S. Surgeon General, in conjunction with the American Medical Association, conducted a study of various weight-loss plans. The study showed that two-thirds of people on these plans gained all of the weight back in one year, and 97% regained all of their weight within five years. A few years later, Ornish showed that, under his plan, patients lost 24 pounds in the first year and kept more than half the weight off for five years. He attributed much of his success to the fact that his patients could eat more food, thereby avoiding hunger pangs and cravings normally associated with dieting.

Ornish then approached insurance companies like Blue Cross Blue Shield, pointing out how much money they could save on payouts for heart bypass surgery if they instead enrolled their clients in his program. In response, the insurance companies put 300 people on his program and saved millions of dollars. The Ornish program for reversing heart disease is now commonly accepted by insurance companies as a deductible expense, a huge breakthrough for the nutrition world. His program recommends a diet largely composed of grains and vegetables, with a formula of 10% fat, 20% protein, and 70% carbohydrates. He also recommends yoga, meditation, and developing a loving heart—"hugging is healthy!"—to keep the arteries clean and clear.

Although this type of diet is high in carbohydrates, when keeping a whole-foods approach, you are getting good carbs. Complex carbohydrates can offer a lot of fiber and nutrients. If these kinds of meals feel simple, play with making your plate full of color and spices. Eating meals consisting of largely grains and veggies may be great for some people's health but might make others feel sluggish.

Vegan Diet

Central Philosophy: Veganism is the practice of abstaining from all animal products, rejecting the commodity status of sentient animals. Followers often extend the ethical principles of veganism into other areas of their lives and oppose the use of animals or animal products for any purpose.

The vegan lifestyle has become increasingly popular these days with help from famous figures like television host and comedian Ellen DeGeneres and actress Alicia Silverstone who make it seem more acceptable and doable. Plus, mega-pop star Beyoncé claims to be a part-time vegan. More companies are also responding to this trend by offering more vegan options, like Ben and Jerry's creating a line of non-dairy, vegan ice creams made from almond milk.

Also known as a plant-based diet, vegans do not eat any food from animal sources, including red meat, chicken, fish, eggs, dairy, or honey. They avoid wearing shoes, belts, or any other clothing made from an animal source as well. A 2016 poll by the Vegetarian Resource Group in the U.S. found that 3% of the country now identifies as vegetarian or vegan, up from 1% in 2009.

While vegan eating probably began in India or Asia, the first known vegan cookbook, *No Animal Food: Two Essays and 100 Recipes*, by Rupert H. Wheldon, was published in 1910 in London.[1] The Vegan Society started in 1944 and created World Vegan Day, which is an annual celebration held in November.[2] The Physicians Committee for Responsible Medicine (PCRM) has recommended a no-cholesterol, low-fat vegan diet since 1991, and they have even created their own food groups: legumes, grains, fruits, and vegetables, to replace the old USDA food groups (meat, dairy, grains, fruits, and vegetables).

People go vegan for many reasons, including health, animal rights, and the environment. From a health perspective, a well-balanced vegan diet greatly increases your intake of fruits and vegetables, and reducing high-cholesterol foods can be helpful for some health conditions. Many people choose to be vegan to live a more activist lifestyle. By choosing not to support the way farmed animals are raised and treated or to eat any animal product, they take a strong stance on living a compassionate life. For some, it's all about helping our environment. Plant-based diets require about one-third of the land and water needed to produce a typical Western diet, according to the Vegan Society.

Many athletes choose to adopt a vegan diet to improve their performance. World famous track star Carl Lewis went vegan to prepare for the World Championships in 1991, running what he called the best meet of his life. He earned 10 Olympic medals over his career, nine of them gold. At age 40, Rich Roll was 50 pounds overweight and completely out of shape. He made some major changes to his diet and lifestyle and became the first vegan to complete an Ultraman competition, finishing in the top 10 males. After tennis star Venus Williams was diagnosed with a rare autoimmune disease she drastically changed her diet to become a raw vegan. She continues to dominate in her sport.

Still, with any strict diet, downsides exist. Vegan diets do not naturally contain vitamin B12, an essential nutrient that contributes to cognitive function and metabolic functions, like enzyme production and hormonal regulation. Since the most usable forms of B12 come from animal sources, many vegans take a supplement to avoid deficiencies. Other potential nutrients of concern include iron, omega-3 fatty acids, and vitamin D.

High-Protein Diets

Central Philosophy: High-protein diets restrict carbohydrates, causing the body to burn its own fat for fuel, instead of carbohydrates. When the body is in this state, many people tend to feel less hungry and, as a result, lose weight.

People love eating protein. It makes us feel stronger and more alert. It increases our sense of power and confidence—two of the most highly prized qualities in our contemporary culture and part of the reason high-protein diets are so popular today. High-protein diets can also lead to significant weight loss, important to many in this time of rising obesity rates. Anne Louise Gittleman, Ph.D., C.N.S., former head nutritionist at the Pritikin Center, and the first to see the downside of a low-fat, high-carbohydrate diet, began to distinguish between "good" and "bad" fats. Saturated fats in dairy products and trans fats in processed foods like potato chips and margarine clog the arteries and contribute to inflammation in the body. Olive oil, avocado oil, omega-3, omega-6, and oils from seeds and nuts nourish the body and prevent the accumulation of cholesterol and triglycerides in our arteries. Ironically, a lack of good fats can actually lead to just the kind of heart disease dangers that low-fat diets are trying to avoid! Omega-3 fatty acids, found mainly in fish oil, are especially effective at clearing the arteries.

Gittleman also pointed out that the average American does not know the difference between healthy and unhealthy carbohydrates. The experts might be talking about the need to eat brown rice, millet, quinoa, wholegrain breads, vegetables, and beans, but most Americans have no idea what these foods are or where to find them. Thinking that all carbohydrates are the same, they eat more refined wheat products, such as bread, pasta, and pizza. In addition, Gittleman warned about the potential dangers caused by gluten in wheat, which may cause allergies, brain fog, candida, and mineral deficiencies in some individuals. Gittleman's contribution to understanding the subtleties and implications of high-carbohydrate diets is significant.

Many people who embrace high-protein diets follow the program prescribed by Dr. Robert Atkins. Atkins began his work in 1972, with the publication of *Dr. Atkins' Diet Revolution*, and died in 2003, at the age of 73.

The title of a recently released biography about Atkins, *The True Story of the Man Behind the War on Carbohydrates*, describes his life's mission well. Atkins's supporters claim that, under his plan, you can "eat delicious meals you love, never count calories, enjoy a cheeseburger when you're hungry, see amazing results in 14 days, reach your ideal weight, and stay there." Dieters can also supposedly eat all the meat and all the fat they want and still lose weight, which may be an attractive option for many people. People who suffer from candida or diabetes, both of which are aggravated by too much sugar consumption, can sometimes benefit from this way of eating for a short time.

The downside to high-protein diets is that too much animal protein may lead to illness, especially heart disease and cancer. Animal meat is full of saturated fats that can spike blood cholesterol levels, has no fiber to aid digestion, and is low in many essential plant-based nutrients, such as antioxidants, carotenoids, and phytochemicals. In addition, there is increasing concern about tainted meat, hormones, and antibiotics in factory-farmed meat. If you decide to go on a high-protein diet, choosing organic animal food when possible can help to cut down on exposure to hormones and antibiotics.

Another problem is that this program doesn't distinguish between animal proteins. In Atkins, eating beef, fish, chicken, or eggs is the same: A protein is a protein is a protein. In reality, each of these has a completely different quality and impact on the body. Furthermore, the body is always trying to maintain an acid and alkaline balance. Protein is a very acidic substance. If you eat a lot of protein, your body may try to create a more alkaline environment in your stomach by leaching minerals from your bones and teeth, which can contribute to bone loss and osteoporosis. People also say these diets lead to constipation, depression, bad breath, and body odor.

The Zone Diet and Glycemic Load

Central Philosophy: The Zone Diet is based on a theory that excess insulin, a hormone that helps control blood sugar levels, makes us gain weight and keep it on. By regulating blood sugar levels with a perfect balance of carbohydrates, fats, and proteins at every meal, the body burns fat more efficiently and has more energy.

The Zone Diet was developed by Dr. Barry Sears in the '90s. He is the author of the bestseller *Enter the Zone*, which is based on more than 15 years of his research in the field of bio-nutrition and the role of diet in hormonal response, gene expression, and inflammation. The Zone is sometimes called a high-protein diet, but it's less extreme than Atkins. The diet's primary aim is to keep you in "the zone," a sports term, describing an almost mystical state of heightened awareness and relaxed intensity in which athletes perform at their best with minimal effort. The goal is to become balanced, relaxed, and well fed so that your energy level is optimal for normal day-to-day living.

The Zone offers a specific meal plan based on each person's gender, activity level, and amount of body fat. It's called "the 40-30-30 diet" because for all of the Zone snacks and meals, you get 40% of your calories from carbohydrates, 30% from protein, and 30% from fat. The theory is that the more you give your body 40-30-30, the faster it will get accustomed to processing this food combination and settle into a specific metabolic state, leading to weight loss.

One of the goals of the Zone is to avoid peaks and valleys in blood sugar levels. A recommendation that I find effective is to eat a meal within one hour of waking up in the morning because that's when your blood sugar is lowest.

The Zone encourages people to eat more fruits and vegetables and reduce bread, pasta, and white grains. The diet is big on drinking water, which I agree with wholeheartedly. I also like the Zone's relaxed attitude about mistakes: No big deal if you fall off the diet, since you are only one meal away from getting back on track.

A downside to the Zone is that, unless you're a scientist, it's very hard to design each meal to be a perfectly balanced 40-30-30. It's also difficult to be on a Zone diet and be a vegetarian because of the diet's strong emphasis on eating protein. In response, the Zone has a plan called "Soy Zone," which recommends eating more soy products. However, many people are allergic to soy or have difficulty digesting it in large quantities, so this is not a viable option for all vegetarians. Critics of the Zone often argue that weight loss on this program comes from restricting calories and not from any biochemical magic induced by the 40-30-30 formula. They also assert that, contrary to Sears's claims, athletic performance may be impaired by reducing carbohydrates.

Paleo Diet

Central Philosophy: Our bodies are designed to thrive on foods that were available to our early paleolithic ancestors from 10,000 years ago.

Similar to traditional ways of eating, the Paleo diet, also known as the paleolithic or caveman diet, harkens back to the eating ways of our ancestors, though this diet first came on the scene in the 1970s, thanks to Walter L. Voegtlin, a gastroenterologist who wrote *The Stone Age Diet*. In it, he argues that humans are carnivorous animals who need mostly fats and proteins and that our jaws and teeth resemble those of other carnivorous animals, like dogs, rather than those of plant-eating animals like sheep. Loren Cordain, author of *The Paleo Diet*, links the movement to a 1985 article in the *New England Journal of Medicine* that claimed the diet could be a reference standard for modern human nutrition.

In 2009, Mark Sisson said you could reprogram your genes in the direction of weight loss, health, and longevity by following the 10 laws (only 2 of which concern food) in his book *The Primal Blueprint*, which outlines a variation of Paleo, allowing more healthy fats and cracking down on the use of artificial sweeteners that other Paleo diet books allow. By 2010, the *New York Times* ran a piece about new-age cavemen, or urban dwellers who follow the Paleo path.

The article chronicled a modern-day renaissance of the diet, following a few New Yorkers who kept large amounts of meat in their freezers and said the diet had helped them clear up health issues. The article also publicized CrossFit, an intense fitness program that combines weightlifting and gymnastics, stating that many Paleo dieters also enjoy these rigorous workouts.

Again, I think any diet with a focus on protein will become popular in the Western world. I do like that this diet focuses on eating whole foods rather than processed foods, and I think many people benefit from this diet simply by removing flour and dairy from their diet, because many people are allergic or have sensitivities to these foods. The downside of this plan, as with many other diets, is that a strict eating plan can be impractical for most people. While it may feel good for a time, many people have a hard time keeping up with such intense food rules.

Raw Food Diet

Central Philosophy: Raw or living food diets are based on unprocessed and uncooked plant foods. Raw foodists believe that eating food above 108 – 116 degrees will destroy vital enzymes in the food and disrupt your body's ability to absorb nutrients from the food.

A raw food diet is one in which people choose to eat food that is not cooked or heated. The basic premise of raw food theory is that we are the only species that cooks our food, which destroys its natural enzymes. In its raw state, fresh food is composed of living cells. Raw foodists view cooked or heated food as dead and lifeless. Heating food changes its basic molecular structure, making it toxic or nutritionally compromised, according to this theory. Interestingly, some nutrients actually become more bioavailable after being exposed to heat. Raw food theory also states that cooked foods are extremely difficult to give up, but once people shift to eating primarily raw foods, they will experience clarity of mind, body, and spirit. Raw foodists believe raw plant food is the only food humans should eat.

Raw food can be very cleansing, healing, and refreshing to the body, and it is especially good for people who have eaten a lot of meat and processed food. Eating raw food may improve digestion and increase vitality. It is an environmentally supportive and ecologically friendly way of eating that can lead to a feeling of deep spiritual connection to nature. Going on a raw food diet can feel like fasting, as it helps remove toxins quickly and effectively from the body and can lead to weight loss. One of the biggest benefits of going on a raw food diet is that it gets people off sugary, processed junk foods. On the other hand, this diet can be too cleansing for people whose systems are weak and in need of regeneration. People with a sensitive digestive tract may find the nutrients in raw food too intense. The cooling effect of raw foods on the body makes this diet difficult to sustain during the winter months. People who are, to use a macrobiotic term, very yin—tall, thin, and/or spacy—may need a more grounding diet, as raw foods are also very yin. Getting adequate protein can be a challenge while following a raw foods diet. Some people can also experience sweet cravings from eating too much sugar from raw fruits. Additionally, a raw food diet can cause digestive distress, especially if you dive in all of a sudden. One approach is to gradually get into this diet to allow the GI tract time to adjust to all that roughage.

Some raw foodists are very adamant in their belief that cooked food is unfit for human consumption. Some eat 100% raw, some 75% raw, and some eat 15% raw. I encourage people to experiment with the percentage of raw food in their diet and notice how it affects them, especially in the summer months, when raw foods are easier for the body to process.

Cleansing Diets

Central Philosophy: You can detoxify the body with a restricted plan of simple, whole foods, through fresh fruit and vegetable juicing, or even a master cleanse mixture of water fasting to boost health. Results from a cleansing diet include increased energy, better digestion, and greater mental clarity, and it can be a very effective method for determining food allergies.

One of the most well-known cleanses today is the Master Cleanser, or Lemonade Diet, a liquid mono-diet consisting of water with fresh lime or lemon juice, maple syrup, and cayenne pepper. Stanley Burroughs, creator of the Master Cleanser, recommends drinking the mixture 6 to 12 times a day for a minimum of 10 days and a maximum of 40 days, depending on a person's physical health. A laxative herbal tea, taken twice a day, and saltwater bathing are also recommended, but no other food is consumed during the cleanse. Directions for coming off the diet include a slow reincorporation of raw fruit, fruit juice, nuts, and vegetables. Burroughs suggests doing the cleanse four times a year for optimum health. The goal of the Master Cleanser is to correct all health disorders. This lemonade drink was first shown to help aid stomach ulcers, and then Burroughs began to recommend it for other conditions. He believes that when we cure one disease, we help cure them all and create vibrant overall health.

Improper diet causes the accumulation of waste, toxins, and poison in the colon. These filter into the bloodstream and circulate throughout the body, inhabiting tissues and cells. The settling of these toxins weakens the cells and the entire immune system, exposing the body to disease. Cleansing the body of this built-up waste rejuvenates its innate healing mechanisms. It then functions at optimal capacity, reducing toxicity, restoring health and vitality, and increasing our life force.

Other people try less extreme forms of cleansing, either with fresh fruit and vegetable juices or simply by eating unrefined, whole foods for a time. Joe Cross helped bring attention to the power of juicing in his documentary *Fat, Sick & Nearly Dead*, which tracked his progress on a 60-day juice fast. He lost nearly 100 pounds and got off his prescription medication for an autoimmune disease simply by increasing his consumption of fruits and vegetables. In 2008, Oprah and her staff embarked on a 21-day vegan cleanse and found amazing results from adopting this diet that is free of all animal products. Even in cleansing, we can see how some people thrive and others struggle with certain ways of eating or eliminating food from their diet, even for a relatively short period of time. Doing a cleanse or simply eliminating coffee, tea, sugar, and comfort foods for a set period of time is a freeing experience. Many people report that cleanses help them lose weight and feel healthier.

It's common for people to decide they are going to fast in the springtime, especially if they've put on weight during the winter months. I've seen this pattern many times. People overeat during the holiday season, and then, when the weather gets warmer and the days get lighter, they announce to everyone they know, "Okay, now I'm going to clean it all up by going on a fast." Being healthy is a daily practice. I do not believe that long-term fasting is an effective weight-loss method. Just by following the simple instructions in this book, you will gradually increase your health and vitality. Sudden fasts are a bit like meditating once a week, instead of integrating spirituality into your everyday lifestyle. The way I see it, I fast half my life. Pretty much every day, I fast from 8:30 p.m. to 8:30 a.m. I break my fast with my morning meal, called breakfast. This process has improved my digestion and my sleeping and allows me to wake up in the morning with a greater appetite for food and for life.

If you really want to fast, the best way is to cut out a specific, selected food, rather than reducing the overall quantity of food you eat. Just eliminating one food from your diet can be a major undertaking. For example, you might decide not to eat sugar for a week. This is a very big deal. Just try it and see. Or, if you know you eat too much chocolate, just cut out this one item, and create a fast this way. You can also fast by adding in food, such as freshly cooked vegetables, every day. This will crowd out other, less healthy foods. If you have success with adding and subtracting things on your menu, you can begin to cut more undesirable foods, one by one, and add more healthy foods, one by one.

When it comes to fasting and cleansing, remember that such valiant activities may appeal to your mind but can wreak havoc on your body. I suggest taking a middle path, doing things in moderation, and realizing that your body doesn't necessarily know what your mind is thinking.

DNA Diet/Nutrigenomics

Central Philosophy: The DNA diet is a customized approach to health and diet that offers specific recommendations for food based on the results of genetic testing.

Foods encouraged or restricted are based on your unique biochemical makeup.

The DNA diet, or nutrigenomics, is a personalized way of eating based on your genetic blueprint. The idea spun out of the Human Genome Project—the government project that identified nearly 25,000 genes in the human body. Many studies have evaluated nutrigenomics and the correlation between diet and genes. Scientists have started using this information to research cures for dozens of genetic disorders, such as diabetes. Testing an individual's personal variations in the genes can provide many answers to health issues, such as heart and bone health, detoxification and antioxidant capacity, insulin sensitivity, and tissue repair. Small differences can influence how your body metabolizes food, utilizes nutrients, and excretes damaging toxins. The idea here is that genetic makeup is the reason why one person can handle a diet rich in sugar, while that same diet will give another person hypoglycemia or even diabetes.

Many biotech labs now offer do-it-yourself testing kits that look at 19 genes to determine a person's future health. You can purchase these kits at a clinic, online, or even at some supermarkets. The kits come with sterile cotton swabs, used inside each cheek to collect cells for the DNA sample. They also come with a lifestyle questionnaire that asks about eating habits and family history. Once all of the information is submitted, it takes about three weeks to get a printed report with details about each of the 19 genes.

Dr. Mark Hyman says that food is not just calories but information. We generally think of food as a means to get energy and fuel our bodies, but he says that food can literally talk to our genes, giving your body instructions on things like how to control metabolism or turning on cancer-protective genes. Nutrigenomics is literally food as medicine—working to turn off certain genes when you eat well or turn on certain genes if you go for foods that are unhealthy to the body, like processed junk foods.

Critics of the diet call it generic advice and say that analyzing 19 of the 25,000 human genes can't provide enough information to identify risk factors, much less specific foods you should eat. They say the advice is nothing more than commonsense information about eating habits that would help anyone lose weight and be healthier, regardless of their genes. The nutrigenomics industry came under further attack when four the leading nutrigenomics companies came out with a line of supplements called "nutraceuticals" that were being sold for close to $2,000 per year and were supposedly tailored to the customer's unique DNA, but upon further examination were shown to be remarkably similar to the multivitamins sold at any local drugstore.

Still, this kind of diet is closer to a bio-individual approach than many of the fad diets out there. It may prove to be effective, simply for offering a personal approach, which can help motivate people. Research in this field has only just begun.

Finding the Right Diet for You

Despite all my years both studying and teaching nutrition, I would never tell anyone how to eat. I think it would be crazy for me to say that there's any one way of eating that works for everyone. It's like saying that rock and roll is the best music and it's been scientifically proven because it has 80 beats per minute. What about jazz or reggae? We have so many styles of music, and, as I've outlined in Chapter 2, we have so many factors that contribute to our health and well-being.

Finding your path with food takes trial and error. It's like making a recipe from a cookbook. You could never make that exact recipe because your ingredients will be gathered from a different place, your oven cooks food at a slightly different temperature, and the environment in your kitchen is going to be different than a test kitchen. You can create something wonderful on your own once you understand all of the elements at play. A recipe may call for you to roast your veggies for 45 minutes, but if you pay attention to other cues, like smell or changes in color, you can see that sometimes the meal is ready sooner than the recipe called for, or maybe it needs to stay in the oven longer than expected.

Dietary preferences are not static. Don't forget that the foods you eat are always changing. Think about what you ate as a kid, what you ate two years ago, and what you enjoy today. It's constantly changing based on your needs. I don't think sending anyone outside of themselves is doing them any favors. Every time I've ever had a conversation with someone about their diet, they intuitively know what would make a difference within minutes. Getting healthy requires you to get curious and committed to your own path. It's not about choosing the right theory. It's about finding what works best for you, then creating your own nutrition theory based on your individual desires and needs. I want you to find what's right for you.

This task is far more challenging than getting swept away by the latest media-hyped fad and jumping on an already-rolling bandwagon. In the end, however, it will be far more rewarding because you will have come to understand your own nutritional needs, and you will arrive at a place of lasting health and physical well-being. It's a very empowering experience to realize you don't need to follow someone else's guidance, but you can control your own destiny and trust your own intuition and intelligence. The result is worth the extra effort.

Exercises

Create Your Own Eating Style

This is an invitation to create your own style of eating. It will help clarify your understanding of how diets work and what works best for you.

1. Get out a piece of paper, and list three major dietary theories that appeal to you.

2. Write down five aspects of these diets that seem the most essential to you.

Example:

I like ______________________ because ____________________.

3. Use these five qualities to create your new personalized approach.

Give your style a name:

The ______________________ Diet.

Be creative! Try finding a name that will catch your imagination.

4. Make up your own rules.

The five most important points are:

a.

b.

c.

d.

e.

5. What results do you expect from following this way of eating?

Chapter 5

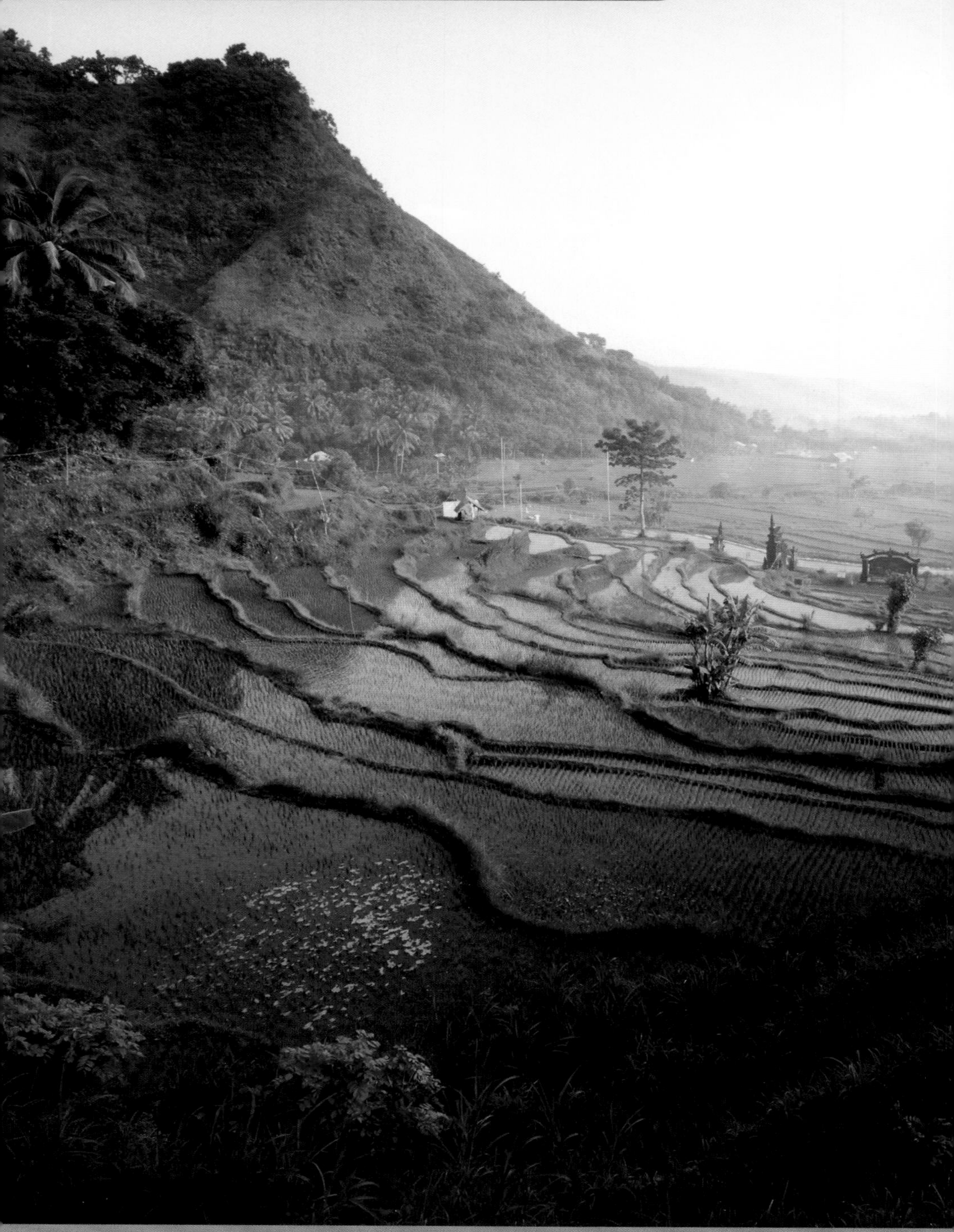

A Global Ripple Effect

> Centenarians never *tried* to live to 100. Longevity happened to them. It was not about discipline or personal responsibility.
>
> — Dan Buettner, author, *The Blue Zones*

When I started IIN, I was just one person with a simple idea that if I could change what people ate, I could change the world. I started by moving to New York City because it's a global melting pot of people. At any time, day or night, you can walk around and experience any kind of food or hear people speaking almost any language. This energy is part of what makes it one of the greatest cities in the world. By living among so many different types of people and experiencing their culture, I felt more connected to the global community. I realized I didn't want to create just a school; I wanted to create a movement.

The phrase "think globally, act locally," coined by the environmental movement, encourages us to understand how our actions can impact the world. With a global mindset, we can create better health and greater happiness. The school's mission is quite similar: "to play a crucial role in improving health and happiness, and through that process, create a ripple effect that transforms the world." One of our core values is to "support each other in the global shift to better health." The world is really set up for this support and connection. At no time ever before have we had such easy and accessible means of communicating through social media platforms, online video calling or chatting, and affordable transportation.

I've already mentioned how the U.S. impacts trends around the world. I think we can also look at local cultures and see how they can influence our thinking about nutrition and health. I think it's fascinating to take a look at what the world is eating and see what's working. People have been eating around the world for millions of years. Each day, we all wake up and have to decide what to eat. We've got a planet of more than 7 billion people who are full of wisdom and customs that we can all learn from. Now that you're familiar with many of the major dietary theories, you can continue to build on the wealth of information gathered from the global community.

It's important to talk about not just the food but the lifestyles and behaviors that contribute to our overall health in the world. I've seen so many cases where primary foods really override secondary foods. When people have a good life, they can often get away with eating whatever they want. Paris is a great example. People always wonder, how can the diet be so high in butter, bread, and rich pâté, and Parisians still be so slim? Well, they eat slowly and enjoy their meals. They talk to each other and give eye contact, rather than constantly checking their phones. I think that eating and drinking in a more balanced and open way also helps them avoid cravings and binges. Many people today order only salads when they are out with friends but spend the night gorging on so-called forbidden foods, like chips or chocolate.

The Secrets to Longevity

More scientific research backs up my idea of primary food—that living well is more than what's on your plate. I first read about the Blue Zones in a *National Geographic* article in 2005. The title of the article was "The Secrets to a Long Life." I thought, "Who doesn't want to know those secrets?" Just look at the market today. We are flooded with products that promise to make us look younger or defy our age. What if we could just live a long, happy life?

Author Dan Buettner wrote the article I read and the subsequent book about these areas of the world that boast centenarians, or people who live to be 100 or more. And they live not just longer but with a better quality of life, having very little disease or stress. As I mentioned in Chapter 1, these areas include Sardinia, Italy; Okinawa, Japan; Nicoya Peninsula, Costa Rica; Loma Linda, California; and the Greek island of Ikaria. What can we learn about these regions of the world that could help boost our longevity?

"In the United States, when it comes to improving health, people tend to focus on exercise and what we put into our mouths—organic foods, omega-3's, micronutrients," Buettner wrote in a 2012 *New York Times* article.

"We spend nearly $30 billion a year on vitamins and supplements alone. Yet in Ikaria and the other places like it, diet only partly explains higher life expectancy. Exercise, at least the way we think of it, as willful, dutiful, physical activity, played a small role at best."[1]

One of the big factors that Buettner emphasizes is social structure. In the Blue Zones, they have different cultural attitudes about getting older—people stay engaged in the community through social activities and family life. Old people are celebrated and talked to rather than shunned or isolated. In Costa Rica they use the term "plan de vida," or life plan, which describes living with a lifelong sense of purpose. Buettner says purpose and love are essential ingredients to the Blue Zones lifestyle.

Some of the other qualities he's found in studying these areas that offer amazing health benefits include eating a plant-based diet, reducing stress in life, participating in spiritual communities, making time for family, and finding your tribe.[2] I know that many students who enroll at IIN feel like they have found their tribe. I speak a lot about finding support in your life and surrounding yourself with people who share your values. Take a nod from the Blue Zones, and start implementing some of these changes in your life.

The Jungle Effect

Along with these longevity hot spots, you can find many places around the world where the diets make you healthier. Family physician Daphne Miller, M.D., traveled to what she calls cold spots—canyons, deserts, islands, frozen lands, and jungles where people have few problems with chronic disease. She decided to learn more about how indigenous diets affect our health for her book *The Jungle Effect: The Healthiest Diets from Around the World*. She found that getting back to the land could create better health for her patients in San Francisco, especially when they followed the diet of their ancestors. Our early ancestors relied on their intuition and experimentation to discover which plants tasted best, along with utilizing the freshest local, natural ingredients.

Miller found clues to solve the diabetes dilemma faced by much of the modern world from the local diet in Copper Canyon, Mexico, home to 50,000 Tarahumara Indians living in remote canyons. Their diet consists of corn, beans, squash, eggs, chicken, chiles, berries, wild greens, cactus, oranges, tomatoes, avocadoes, and the occasional wild game or fish. She was surprised that their diet was quite high in carbs, but they were unrefined and homemade. She learned that the glycemic index of corn is reduced when combined with beans and squash. Plus, many of the healing spices and plants in Mexico, including cactus, have been shown to help lower blood sugar. She realized that the high rates of diabetes in Latino populations living in the U.S. could be explained by losing these parts of the traditional diet, along with the adoption of highly processed, sugary foods.

In Iceland, people have low rates of seasonal affective disorder and depression, even though they have periods of winter with no sunlight and not a lot of vegetables growing on the island. People do, however, eat wild fish and game, fresh milk, and wild berries. In fact, Icelanders eat more fish per capita than anywhere in the world, according to Miller.[3] And even foods like lamb have high amounts of omega-3 fatty acids in them because the lamb eat tundra grass.

"They are able to get their antioxidants through surprising ways, like waxy potatoes, cabbage, and wild berries," Miller wrote. "I suppose they could import more greens, but they prefer their traditional foods. There is a feeling that this is what we do and we keep healthy." This example shows that the secrets to good health are really all around us when we choose to tune into our environment.

Miller also explored her own Ukrainian grandmother's recipe for borscht, which was made with canned sweetened beets, generous amounts of sour cream, and store-bought chicken broth. After a little digging, she found the recipe for borscht in her grandmother's hometown of Chodorov. Turns out the original recipe used fresh grated beets, light chicken stock, salt, pepper, and a spoonful of yogurt or clotted cream.

Putting these two soups side by side, you may not notice the difference, but think of all of the potential nutrients lost when we switch from homegrown beets to canned beets with added sugar. Sometimes in our quest for convenience, we lose our traditional foods and the nutrients that came with them. You don't have to have a Ph.D. in nutrition to see how the modernization of these indigenous diets could create health problems around the world.

Sometimes the best recipe is to keep it simple and nutritious and use whatever foods are freshest in your area.

"Studies suggest that indigenous groups get into trouble when they abandon their traditional diets and active lifestyles for Western living," according to a *National Geographic* magazine article written by Ann Gibbons, a science writer who specializes in human evolution. She cites examples of the Maya in Central America who saw virtually no rates of diabetes until the 1950s, when their diet switched to a more Western style with more refined sugars. Similarly, Siberian nomads ate diets loaded with meat and had almost no evidence of heart disease until the early '90s, when, during the collapse of the Soviet Union, many resettled in towns and ate processed foods instead of wild foods. Today, many of these former nomads are overweight, and about a third have hypertension.

A Country Without McDonald's

While many fast-food chains are rapidly expanding throughout the globe, there's one country in South America where McDonald's did not survive. In Bolivia, people prefer their traditional foods to Big Macs. Citizens still love hamburgers, but they prefer to buy them from indigenous female street vendors called cholitas. The fast-food chain closed all locations in 2002 because it was simply not profitable. The failure piqued the interest of filmmakers, who made a documentary in 2011 called *Why did McDonald's Bolivia Go Bankrupt?*[4]

"Fast food represents the complete opposite of what Bolivians believe a meal should be," according to the blog El Polvorin.[5] "To be a good meal, food has to have been prepared with love, dedication, certain hygiene standards, and proper cook time."

What I find most interesting about Bolivia is the fact that community values prevail. Bolivia's population values their food systems, food producers, and ecosystems so much that food sovereignty laws continue to pass in the government to ensure that they preserve their food traditions and put less economic pressure on commodity crops. The country's first indigenous president, Evo Morales, even called U.S. fast-food chains "a great harm to humanity" at a United Nations General Assembly meeting in 2013. Talk about a slow food nation. I wonder what would happen in other countries if more of the population embraced longer, slower meals, rather than quick, convenient foods.

The Healthiest Regional Cuisines

We now live in a global food market. Imagine if you no longer had access to lemons or coconut oil because they weren't available in your local economy. Think about coffee and tea or the spices you use to flavor your food. When it comes to our food today, much of what we consume comes from this global interaction. Merriam Webster defines globalization as "the development of an increasingly integrated global economy." We have gained so much from the many food traditions throughout the world that we don't even think about. At the same time, we are at risk of losing our deep connections to our ancestors' diets. These foods provided sustenance and kept those people healthy for thousands of years. Local cultures and food traditions are disappearing, as multinational food corporations are increasingly providing more and more food without much thought to the regional foods of the world.

"Diets evolve over time, being influenced by many factors and complex interactions," according to the website of the World Health Organization.[6] "Income, prices, individual preferences and beliefs, cultural traditions, as well as geographical, environmental, social, and economic factors all interact in a complex manner to shape dietary consumption patterns."

Many regions of the world are less reliant on processed, convenient foods and, instead, have amazing regional foods and customs that keep people healthy. Here are a few examples.

Africa

This large and diverse continent is home to root vegetables, leafy greens, beans, and wild meats and fish. Okra and watermelon are native to Africa. The main grains found in Africa are couscous, sorghum, millet, and rice. Researchers have found that North Africans may have been making yogurt around 7,000 years ago.[7] Pottery shards were discovered with traces of fat from a fermented dairy product, and scientists believe this method made it more digestible. Traditional Central and Western African meals are often based on hearty and aromatic vegetable soups and stews served over tubers or grains. Fufu is a dish made from starchy foods like cassava or yams, usually served with grilled meat. Eastern Africa serves up more whole grains and vegetables, especially kale, cabbage, and maize (cornmeal). Ethiopia and Somalia feature flat breads like injera (made out of teff or sorghum) and spicy beans like lentils, fava beans, and chickpeas.

Australia/New Zealand

Traditionally, the diets in these island nations took their roots from the English diet, with stewed meats, puddings, and pies. Dinners typically consisted of lamb, beef, or chicken with potatoes or root vegetables. Seafood is certainly abundant in coastal areas. The indigenous Aborigine in Australia enjoyed meat from kangaroo, crocodiles, and turtles, along with shellfish and native fruits like wild peach or riberry (similar to cranberry). The Maori in New Zealand took advantage of the many wild plants and roots like kumara (sweet potato) and taro. The world knows these areas for Marmite and Vegemite, food pastes made from yeast extract and used to spread on toast and sandwiches. With an intense flavor, these spreads are rich sources of B vitamins, niacin, and folic acid.

Caribbean

Many local fruits and vegetables offer tons of nutrients and energy to the Caribbean lifestyle. Guava is a small, oval-shaped fruit with a rough outer skin but with a sweet and sour taste inside that's high in fiber, potassium, and vitamin C. Breadfruit can be boiled or mashed much like a potato, and it's an excellent source of fiber and potassium. Beans are another staple in the Caribbean diet, including lentils, chickpeas, kidney beans, black-eyed peas, and split peas. Callaloo, the national dish of Trinidad and Tobago, consists of a stew made with green leafy vegetables, usually some kind of spinach variety.

India

India is famous for its aromatic cuisine. The country has some of the lowest rates of Alzheimer's disease in the world, thanks in part to some of its healthy spices. Curcumin, responsible for the yellow color found in curry spice, continues to be studied for its health benefits that include cancer prevention and anti-inflammatory properties that help ward off the onset of Alzheimer's. Other spices, like ginger, chilies, and cardamom, are also great for you. Indian dal is made with lentils and veggies, is full of magnesium, and can even help stabilize blood sugar. Indian surveys show that about 40% of the population is vegetarian, but demand for meat seems to be rising in recent years, along with more of the health issues associated with it.[8]

The Nordic Region

Citizens of Sweden, Denmark, and Norway boast some of the lowest obesity rates in Europe, perhaps because their diet is full of cold-climate veggies like kale, cabbage, and cauliflower. Their bread is made with rye grain, which is easier to digest than wheat and has more soluble fiber, helping to lower cholesterol and glycemic load. A small, randomized study from 2010 tested the health of the Nordic diet using local foods like herring, rapeseed oil, and berries on people with metabolic syndrome (a precursor to diabetes). Researchers found that those eating the healthy Nordic foods had significant improvements in their bad cholesterol/good cholesterol ratio and also in a marker for inflammation, which could result in a 20% to 40% decrease in likelihood of developing type 2 diabetes.[9] While scientists felt confident the diet had health benefits, they also recognized it might be hard to replicate the diet outside of Nordic countries. It's just another testament to the power of local, whole foods.

The Middle East

Another region of the world known for its spices and healthy dishes is the Middle East, including countries like Turkey, Israel, Iran, Iraq, Lebanon, Palestine, Jordan, and more. Some of the most common ingredients here are olive oil, chickpeas, sesame seeds, dates, and herbs like mint and parsley. This region is known for hummus and other healthy dips served with plenty of vegetables. Sumac, a dark red spice made from wild sumac berries, offers a tart flavor used as a rub on meats and kebabs, as well as in marinades, dips, and stews. Traditionally, the spice had medicinal purposes, too, helping promote good digestion, easing stomach pains, and even reducing fevers. Sumac berries contain antioxidants and antimicrobial properties. The spice is used in a spice blend called za'atar, which also includes wild oregano, thyme, toasted sesame seeds, and salt. This health food dates back to the 12th century when the Spanish Jewish philosopher Maimonides is said to have used it with his patients to treat many ailments.[10]

Philippines

The Filipino diet includes rice with almost every meal, along with lots of fresh seafood and local vegetables, like water spinach, eggplant, and bitter melon. People tend to eat three meals a day, along with a morning and afternoon snack. The food prep is usually quite simple—grilled, steamed, or raw. Fish and veggies typically receive a marinade of vinegar or lime juice. More recently, American-style fast foods like hamburgers and pizza have become more popular, creating a similar rise in overweight and obese people, as in the U.S.[11]

Japan

Japan is another place where obesity rates are low, and people who live in the Blue Zone region of Okinawa live to be 100 or more. Food prep is usually light steams and quick stir-fries with fresh vegetables and fish. Of course, sushi is also easy to digest and can be high in heart-healthy fish oil. Some of the staple foods that contribute to that health are calcium-rich greens like bok choy, shiitake mushrooms, sea vegetables, and antioxidant-rich green tea. Miso, tempeh, natto, and other fermented soy products are easy to digest and offer increased nutrition as rich sources of iron, magnesium, and zinc.

South America

Another diverse continent, South America makes use of fresh vegetables, beans, and fruit. A high-protein seed that cooks up like a grain, quinoa, is a superfood that grows abundantly here. Some areas like Brazil and Argentina are known for steaks and meat but also have healthier dishes like ceviche—a mixture of raw seafood, citrus juice, and tomato. And the most basic South American meal of rice and beans with fresh cilantro and chili peppers is another healthy dish.

Southeast Asia

Fresh herbs, vegetables, and fish prevail in this area. Using more water and broth for cooking is an easy healthy habit to take from Southeast Asian kitchens. Flavorings like cilantro, mint, ginger, tamarind, and chilies are all great for digestion and help fight inflammation in the body. In Vietnam, you find pho, an aromatic noodle soup full of antioxidant-rich spices. Researchers at Thailand's Kasetsart University have studied the immune-boosting qualities of Tom Yum Goong, a soup made with shrimp, mushroom, coriander, lemongrass, ginger, and other herbs and spices. Incidences of digestive tract cancers are lower in Thailand than anywhere else in the world.[12]

Spain

Spain is synonymous with tapas—small plates of veggies, fish, or meat. The rest of the world could certainly benefit from this ritual of eating smaller portions during a long, leisurely meal. Spanish food features fresh seafood, vegetables, and olive oil, a darling of the Mediterranean diet. Particularly healthy dishes like gazpacho are full of antioxidants, like lycopene, known for its cancer-fighting properties. Paella is another great meal with seafood, rice, veggies, and spices.

Wherever you are in the world, it's important to look at the whole picture and find balance with both primary and secondary foods. Healthy ingredients are great, but many people who eat relatively healthy still don't have the energy and zest for life of people who feel truly fulfilled in their lives. It's not just the food but also the lifestyle that contributes to the health of families, the environment, and ultimately the planet.

Superfoods of the World

As I mentioned in Chapter 1, many unhealthy habits get exported around the world. But a new trend has emerged around superfoods, or foods that are nutritionally dense and thought to possess super immune-boosting properties. It's a relief to see more nutrient-rich foods getting imported, exported, and integrated throughout markets in the world. But as with any trend, be curious about where your food comes from, and don't forget your unique nutritional needs. We are all bio-individuals, even when it comes to superfoods. Some exotic berries or seeds might contain super nutrients, but the foods that grow right in your neighborhood usually contain the best nutrients for you.

The word "superfood" is not a scientific or regulated term. You might notice that many lists rate the top superfoods in the world with as many as 50 or 100 foods, including everything from blueberries to seaweed. Don't forget the basics. Any food can become a superfood if it gives you energy and vitality. Eating a glamorous superfood every now and again cannot make up for nutritional or lifestyle mistakes happening day in and out. Right? You can't get by on a few hours of sleep and hope that a shake of superfoods will repair the damage. So don't get too swept away by these foods, and remember to always listen to your body.

Technology today has allowed for the exchange of information and ideas at a more rapid pace than ever before. People learn about superfoods and nutrition from articles on the Internet or a friend's recommendation on Facebook. We have seen some of the disadvantages of exporting certain foods, as the SAD diet has increased heart disease and obesity to the areas of the world that have embraced it.

But we also have the potential to improve the world's health by spreading more positive messages about food. Perhaps TEDx says it best with their mission of "ideas worth spreading." Understand that just one person—one person reading this book, just like you—can make an enormous difference for the health of yourself, your family, and your community.

U.S. President John F. Kennedy said, "Ask not what your country can do fosr you. Ask what you can do for your country." Well, it's time to expand this thought, as we are so well connected. It's time to think about what you can do for your world.

Global Superfoods

Please note: These are powerful and very nutritious foods. But if you are on medications like blood thinners or are pregnant or breastfeeding, talk to a medical professional before adding these foods into your diet.

Acai — Region: Brazil From the rainforests of Brazil, this small, bright-purple berry is one of the most nutritious foods found on the planet. It's packed with antioxidants, amino acids, and healthy fats. You can find it in powder or frozen form, which you can add to smoothies and juices for an extra punch of nutrients.

Bee Pollen — Region: Worldwide Found wherever bees roam, bee pollen is used throughout the world as a holistic remedy and superfood. It's the result of the accumulation of flower pollen, nectar, and bee's salivary substances. It's rich in amino acids, B-complex vitamins, and folic acid.[13]

Cacao — Region: Mexico and the Americas Native to the Americas, the cacao bean was first cultivated in Mexico in 1500 B.C.[14] Now people use it to make raw chocolate or cacao powder because of its antioxidants and high amounts of magnesium, fiber, and iron.[15]

Camu Camu Berry — Region: Amazon Rainforest This berry, which in its whole form looks more like a cherry, is one of the highest sources of vitamin C on the planet and a great source of anthocyanins, a powerful antioxidant. Camu camu berry helps to reduce inflammation and decrease oxidative stress. It has a tart flavor and is usually found as a powder that you can add to smoothies or prepared dishes.

Chia Seeds — Region: Mexico and the Americas Aztecs and Mayans used chia seeds to gain strength and stamina starting around 3500 B.C. The nutrients offered by these small, dark seeds include antioxidants, fiber, calcium, and Omega-3 fatty acids.[16]

Goji Berries — Region: China This berry is also known as the wolfberry and is a small red berry known for its high level of carotenoids, which can help boost the immune system.[17] It has been used in traditional herbal medicine for about 2,000 years, and in China they hold a strong belief that this fruit can significantly extend life.[18]

Hemp Seeds — Region: Central Asia The hemp plant originated in Central Asia as a food crop, but today it is grown all over the world. The seeds come from a variety of cannabis plant, but it contains very little THC—the part that is considered a drug in most countries. It's similar to the amount of opium in poppy seeds. Hemp seeds are very high in Omega-3 and Omega-6 essential fatty acids and are an excellent source of protein.[19]

continues

Global Superfoods *(continued)*

Quinoa — Region: South America The Food and Agriculture Organization of the United Nations (FAO) declared 2013 "The International Year of the Quinoa."[20] This seed is very high in protein but cooks up like a grain, making it a great option for those looking to cut back on carbs. It's full of antioxidants, fiber, and minerals like manganese and magnesium.

Maca — Region: South America A staple in the Peruvian Andes for thousands of years, this root vegetable helps increase energy, endurance, fertility, and libido. Usually found as a dried powder, this superfood may support cognitive function, protect from osteoporosis, and help reduce blood pressure.

Manuka Honey — Region: New Zealand This honey, native to New Zealand, comes from bees that pollinate the Manuka bush. Honey has a healing reputation, but Manuka honey has been effective in scientific studies when used on top of wounds. It's also effective in fighting infection and promoting healing.[21]

Moringa — Region: Africa/Asia The leaves of this tree are thought to be a superfood because it's one of the world's most nutritious plant species, with more than 92 types of nutrients and 46 types of antioxidants. It also contains protein and is a great source of iron—100 grams of dry moringa leaf contains 25 times the iron of spinach. It's usually available in powder or capsule form and can be brewed into a tea or added to a smoothie.

Sea Vegetables — Region: Worldwide Found seaside in any part of the world, sea vegetables, like nori, kelp, and dulse, are rich in nutrients drawn in from the ocean and sun. Sea vegetables are full of nutrients, like iodine, magnesium, calcium, and potassium. They also help support immunity, reduce cholesterol, decrease the risk of cancer, and can be especially beneficial for thyroid and hormone function.

Spirulina — Region: Africa This microalgae gets its name from its spiral shape, thriving in fresh and salt water throughout the world. It is rich in protein, vitamins, minerals, carotenoids, and antioxidants.[22]

Exercises

1. Think Globally, Act Locally

With a global mind-set, we can create better health and greater happiness for all. Consider how your actions impact the world, and think about what you can do to get more of your food locally.

Which foods are local to your country or community? Create a recipe using as many local ingredients as possible. Recreate a favorite family dish, or try something new. Entrees, side dishes, smoothies, and juices all count. How do you feel after cooking with local versus store-bought, out-of-season ingredients? How do local ingredients affect the taste?

2. What Makes a Superfood So Super?

Find a food labeled as a "superfood," and then compare it to an unlabeled whole food from your local market. Example: chia seeds versus brown rice. How do the cost and nutrition compare? Do a little research on both. How do these foods make you feel? Can you incorporate one superfood each day, regardless of the label?

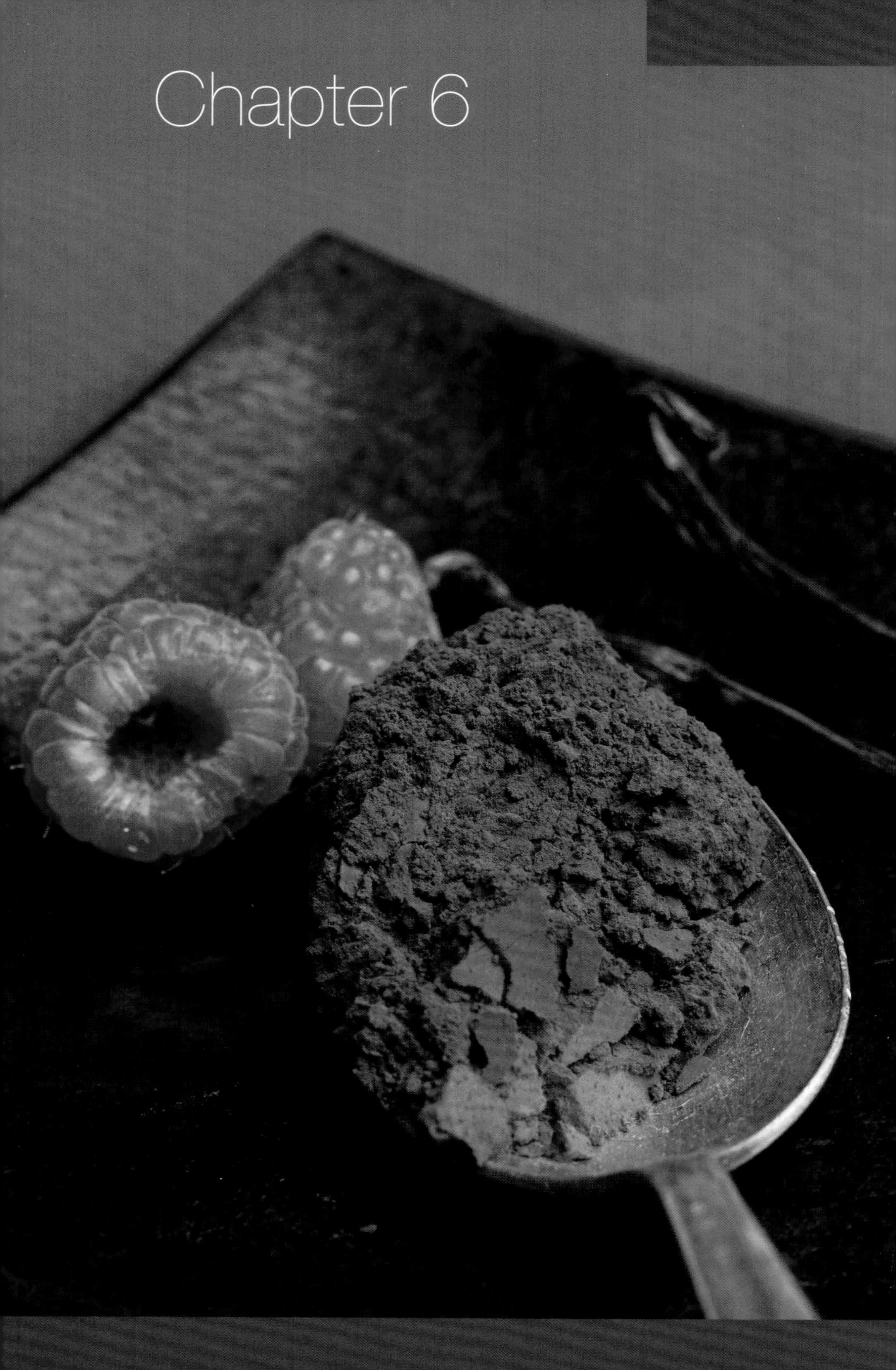

Chapter 6

Deconstructing Cravings

> Cravings indicate imbalances in the body and are actually incredibly helpful in guiding you to ideal health ... kind of like a smoke alarm.
>
> —Joshua Rosenthal, from *Crack the Code on Cravings*

Chocolate, bread, steak, eggs, French fries, candy bars, ice cream—it really doesn't matter what you crave. The important thing is to understand why you crave what you crave. Most people believe cravings are a problem, but I have a different perspective. Once we realize that the body is a reliable bio-computer that never makes mistakes, it's much easier to conclude that cravings are critical pieces of information that help you understand what your body needs.

I've been craving ice cream since I was a child, with a special sweet spot for Ben and Jerry's Cherry Garcia, the perfect blend of dark chocolate, sweet vanilla, and tart fruit. I noticed that on Sunday nights, after teaching class all weekend, it seemed like an alien force would take control of my body and drive my car directly to the convenience store to buy a pint. As I watched myself eat all this ice cream, I wondered, between delicious mouthfuls, "What am I doing in my life that might trigger such an extreme craving?"

At the time, I was teaching many hours, eating a primarily macrobiotic diet, and drinking hot peppermint tea throughout the day to stay grounded and focused. When I started investigating the craving, I noticed that my body felt hot and tense when I had the tea, and shortly after, I began to daydream about chocolate-covered cherries smothered in rich, cold vanilla ice cream. The hot tea was causing my craving for cooling foods. I started drinking more water, stopped asking for water without ice at restaurants, and increased my intake of vegetables, which have a cooling and relaxing effect on the body. I also realized that after gorging on ice cream, I felt extremely satiated. Knowing that fat is what makes us feel satisfied and that my macrobiotic diet did not contain much fat, I incorporated more olive oil into my cooking to provide an alternative source of fatty satisfaction. Long hours of teaching can be stressful, and the fact that I was having these cravings on Sundays indicated that I was using the ice cream as a reward or de-stressor after teaching all weekend.

Lo and behold, within a few weeks of making these changes, my cravings passed, and my Sunday night ice cream binges ended. Of course, I still look forward to a few bites every once in a while, but the days of empty pints in the backseat of my car are long gone. By observing my own behavior and trusting that my body needed something from the ice cream, I was able to modify my diet and lifestyle to get what I needed in a more health-supportive way.

A food craving can be defined as an intense desire for a particular food (or type of food) that is difficult to resist."[1] Almost everyone has had a craving at some point in their lives—about 97% of women and 68% of men have experienced cravings, according to research.[2] Still, the conventional approach to cravings is usually centered on conquering and suppressing these desires. Doesn't that seem odd? Almost everyone is craving something, and we're often told to squash those cravings.

I think cravings are important messages from your body. They are one of the most natural ways your body speaks to you about what you need and how to stay in balance. Once you start to see your cravings in a new light, you will be amazed at what you can uncover. Your body has a specific message just for you. Are you willing to listen?

Along with the information in this chapter, I wrote an entire book on cravings called *Crack the Code on Cravings* for those who want to explore this topic further.

Sugar Addictions

Many years ago, a successful female dentist came to me for help with her sugar cravings. She confessed that all day long she told clients to avoid sugar, but every afternoon she would sneak into her back office and secretly binge on sweets, particularly candy bars: Butterfingers, Snickers, Milky Ways, or Twix bars. She was a sincere, intelligent woman who knew that consuming large amounts of sugar was not good for her teeth, but she was helpless when it came to her own cravings. She was puzzled and felt helpless, not for a lack of understanding or discipline, but because willpower is often not enough when it comes to food dependencies, especially those involving sugar.

"I'm addicted, and I feel like an absolute hypocrite," she told me.

"You're not a hypocrite," I said. "Humans naturally crave sweet flavors, but there is something you can do about it. Let's get some milder sweet foods into your diet on a more regular basis to avoid these afternoon binges."

I explained the distinction between simple and complex carbohydrates, advising her to reduce processed foods—except pasta, which she loved—and increase grains and vegetables. I knew, however, this alone would not be enough to beat her intense sugar cravings. So I supported her to find some less processed options and told her to experiment with what worked best when she was craving something sweet. Could she try organic dark chocolate squares as a substitute for commercial candy bars? Could she make her own cookies rather than eating ones from a box? In two months, her sugar cravings had diminished remarkably.

These days, a lot of natural options can help you transition from refined, processed sugars, and more research is addressing how much we all need to make the leap. At the forefront of the research is Dr. Robert Lustig, a pediatric endocrinologist from California, who believes sugar is downright toxic and addictive. He's authored dozens of scientific articles, but in May 2009 Dr. Lustig made headlines with a lecture he gave called "Sugar: The Bitter Truth," which was later posted on YouTube and has been seen by almost 7 million people. In it, he argues that sugar is the primary cause of our worldwide health crisis due to its potential for abuse, its toxic nature, and its growing prevalence in the Western diet. He brings to light that sugar is hidden in almost all processed foods today, from bread to peanut butter to canned sauces and dressings, especially in the form of high fructose corn syrup.

Dr. Lustig says evolution has taught us that sweet things are safe to eat. But fructose, the naturally occurring sugar in fruit, comes with fiber and other important nutrients, which is a far cry from the sweet stuff we are consuming today. One study linked increased sugar consumption with increased rates of diabetes in 175 countries worldwide.[3] Researchers found that increased sugar in a population's food supply was linked to higher rates of diabetes. As sugar has become a bigger part of the daily diet around the world, so have chronic diseases.

Simple and Complex Carbohydrates

Nearly everyone craves sugar. When experiencing such cravings, most people go right for the most accessible sweet treat: candy, chocolate bars, or cookies. But what these people don't realize is that many healthy alternatives can help alleviate sweet cravings.

A sugar craving is simply the body asking for energy. When sugar is digested, it becomes glucose. Glucose is fuel for all of the body's cells. When you eat sugar, it enters the bloodstream and is converted into glucose at different rates, depending on the type of sugar you consume. All carbohydrates contain sugar, but depending on their chemical structures—simple or complex—they are processed differently. Most simple carbohydrates are highly processed, contain refined sugars, and have few vitamins and minerals. Processed foods contain short chains of sugar, which enter the bloodstream quickly after they are ingested. This causes a rapid rise in the glucose levels in the body—a sugar rush. The rush is shortly followed by a crash. The body sees the high level of sugar as an emergency state and works hard to clear it as quickly as possible. Then blood sugar drops precipitously. Whole foods, like fruit, contain naturally occurring simple sugars. Fruit is high in fiber, which helps slow digestion, limiting the amount of sugar that is absorbed at once.

Carbohydrates that appear in whole foods like vegetables and whole grains are considered complex because they are composed of long chains of sugars. The body processes complex carbohydrates by breaking the chains to create simple carbohydrates, which can then be absorbed and utilized for energy. Since metabolizing complex carbohydrates involves more steps, sugar is absorbed into the bloodstream at a slower and steadier rate, allowing us to regulate our blood sugar levels more closely and avoid spikes.

If you eat a whole grain—which contains fiber, a type of complex carbohydrate—for breakfast, you will likely feel satisfied throughout the morning and then experience a mild dip around noon, signaling that it's time for your next meal. Fiber helps to slow digestion and increase satiety, which helps us feel satisfied for a longer amount of time. If you eat a cookie or white bread—which contain mostly simple carbs—the bloodstream becomes overloaded with sugars, providing a quick burst of energy, but also requires a more concerted effort to be cleared, which becomes taxing on the body. After consuming foods high in simple sugars and lacking fiber, your blood sugar dips, creating an extreme shift in a short amount of time, which leaves you hungry again. Since your body wants to maintain balanced blood sugar, it is signaling for you to eat something else to bring your blood sugar back up. Most people go for more sugar, which makes sense since it provides a quick source of energy, but it supports a cycle of energy ups and downs throughout the day. Blood sugar often drops around 3 p.m., a few hours after lunch—the time when most people seek sugar or caffeine to get them through the rest of the afternoon.

In today's modern nutrition world, high-protein diets are fashionable and "carbohydrate" is more of a dirty word, associated in many people's minds with the obesity crisis. But not all carbs are created equal. The right carbohydrates provide the energy needed for normal body functions and even provide energy to our brains. Carbohydrates are in everything from candy bars to grains and even vegetables, which is why it's important to make the distinction between carbohydrates of high and low nutritional value. The problem is that people are not eating the types of carbohydrates nature intended. They're eating carbohydrate-rich foods that have been deformed and highly refined. Refined sugars can lead to weight gain because our cells do not require large amounts of glucose at one time, and the extra sugar is stored as fat. The anti-carb movement should really be an anti-refined sugar movement.

Let's talk about fruit for a moment too, because it can also get a bad rap. Unlike sugar or most processed foods with added sweeteners, fruit is a good source of fiber. Generally, fresh fruit doesn't cause as sharp a spike in blood glucose levels. Fresh fruit is also a source of antioxidants, vitamins, and minerals, offering much more nutritional value than simple energy.

Overconsumption of refined forms of sugar has led to an abundance of hyperglycemia (when blood sugar is too high). Too much sugar in the diet disrupts our body's ability to manage sugar effectively. Over time, this condition leads to the risk of developing metabolic syndrome and increases overall inflammation in the body. People also experience more hypoglycemia, which is when the body's blood sugar gets too low. It's common among people with diabetes but can also be caused by an overload of sugar, alcohol, caffeine, and stress. A person with hypoglycemia may feel weak, drowsy, confused, dizzy, and hungry, especially around 3 p.m., when blood sugar is naturally at its lowest. When your blood sugar is low, you are vulnerable to cravings because your body urgently needs something to spike its glucose. Again, both conditions can be prevented when we focus on real foods over sugary snacks.

Sugar cravings are as natural as our desire for air. Throughout two million years of evolution, humans have been programmed to desire sweet-tasting foods. Long before food processing, the only source of sweet tastes was plant foods, such as squash, tubers, and fruit. In order to get the sweet taste their bodies desired, people had to eat plants. It is no coincidence these sweet foods are also great sources of nutrients, energy, and fiber—everything we need to maintain our health. So, the best way to curb or alleviate intense sugar cravings is to provide the body with the sweetness that it needs by regularly eating naturally sweet foods.

Hungry for Nutrition

A student of mine once talked to me about her "problem child," Kevin, who was addicted to processed foods, like sugary cereals, peanut butter and jelly on white bread, pizza, fast food, and all kinds of sodas and salty snacks. The more Kevin ate, the hungrier he got. This ravenous 11-year-old was clearly eating too much and was overweight as a result.

"Maybe he's not hungry for calories," I said to her. "Maybe he's hungry for nutrition."

"What do you mean?" she asked. "I'm feeding him all day long. I would think he's getting too much nutrition."

I explained that the food he was eating was all processed and rich in simple sugars but deficient in nutrients. Sugar is fuel for cells, but they need vitamins and minerals to do their jobs properly. He was fueling his body, making his cells work but not giving them the raw materials they needed. Kevin was craving more and more food because his cells were starving for vitamins and minerals. He was suffering from malnutrition, which some refer to as the obesity paradox because you can be undernourished but overweight. Even with an abundance of calories, your body still craves nutrients.

"He's on a very inefficient diet and needs to eat a lot of food just to get enough nutrients to operate his body," I told her.

"But what can I do?" his mother asked, looking a bit stunned.

"He's got to reverse the formula," I said. "Eat foods that are rich in nutrients and low in calories, the exact opposite of what he's doing now."

I then laid out a program for her son that did not take out any of his foods, but rather added nutrient-rich foods, especially vegetables and whole grains, to his diet and suggested plenty of exercise. I spoke to her about making home-cooked food that might appeal to her 11-year-old. He could still have his favorite peanut butter, but on a celery stick instead of white bread with sugary jelly. He could still eat pizza, but homemade pizza with vegetable toppings. She had to take it slowly. Kevin wasn't going to immediately start loving collards and brown rice. Getting a child who is hooked on sugar and processed foods to eat natural foods can seem impossible. His taste buds were accustomed to artificial flavors. Natural foods would probably taste bland.

I sometimes tell students to pour chocolate sauce on greens at first, if it will get their kids to actually eat them. Do whatever it takes to get kids accustomed to natural foods. It takes most people, both children and adults, three times of trying a food before they really begin to enjoy it. I suggested that Kevin's mom make greens and have him eat just a few pieces the first time, the second time, and the third time. After that, he was helping himself to the greens. Six months later, Kevin had lost 30 pounds.

Like a lot of people, Kevin was stuffing himself with sugary foods and becoming sick and overweight. He kept eating because his body was craving nutrients, not simply food mass.

The body is smart. It tells you when you are not feeding it properly. If you feed it fats, low-quality oils, and sugar, it is going to send you messages that needs aren't being met. It needs protein. It needs vitamins. It needs minerals. But if you are not accustomed to eating vegetables, whole grains, and other nutrient-dense foods, you're not going to decipher this message as a specific craving for something healthy. So Kevin, for example, was just getting the hunger signal and grabbing the foods he'd been brought up on: meat, pizza, bread, sugar, Big Macs, or whatever.

A heartbreaking number of children in the U.S. and around the world are struggling with their weight and obesity. They are addicted to sugar and processed food. Most people don't realize that they keep eating because their bodies are hungry for nutrition.

Contracting and Expanding Foods

Your body naturally wants to be balanced. The food you eat is a major contributing factor to the overall balance of the body. Certain foods, such as vegetables and whole grains, have mild effects on the body. Other foods, such as meat, milk, sugar, and salt, have more extreme effects on the body, throwing off its natural balance. This struggle eventually leads to a craving for whatever the body needs to regain balance. I call these foods extreme foods, and I divide them into two categories: contracting and expanding. This idea is based on macrobiotic philosophy.

Contracting Foods

The most common and powerful contracting food is salt, which many of us consume regularly in large quantities. Salt is used commonly as a preservative, especially in artificial junk food. Other extreme contracting foods are animal foods, including beef, pork, ham, hard cheese, eggs, chicken, fish, and shellfish. The main benefit of animal foods is that they are rich in protein and give us feelings of strength, aggressiveness, and increased physical and mental power. However, when we eat too much of these foods, we create an imbalance and quickly feel bloated, heavy, sluggish, and mentally slow. The more contracting foods we eat, the tighter our bodies become. As a result of eating contracting foods, the body naturally craves expanding foods as a way of maintaining balance.

The 8 Primary Causes of Cravings

1. Lack of Primary Food Being dissatisfied with a relationship, having an inappropriate exercise routine (too much, too little, or the wrong type), being bored, feeling stressed, being uninspired by a job, or lacking a spiritual practice can all contribute to emotional eating. Eating can be used as a substitute for entertainment or to fill the void.

2. Water The body doesn't send the message that you are thirsty until you are on the verge of dehydration. Dehydration presents itself to us as mild hunger, so the first thing to do when you get a strange craving is to drink a full glass of water. Excess water can also cause cravings, so make sure you find balance with your water intake.

3. Yin/Yang Imbalance Certain foods have more yin qualities (expansive), while other foods have more yang qualities (contractive). Eating foods that are either extremely yin or extremely yang causes cravings in order to reestablish balance. For example, eating a diet too rich in sugar (yin) may cause a craving for meat (yang). Eating too many raw foods (yin) may cause cravings for heavily cooked foods and vice versa.

4. Inside Coming Out Oftentimes, cravings come from foods that we have recently eaten, foods eaten by our ancestors, or foods from our childhood. A clever way to satisfy these cravings is to eat a healthier version of one's ancestral or childhood foods.

5. Seasonal Often, the body craves foods that balance out the elements of the season. During warm months, people typically crave cooling foods, like fruit, raw foods, and ice cream, and as the weather cools, people crave grounding foods like squash, onions, and nuts. Other cravings, such as turkey, eggnog, or sweets, can also be associated with the holiday season.

6. Lack of Nutrients If the body is getting an inadequate amount of nutrients, it will produce odd cravings. For example, inadequate mineral levels produce salt cravings, and overall inadequate nutrition produces cravings for non-nutritional forms of energy, like caffeine.

7. Hormonal When women experience menstruation, pregnancy, or menopause, fluctuating testosterone and estrogen levels may cause unusual cravings.

8. Devolution When things are going extremely well, sometimes a self-sabotage syndrome happens, where we suddenly crave foods that throw us off balance. We then have more cravings to balance ourselves. This often happens from low blood sugar and may result in strong mood swings.

Expanding Foods

The predominant expanding food is refined white sugar. Expanding foods provide feelings of lightness, elevations in mood, and relief from blockages and stagnation. However, refined white sugar also causes rapid elevations in serotonin, followed by rapid declines. When serotonin levels fall, we typically experience feelings of depression, low energy, anxiety, and loss of concentration. We crave extreme contracting foods to balance the equation and again find ourselves in the throes of the ping-pong diet, using one type of extreme food to alleviate the effects of the other.

Our bodies can enjoy a certain quantity of extreme foods without creating too much imbalance. But when we exceed our personal limit—and it varies with each individual—there are consequences. If you eat extreme foods daily, your body will become exhausted and depleted as it frantically tries to rebalance itself. To get out of this cycle, you need to deconstruct what you are craving and seek out less extreme, healthier alternatives to satisfy you.

Hunger and Binging

Sometimes cravings come as the result of extreme hunger. You don't know what you're hungry for; you just know that you're starving. Most people avoid hunger at all costs, and many develop habits of overeating and/or constant eating just to avoid ever feeling hungry. When we habitually overeat, a high proportion of our available energy is always directed toward digestion. If we eat when we are not hungry, we compromise our digestion of the food. You may want to consider the idea, almost heretical in this day and age, that it's okay to be hungry now and then. I'm not talking about a drastic form of starvation dieting—just an experiment to see how it feels. It's not going to kill you, and it may make life more interesting.

On the other hand, many people today try to go hungry all day, ignoring the body's cravings for food. This habit creates a backlash, which I call the "binge eater's diet." In an attempt to lose weight, these people skip breakfast, go off to work, maybe grab a mid-morning cup of coffee to keep going, and then settle on a salad for lunch. Somehow they make it through the afternoon, but by the time they get home in the evening, they discover that they are ravenous. The hectic activity of the workday may have distracted them from urgent messages emanating from their stomachs, but as they slow down, they realize, "I am so hungry!" Then they overeat heavy foods at dinner, until they feel stuffed and uncomfortable. The next morning, they start the cycle over again, not eating breakfast because they feel full from last night's binge.

I do not believe in trying to override natural instincts. Of course, it helps to have discipline around food, but trying to control the body by using the mind is very challenging in the long term. For one thing, the head often makes mistakes. Remember when you went shopping for a fabulous new outfit and spent a lot of money but never wore the clothes? Another mistake your head can easily make is to decide, "This is the right diet for me. I can handle this one." Our bodies don't really care what our heads think. Our bodies are built to survive and thrive. Your head can say, "I am not eating this food because it is fattening," and your body may cooperate for a while. At some point, though, it will start murmuring quiet messages like, "Hmm, we definitely need some more fat in here, to keep the brain thinking and make me feel satiated." The next thing you know, you're holding an empty pint of ice cream.

Learning to listen to your body is essential. The longer you ignore your body's messages, the more extreme the backlash. Just as a crying child will use increasingly extreme measures to get attention, the body will heighten your cravings and create disease if you don't listen to it.

Crowding Out

One solution to cravings that I've found to be quite effective over the years is to add more to your diet rather than taking away from it. For years, I did not eat bread at home. I just ate whole grains. But when I was in restaurants and they put bread on the table, I would wolf it down very quickly. I realized that bread was a part of my upbringing. It was what my parents grew up on and what I grew up on. Rather than have the white bread version at restaurants, I started to incorporate hearty sourdough breads at home. Now when I'm out eating, I can take the bread or leave it. It's no longer as if I have a parched throat in the desert, and bread is my water. Bread is now just another food.

Many people are turned off by nutrition because they think it means they have to be on a restrictive diet. People think they'll have to give up their regular diet and start eating things they know are "good for them" but that they don't enjoy. Taking away people's favorite foods is like taking heroin away from a heroin addict. The food is giving them something they need. I have found that one of the most effective methods to overcome habitual consumption of unhealthy foods is to simply crowd out these foods. It's hard to eat five fruits and vegetables a day and binge on ice cream at the end of the day. The body can only take so much food. If you fill your body with healthy, nutrient-dense foods, it is only natural that cravings for unhealthy foods will lessen substantially.

By eating and drinking foods that are good for you earlier in the day, you will naturally leave less room and desire for unhealthy foods. This method is most evident when you increase your intake of water. Fill a water bottle or pitcher with clean, filtered water, or buy a liter of pure spring water, and sip it steadily throughout your morning. As the day continues, you'll have less room for sugary drinks. Really, it's that simple. You will immediately begin to cut down on other liquids if you keep yourself well hydrated. You may need a second bottle for the afternoon. People's need for water varies, so you should listen to your body to determine how much you need to drink in a day. Not only will water crowd out more unhealthy drinks, but it may also improve your health in other ways.

Just as drinking water crowds out unhealthy beverages, eating healthy foods can crowd out junk foods. Vegetables are high in vitamins and minerals, and you can eat a lot of them. When you increase your intake of nutritious foods, such as dark leafy greens and whole grains, your body will have less room for processed, sugary, nutrient-deficient foods. And the beautiful part is that once you start adding these foods into your diet, your body will naturally begin to crave them. The trick is to organize your life so that you have access to these healthful foods at all times, especially when you feel like snacking at work or when you are traveling. Then you can make it to your evening meal without impulsively eating junk food because that's the only thing available. It takes a little practice to make this happen, but it's definitely possible.

Cravings Are Not the Problem

The lesson here is to look for the foods, deficits, and behaviors in your life that are the underlying causes of your cravings. Many people view cravings as weaknesses, when in reality they are important messages meant to help you maintain balance. It all comes down to trusting your body, instead of thinking of your cravings as an enemy to be ignored or defeated.

How much do you trust your body? When I ask people this question, most tell me, "Not very much."

"Why not?" I ask.

"Because it's always craving foods that get me into trouble," they say, shaking their heads sadly, disappointed at their own perceived weaknesses.

"What do you mean?" I ask.

"Well, whenever I'm on a diet, my body wants foods that I'm not supposed to eat, foods that make me fat or sick."

"Why do you think your body craves such foods?" I ask.

"I don't know," people say, genuinely puzzled. "I guess I've got some built-in flaws. I can never do the right thing when it comes to food."

We have been taught to believe that our inability to stick with a diet is our fault, a flaw of our body and our will. This is absolutely incorrect. Diet book authors claim that, if we want to lose weight and regain health, we must conform to their rules and control our cravings for foods they deem unhealthy. To do this, we must develop deep discipline over our natural instincts. We accept these ideas even though every other diet we have been on was unsuccessful. We start the newest program with the best of intentions, determined to make good this time. Again and again, we repeat this cycle, blaming ourselves when the part of us that directs our food choices asserts itself, showing once again that it cannot be disciplined, controlled, suppressed, or denied.

Increasingly, we find ourselves craving "illegal" foods until one day we fall off the diet, giving in to our cravings for whatever foods have been forbidden. Afterward, we feel guilty and worthless and blame ourselves for failing to stick to the diet, which seemed so simple, so promising just a few weeks ago. It's never the program's fault; it's always our fault. Or so we think. It never dawns on us that there's nothing wrong with us, that maybe the diet itself is flawed—that it actually sets us up to fail and then unfairly lays the responsibility on our shoulders when we do.

Why is the human instinct that determines food choices so powerful and unruly? Why can't it be easily controlled and disciplined? And what motivates these choices and cravings? Clearly, this is not a cerebral process. So what is it?

In my experience, the part of us that cannot be controlled is actually our inner guide to health and happiness. This innate wisdom is always trying to make us feel better by urging us to eat foods that will dissipate, at least temporarily, our physical tension, give us more energy, and lift our moods. In essence, this part of us is always monitoring our physical, emotional, and psychological conditions and struggling to create balance, harmony, and happiness. Cravings are the body's solution to underlying imbalances, and food becomes a kind of medicine to regulate our current inner state.

Let me give a few examples. When we don't sleep well and wake up feeling lethargic, we often crave coffee to boost our energy and clear our minds. If we experience loneliness or mild depression, we often reach for chocolate or some other sweet food to boost our mood. After a stressful day, many of us want to eat something sweet or drink an alcoholic beverage to release tension. Afterward, we often feel weak and empty and want something nutritious and strengthening. We crave eggs or steak, which can leave us feeling bloated and heavy. It's a vicious cycle as we ping-pong from sweet, processed foods to excessive amounts of animal foods, from one extreme food group to another. Our minds, bodies, and spirits are drained of energy with no apparent way out.

Trust Your Crazy Cravings

When your body is craving something, pause for a moment and wonder, "What's really going on here?" Whenever you find yourself impulsively reaching for something you know is not good for you, take a moment to slow down, breathe, and reevaluate the situation. Consider what your body is really asking for. Start with the flavor.

Are You Craving Something Sweet?

Sweet foods vary widely in nutritional content, from chocolate, cookies, and pastries to sweet vegetables, fruit, and fresh juice. As much as possible, try to satisfy your desire for sweet flavor with a milder, less extreme food that doesn't contain refined white sugar. Try making a smoothie with a mix of fruit and nut butter. If something stronger is desired, try various cookies or pastries made traditionally from whole grain flour that are minimally sweetened.

Certain vegetables have a deep, sweet flavor when cooked, like corn, carrots, onions, beets, winter squash (butternut, buttercup, delicata, hubbard, or kabocha), sweet potatoes, and yams. Eating a lot of sweet vegetables may help satisfy your natural cravings for sweet foods and reduce your cravings for sugary, processed junk food.

Natural sweeteners can also help with sugar cravings. My favorite, and the favorite of most of my students, is raw wild honey, which is made from the pollen of plants and trees. Unprocessed honey is a rich source of antioxidants with a plethora of health benefits. Due to the presence of live enzymes, raw honey is easily digestible for most humans. It's great to have around the house to use in tea or salad dressings, or when baking.

When choosing a sweetener, it is always best to understand how it got from the source to you, because oftentimes the marketing of products can be misleading. Other popular alternatives to sugar are coconut sugar and stevia, an herb native to South America. All of these can be found in your local health food store. Try them, and find the ones that work best for you. For a complete list of sugar alternatives, see Chapter 10.

Quality also makes a big difference. If you decide to have an extreme sweet food, choose the best quality you can buy, and chances are good that you'll be satisfied with much less. Eat the food consciously, chewing it slowly and thoroughly enjoying it. Take chocolate as an example. Many of us crave chocolate and end up inhaling a package of M&M's while on the run or during a crunch time at work. It's a much different experience to quietly indulge in a small piece of organic dark chocolate, thoroughly chewing each morsel. If you're a chocoholic, check out the chocolate section of your health food store, and you will find many brands of organic chocolate, with many wonderful flavors, such as ginger, currant, and, my personal favorite, lavender.

Are You Craving Salty Foods?

Cravings for salty foods often indicate mineral deficiency; however, sodium deficiencies are rare—especially in the U.S. Natural sea salt contains 60 different trace minerals, which are the basis for the formation of vitamins, enzymes, and proteins. Many people use common table salt, which has been refined and stripped of these minerals. People's diets are generally lacking in minerals because much of our food has been highly processed, hence the popularity of salty foods. Before you go out and have a bag of pretzels or chips, try eating a wide variety of vegetables, especially leafy green veggies, which are very high in minerals. These foods often satisfy the craving for salty foods. You may also want to purchase a high-quality sea salt to use in your cooking and incorporate sea vegetables, which have a naturally salty flavor and are high in minerals.

Are You Craving Bitter Foods?

Remember the old saying, "It's the bitter pill that cures you?" Well, this is a good rule to live by, especially because most modern diets don't contain many healthy bitter foods. Bitter foods enhance digestion and stimulate the production of digestive juices, so a craving for bitter flavor may actually be a craving for nutritious foods to help break down fat. Most people satisfy bitter cravings by drinking coffee and dark beers. If you find yourself craving bitter tastes, try eating dark leafy greens, such as dandelion, mustard greens, arugula, kale, and collards. These greens will promote healthy assimilation and elimination.

Are You Craving Pungent Flavors?

Chinese cooking often incorporates pungently flavored foods that act as digestive aids. In Traditional Chinese Medicine, ginger is an herb for the large intestine and lungs. It enhances the function of, and promotes healing in, both organs. So, if you have a craving for heavy, saucy Chinese food, it may be your body asking for the healing properties of pungent flavors. When this happens, try grating fresh ginger on your vegetables or in your soup. Other foods that will quench this craving are cayenne, scallions, onions, leeks, garlic, and pepper.

Are You Craving Spicy Foods?

Are you looking for an array of flavors, both subtle and strong, or are you looking for hot spices? So much processed food is lacking in flavor because it's been on the shelf for such a long time. This kind of food lacks vitality and includes added fat. When people eat this kind of diet for years, the body can become overweight and stagnant. Blood becomes thick, or viscous, and circulation slows. As circulation weakens, organs and extremities become cool. At this point, the body may start craving spices.

When people crave spicy foods, they often turn to pizza or hot Mexican spices. These extreme foods warm the body but also create a lot of stressful, chaotic energy. Instead of eating a pizza, with its dry, hard crust and heavy cheese, or refried beans and hot jalapeño peppers, try a bowl of rice noodles mixed with green vegetables and a nice marinara sauce with oregano, basil, red pepper flakes, onions, garlic, and celery.

You can use a variety of spices and condiments to add kick to your food. Two popular choices are ground cayenne and hot pepper sesame oil, both of which you can find at any health food store. You can also chop jalapeño peppers and add them to a salad or stir-fry for that extra bit of spice.

What Texture or Consistency Are You Craving?

When craving something creamy, consider whether you've had a lot of bread, crackers, or other baked flour products recently. When eaten in excess, these foods create feelings of dryness and can also make us feel stuck, hard, and irritable. When we reach that state of imbalance, we very often crave creamy, relaxing foods, such as ice cream, milk products, or oily foods. Try eating porridge made from whole grains, such as amaranth or brown rice. You can also make cream of broccoli soup or cream of watercress soup and use oatmeal rather than cream to get the consistency you desire.

If you are craving chips or pretzels, it may be the crunch that you actually desire. I think when the body wants crunch it's probably because you're not chewing enough. The act of chewing actually enhances digestion. Instead of grabbing processed snack products, try satisfying your crunchy cravings with raw carrots and celery, nuts, or organic versions of potato chips and hard pretzels without added sugar. And don't forget to chew all your foods to assure proper digestion.

Are You Craving Something Moist or a Liquid?

When craving liquids, ask yourself if you've been eating an excessive amount of salty foods or dry crackers. Do you feel dry or tight? Are you thirsty? Many physical problems, including headaches, urology problems, and kidney stones, are the result of chronic dehydration. People typically just don't drink enough water. Instead of quenching thirst with sugary and caffeinated beverages, try drinking water. Put a bottle or a cup of pure spring water on your desk, and sip it throughout the day. As you drink, notice how your body responds. If you suddenly awaken to how thirsty you are, then you know you've been ignoring your thirst. If you don't want the water, you will feel your body resist it, signifying that you are well hydrated.

Are You Craving Something Crispy and Dry?

If you are craving something crispy and dry, you may be drinking too many liquids. If this is the case, try to keep away from chips because they are rich in fats, especially saturated and trans fats. Avoid crackers that are highly processed, as they will elevate both glucose and insulin levels. To fulfill your craving for crispy and dry foods, choose rice cakes, high-quality crackers without oil, or sugar-free sesame sticks. You can also bake your own sweet potato or veggie chips, which tend to be healthier than the store-bought versions.

Are You Craving a Light or Heavy Food?

If you crave heavy foods, ask yourself whether you've been eating a lot of salads or fruit. Are you cold, especially your hands and feet? Salads, fruit, and other raw foods make the body feel light. They also cool the body and may give rise to cravings for heavier, warming foods, such as fish, beef, or hard cheese. Fish is rich in protein, low in fat, and high in omega-3 fatty acids, which boost immunity and prevent heart disease.

Sometimes when you are not hungry enough for a meal but need something light to eat, you'll go for a snack. The snack food shelves at supermarkets and even health food stores are full of tantalizing items chock full of sugar. When you're craving a light snack or meal, why not eat some raw or steamed vegetables instead of a sugary snack? If you are hungry, and nibbling on a raw carrot doesn't satisfy, try a handful of trail mix, an avocado sandwich, or a fruit smoothie.

Are You Craving a Nutritious Food?

When I check in with my body to see what I am actually craving, I often realize that what I really want is something nutritious, something of substance, especially when I am working hard and utilizing the nutrition my body is getting from my diet. This craving also happens when I travel and my routine of eating home-cooked food becomes unavailable. At these times, I long for plain vegetables and simple foods.

Non-Food Cravings

Sometimes we also crave food for emotional reasons. Maybe we are looking for excitement in our lives or looking for comfort after a stressful situation. This nourishment is a kind of emotional feeding. It's not really about the food but about the emotion it creates.

Are You Craving Entertainment?

We often use food to distract us from boredom. It's important to decipher true cravings from eating as a form of entertainment. If you are bored, try to deal with the issue directly rather than distracting yourself by snacking and munching to fill time. Boredom is a challenge to be more creative with your life. The prime example of this craving is at work. Many people snack or eat just to take a break from staring at the computer. The next time this happens, try taking a walk around the block with a coworker. Or close your office door, and stretch for five minutes.

Are You Craving a Hug?

One of the biggest problems with diets today is that people attribute their cravings to appetite and hunger, when these cries are usually from another part of their being that is starving. These cravings have nothing to do with physical nutrition. They are for love, affection, and fulfillment. Food can fill you but not fulfill you. Touch is an important part of the human experience. Don't be afraid to ask for a hug when you need it. Try it with your friends, your kids, your sisters or brothers, or whomever you are close with in your life. You might be surprised at how many hugs you've been missing.

Are You Craving Movement?

Stress, hard work, and lots of thinking create tension in the body, which can lead to chronic aches, tightness, and constipation. Many people try to alleviate these symptoms with alcohol and sugar, which only serve to dampen their unease and anesthetize the body. Exercise is an ideal way to release a buildup of physical tension. Developing a regular exercise program to suit your particular body type and lifestyle will have numerous rewards. Start small. Go out for a walk, or check out a gentle yoga or karate class. Listen to your body about what kind of movement it desires.

Your Body Loves You, Unconditionally

Physical health is the foundation of our lives. Once we free ourselves from extreme foods, the healing mechanisms of the body can be harnessed to overcome our deeper physical and emotional issues. That's when healing miracles happen. When people learn how to deconstruct their cravings, they can reclaim the sense of balance and bodily harmony that they were haphazardly seeking through indulgence or willpower.

Our bodies are like crying babies. The child is crying, but it can't talk, so the mother has to figure out what has disturbed her child. Did it hurt itself, not get enough sleep, or wet its diaper? Is it teething, or does it have allergies? The mother goes through a process of elimination until she finds the real problem. It's a similar situation with your body. Your body can't talk, but it can send you messages through discomfort or food cravings that need to be decoded. If we acknowledge and accept our cravings, they will point us toward the foods and lifestyles we need. For example, if you have a headache, try to figure out what caused it. Did you work too much in front of the computer yesterday? Did you not drink enough water? Did you drink too much wine at a party? Did you sleep with the window closed and need some fresh air?

We can, and must, develop dialogue with our bodies. They're talking to us all the time, and their messages are too important for us to ignore. And please remember, your body loves you. It does everything it can to keep you alive and functioning. You can feed it garbage, and it will digest it for you and turn it into energy to fuel your life. You can deprive it of sleep, but still it will get you up and running the next morning. You can drink alcohol, and it will process it through your system. It loves you unconditionally and does its best to allow you to live the life you came here to live. Working to understand your cravings is one of the best places to begin to build a loving relationship with your own body.

Exercises

1. Craving Inventory

For one week, keep a journal of every food you crave each day. Rate the craving on a scale of 1 to 10, with 10 being the strongest level of desire. Write down your thoughts next to each entry on how that craving is a response to an imbalance somewhere in your diet or life.

Craving rating:

Time of craving:

Type of craving:

Thoughts:

2. Dearest Body of Mine

Write a letter to your body, announcing your intention to listen more carefully to its messages and to act in a more loving way toward it. The following list of suggestions may be helpful to include, but be sure to make your letter personal to your own body. Set a specific period of time aside when you can sit quietly by yourself, undisturbed and in pleasant surroundings, and then begin to write. You don't need to complete the letter in one session. It is sometimes helpful to come back to your letter after a day or two, review the contents and make additions or subtractions. Write from your heart, as well as from your mind.

Dearest body of mine,

After careful thought and consideration, I hereby promise to:

Accept you and be grateful for you just the way you are,

Love and appreciate you for what you do,

Offer you healthy foods and drinks,

Realize that laughter, play, and rest help you feel good,

Exercise regularly and appropriately for my body type,

Understand that my unexpressed emotions and thoughts affect you,

Listen to the messages you are sending me when you are tired or sick,

Realize that you deserve to be healthy,

Honor you as the temple of my soul.

I love you so much,

____

Please Sign here

Chapter 7

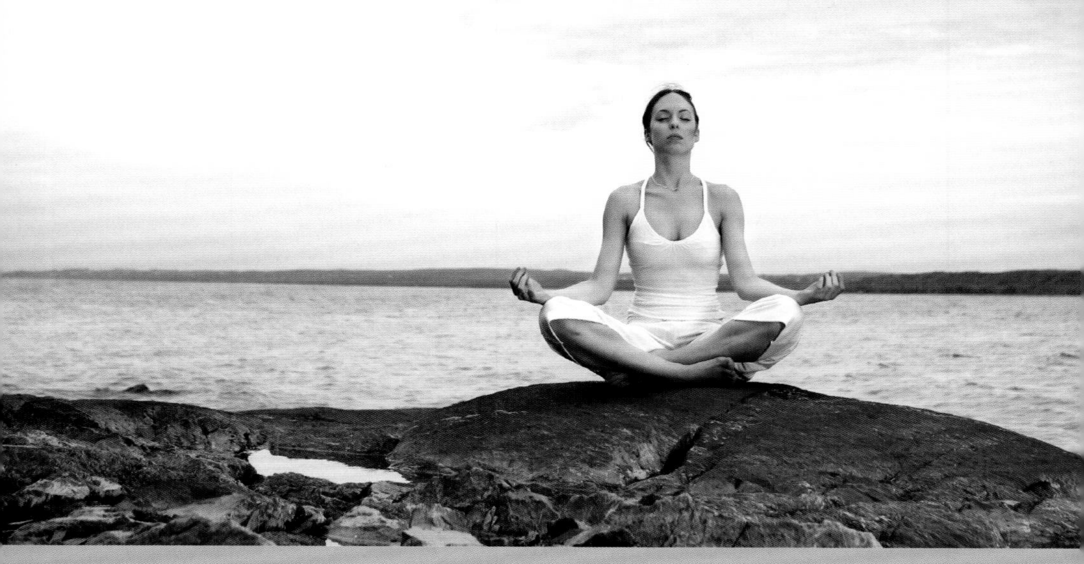

Primary Food

> Just as food is needed for the body,
> love is needed for the soul.
>
> —Osho

This chapter explores the differences between ordinary food and what I call primary food. Recall from Chapters 1 & 2 that primary food is more than what is on your plate. Healthy relationships, regular physical activity, a fulfilling career, and a spiritual practice are the four core areas that can fill your soul and satisfy your hunger for life. When primary food is balanced and satiating, your life feeds you, making what you eat secondary.

We hunger for play, fun, touch, romance, intimacy, love, achievement, success, art, music, self-expression, leadership, excitement, adventure, and spirituality. All of these elements are essential forms of nourishment. When we create nourishing lives for ourselves, then we are truly living a fulfilling life. At the end of this chapter, you'll have an opportunity to check in on your primary foods and use the Circle of Life tool—one of my favorites!

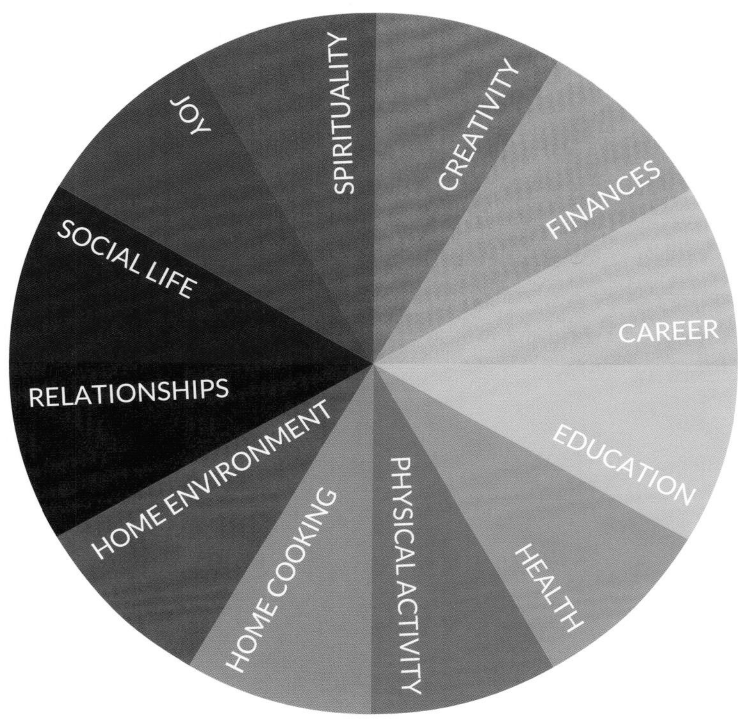

The concept of primary food became clear to me while working in a small natural food store. All day, every day, I watched customers moving through the aisles, shopping, asking questions, giving great care and attention to the quality of the foods they would be consuming. Then, after work, I would often go out into my neighborhood to chill out. Sometimes I would go to the movie theater next door, where many of the popcorn-munching, soda-gulping moviegoers were laughing and enjoying themselves with their friends or a romantic partner. I began to notice that the people I saw in the evening often looked healthier, happier, and more alive than the people shopping in my store. This discrepancy got me thinking it wasn't just about the food.

One time a client came to her coaching session crying about her marriage. While working with her, I saw that eating more fruits and vegetables was not going to make the issue disappear. And then later I found other clients who made great improvements in their health by smoothing out their relationship issues. Creating more positive relationships made them happier and healthier than any dietary change could have made them. The idea of holistic health is to look at the integrated system rather than one or more separate parts, which includes the physical, mental, spiritual, and emotional parts of life. I encourage you to look beyond the food on your plate and consider these other forms of nourishment that truly feed you.

Relationships

During the course of a lifetime, we have relationships with parents, grandparents, children, husbands, wives, boyfriends, girlfriends, extended family, friends, teachers, coworkers—the list is endless. The quality of these relationships explains a lot about the quality of a person's life and his or her health. Just as no one diet is right for everyone, no one way of relating works for everyone. What's important is to cultivate relationships that are healthy and that support your individual needs, wants, and desires. In fact, a 75-year-long Harvard study[1] followed two sets of men throughout their lifetimes and found health benefits associated with relationships. Men who described having close relationships with family, friends, and community lived longer than those who did not. The men who felt lonely in the study reported more health issues, such as sleep problems, and said they felt less happy, reporting more mental health issues.

Friendships

I believe a key ingredient in personal fulfillment is community. Today, people in the modern world lead overly isolated lives, spending large amounts of time with media. The extended family is gone. You can eat all the broccoli and brown rice in the world, but if you feel isolated and lonely, you are not going to be living life at full capacity. Having high-quality friendships adds depth and meaning to life. Friends who truly listen and care and are open to new ideas can be difficult to come by, but you can take steps to create a positive, supportive community.

I invite you to look at your relationships the same way people look at their wardrobes. You've probably kept many clothes hanging in your closet that you haven't worn for years. Maybe you are hoping they'll come back into style, or maybe they don't quite fit, but you keep them in the back for sentimental reasons.

It's the same with friends. If you think of everyone you know, chances are you will find at least a few people from your past who don't really belong in your present. In fact, if you're honest with yourself, you'll admit you find their company draining, but you keep them in your wardrobe of friends even if they have little to offer in return. They could be past lovers who keep hanging around or people whose lives are always in crisis, requiring large amounts of time or energy from you, never to return the favor. Remember, you're their friend, not their therapist.

I suggest you determine which of these people you can let go of. If breaking off all contact seems too drastic, you can downgrade your relationships with them. You can see them less often, give them less of your energy, or stay in touch by email. If this seems scary, don't worry. You'll maintain your quality friendships while at the same time clearing space for new people to come into your life.

I once had a client who was struggling with low self-esteem and confidence due to her upbringing in a dysfunctional family setting. Most of her friends did not treat her very well. Then one day, through our coaching, she woke up and saw the whole picture. She had unconsciously recreated her parents in her circle of friends. She was always the one calling to set up times to meet; she was the one who was listening to most of the problems. The friends were the ones canceling at the last minute or asking for favors, and it just wasn't working for her.

So, step by step, for months, she let go of people. She removed their numbers from her cell phone, stopped sending them email, and created a vacuum in her life. At first it felt lonely. Then, eventually, it felt new and exhilarating to have free time to think and feel. Slowly but surely, she found herself meeting new people and making friends with inspirational people she admired.

Please think of two or three people you would enjoy spending more time with—people who are more of a contemporary mirror for you and have qualities with which you resonate. Maybe you're thinking of someone outside your social strata, but you are excited by the idea of spending more time with them. Contact them. One of the easiest ways to do this is to invite them out for tea or lunch. The worst that could happen is that they say no, but if you set an intention, the universe will deliver. Once you are clear about who they are, be proactive and take initiative to see them more often.

Like all relationships, friendships take work, yet they can also be hugely rewarding. Remember, friendship is primary food. It should nourish you.

Love and Intimacy

We all have a need to give and receive love. Love is food for the soul. Love nourishes body, mind, and spirit. To bring more love and intimacy into your life, I suggest improving connections with everyone. Being well connected with others is an essential part of life. We all feel a sense of comfort, safety and connection when we are free to express our hopes and dreams, fear, and anger, joy and struggles with others.

When examining relationships, try to understand your personal preference with regard to how much intimacy you want in your life. Some people love being alone; they feel energized by the experience and require plenty of time to catch up with themselves. These people are relatively introverted and develop ways to be on their own with great ease. They usually prefer to relate with one or two people and are finicky about their choices in friends. At the other end of the spectrum are those who love being around people. They are more extroverted, become energized by social interaction, and often create an extended family and a network of friends. They have hundreds of people on speed dial, and their email list is extensive. They look forward to seeing everyone at parties, holidays, and group events.

Most people fall somewhere in the middle. It may be helpful to think about your own social needs and preferences on a scale of 1 to 10. Where do you fall on this scale? Please avoid making judgments about what is socially acceptable or superficially desirable, and take time to reflect about who you really are and what style of relating works best for you. No rules, just what is genuinely true for you at this point in your life. Vive la différence!

When I suggest improving the quality of your relationships, I am not suggesting everyone should be more social or get married. I am saying find a type of love and intimacy that is appropriate and nourishing for you. It's a bit like establishing the amount of protein, vegetables, or exercise that is appropriate for your body. Each person needs to find the right balance of togetherness and aloneness and to know that these needs will change with time, just as dietary needs change and just as everything in life changes.

For single people who are dating, experiencing love and intimacy can be tricky because you don't have a set agreement with one person or an established routine. Each person is new, and you have to navigate these new relationships. In these new situations, be clear with yourself about what you are looking for. Confusion often arises when one person is looking for a life partner and the other person is looking to meet a lot of different new people. Wouldn't it be so much easier if you were honest about this up front? It greatly reduces confusion later.

For singles: Take some time to get as clear as possible with yourself about what kind of experience you want to have with dating. Are you looking to meet a lot of different people? Are you looking for deeper intimacy but only for a short period of time? Are you looking for a life partner? As you are dating, what you want will probably change, so keep checking in with yourself about your priorities. This is much more effective than just throwing yourself out there to see what happens or going along with whatever your friends are doing or whatever your date wants. When you are clear about your priorities, you can communicate them clearly to the people you date. In the end, you will find yourself spending time with the person or people who want the same kind of relationship or relationships that you do. Also, spend some time assessing your personal boundaries. What are some healthy expressions of love that you want to experience? What kinds of behaviors and attitudes are you not comfortable with? The better you understand your own boundaries and desires, the more you'll be able to make healthier choices for yourself.

People with boyfriends or girlfriends often feel they have a "go-to" person to experience love and intimacy. In my opinion, open communication is extra important at this stage of relationship. Everyone has different ideas of what it means to be in a relationship—how much time you spend together, how serious you are, when to meet the parents, etc. Often our ideas come from our families or from the media, but your ideas about relationships may differ drastically from those ideas. So, be open, and share your needs and ideas with your partner. Some couples like to set timeframes. For example, they might say to each other, "This seems like it's working—let's do this for three months and then check in again." Sometimes it's going great; sometimes it's not working out, so they make some changes and keep going, while sometimes they separate. In all those cases, both partners know what the other one wants and needs in order to enjoy and be nourished by the relationship. Whether you are with your boyfriend or girlfriend for three months or three years or forever, talking things through in a gentle, honest, and caring manner will make the whole experience more loving and less stressful.

People who are married often have a bond that goes beyond personal needs. They often have children together, have a community of friends in common, and share ownership of cars, houses, or businesses. I've noticed many married people may care strongly for one another but have no time to spend together, or they get stuck in what feels like a rut. They may have "lost that loving feeling" and focus solely on the external trappings of their relationship. In the U.S., only about 50% of marriages last. Marriage relationships need to be nurtured by both partners. I strongly encourage married people to find time to spend alone together and to find more time to have fun. Sit down every so often, and evaluate how things are going and whether any changes need to be made. Small resentments that build up over time can erode the foundation of any relationship.

Flexibility and growth in long-term relationships is important. It's kind of crazy to expect the person you married (or live with) to stay the same for 5, 10, or 20 years of marriage or to expect this person to fulfill all of your needs. Many couples live together, vacation together, go out to eat together, and spend all their free time together. No matter how much you enjoy one person's company, over time you can grow tired of one person if you are constantly together. Work to find balance between activities you enjoy together and activities you can enjoy with other friends or on your own.

It is natural and healthy for everyone to change and grow. If one partner is not open to growing and learning new things, or if only one partner is putting energy into the relationship, it might be healthiest to reassess. But often, you can find a way to work it out. Many, many resources are available for learning how to communicate well and deepen intimacy. If you are concerned about your relationship, find a coach you like who specializes in helping people in long-term relationships. If you don't make progress with one, you may want to try another one before giving up on the process. Take the initiative to create the relationship you really want.

For people at any stage of a relationship, you can increase the level of love and intimacy in your life simply by setting new intentions. Explore what you really want from your relationships. You can journal, meditate, or talk to a trusted friend about it. Make a list of what you are looking for from your current relationship or from a new relationship. Look at your list every day, and know that you are a unique being who is worthy of love and intimacy. When we are clear about our intentions, the universe very often delivers.

Touch, Hugs, and Cuddles

Children who aren't held and touched enough won't grow to their full potential. Babies thrive on human touch, and holding them helps them become healthy, happy, and well adjusted. The same holds true for adults as well. Most of us feel nourished by human touch, warmth, and intimacy. Yet most adults are touch starved. We can get along without it, but in time we will feel the lack and crave connection.

It feels good to be touched, to be massaged, to feel physically connected to other people. We even release a specific hormone from physical touch called oxytocin,[2] sometimes referred to as the "cuddle hormone." Our oxytocin levels increase from activities like holding hands, hugs, and massage, which helps us feel relaxed and more bonded with the people around us. However, our society tends to confuse touching with sexuality so much so that many people today actually fear touch. In certain cultures, it's common for women to walk arm-in-arm and for men to hold hands, but in Westernized countries this behavior is much less acceptable.

Sexual concerns aside, touching makes many people feel uncomfortable because it is an open expression of love, care, and appreciation. If someone is not accustomed to expressing their feelings or to giving and receiving love, a layer of embarrassment and awkwardness around physical contact may exist. You've probably noticed this barrier even between family members or close friends.

You can break through this social barrier by finding comfortable, non-threatening ways to connect. Human touch helps us realize we're all in this crazy modern world together. Think of it in the same way as a supplement. Be sure to get your recommended daily allowance of positive human interaction and touch. It's not as difficult as you may think. You can find people who are aware that modern life is increasingly isolating and who want to connect and say hello in a warm way. Talk with one or two people you currently feel close to, such as a partner or friend, about exchanging neck and shoulder massages. Even a five-minute neck rub can have a positive impact on your day. A little touch goes a long way.

Sensuality and Sexuality

Another level of physical contact, beyond massage, hugs, and cuddling, is sensual touch and sexual interaction. These experiences can be very nourishing, and it is important that people understand what they're looking for in these delicate areas. Sex is a major part of life, but issues around sensuality, sexuality, love, and relating are rarely discussed in an open, intelligent manner.

None of us would be here without sex. Sex created me. Sex created you. So, it's completely natural and normal that most of us are fascinated by sex. It doesn't mean there is anything wrong with us. If we weren't meant to enjoy sex, we would just touch index fingers or lay eggs to make babies. Or, at the very least, we would not be so full of hormones that from adolescence on we feel continually drawn toward sexual contact. Indeed, within the deepest and most primal part of our brain, we are programmed to seek pleasure.

For many centuries, sex has been considered primarily a means of reproduction. The idea of sex as a nourishing, pleasurable, and recreational experience, unrelated to childbirth, is relatively new, especially for women. Since the Women's Movement, women have more independence and access to birth control and the right to choose. Sex is not just for making babies. Sex can be fun. Sex doesn't even require a partner. People have always pleasured themselves but usually in secret and cloaked in guilt. Recently, this has expanded to include full permission to spend time alone, finding ways to create sensual and sexual pleasure.

The freedom we now experience in the 21st century has given us more opportunities to feed our bodies and souls with positive sexual experiences,

At the same time, our communication skills about sex haven't quite caught up to our freedoms. People are often confused about what they're looking for in terms of sex and relationships. This confusion increases the likelihood of misunderstanding, exploitation, and frustration.

Sexuality and sensuality are exciting parts of the human experience and can be deeply nourishing if you are clear about what you want. Whether you are casually dating or in a serious relationship, take some time to investigate what you want and need. If there is something you need that you are missing, ask for it. If you often find yourself in unhealthy situations, I encourage you to determine what boundaries you need to set for yourself and others and to stick to them. Once you start speaking about your needs in a clear, kind, and mature manner, you will see that it is like discussing any other topic. Don't be afraid to express yourself. Others will appreciate your good communication skills and respond to your needs.

It may seem strange to be talking about sex in a book on nutrition, but we can eat an awful lot of green leafy vegetables and not get anywhere near the healing effects that come from having great sex.

Communicating in Relationships

When it comes to relationships, especially intimate relationships, effective speaking and listening are key in staying connected and nourishing one another. But you've probably noticed that it's very rare to have a conversation with someone who actually listens to what you're saying, without interruption or judgment.

Most people live in their heads, thinking about what they have to do tomorrow, what happened yesterday or an hour ago—pretty much anything except the present moment. Have you ever been to a party where someone asked you a question and then didn't listen to a word of your response? These interactions happen all the time. It is equally unusual that we listen to another person without interrupting them, judging, or planning what we're going to say next.

We are all starving to be heard. Healing occurs when people listen to us and when we listen to them. By harnessing the power of listening, you can greatly improve all of your relationships. When in conversation with others, try to concentrate and listen to what they are saying. While they are speaking, put all thoughts about yourself out of your head, and be present for them. The other person will feel heard and appreciated. This habit will greatly improve the quality of your communication.

Many, many loving and caring couples struggle in their relationships because of communication problems. Sometimes one partner does all the talking, and the other partner does all the listening. Perhaps they only talk about their problems and not about what they love about the other person. Maybe they never talk about their problems but save them up until one day it all comes out in a hurtful manner, and the relationship ends. A helpful exercise for any couple is to speak regularly about the positive and negative elements of their relationship and to practice listening to one another.

I recommend scheduling a specific time when both people have enough time and space to discuss delicate issues in a calm and sincere way. You should plan to talk in a space that feels private and safe. You can help establish a healing, positive environment by lighting a candle, playing your favorite music, or sharing a meal together.

Begin by looking at the positive. Take turns. Each partner should speak, uninterrupted, for as long as he or she wants about everything that is going well in the relationship. Some things to mention might be how the other person makes you feel, qualities of your partner that you appreciate, gratitude for specific ways in which your partner has supported you lately, and admiration of the other person's appearance. Brag about all of the aspects of your relationship that are going well, and allow yourself to fully verbalize and appreciate the other person. One partner should listen carefully and take in all that the other person is saying without interrupting. Then switch so that each person has a chance to speak and to listen.

Take as much time as you want to cover everything that is going well. The bond you share is something worth acknowledging and celebrating. When you have both spoken, take a short break. Sit silently for a few moments, absorbing what each person has said.

Next, take note of one or two aspects of your relationship that you would like to improve. Maybe it's something simple, like household responsibilities, or maybe it's something deeper and sensitive, like wanting more quality time for intimacy and togetherness, or the opposite, maybe a little bit of space would be refreshing. Repeat the same structure as above, allowing one partner to speak openly about his or her feelings and perspective while the other partner listens carefully, and then switch. You can remedy problems more easily once each of you clearly understands what the other wants.

During this exercise, practice communicating without blame to offer solutions and to explain how you would like your relationship to grow. Remember, the aim is to strengthen the flow of nourishing energy that passes between two people. You are each other's primary food, and you are fine-tuning the recipe for long-term satisfaction.

Sometimes a partner may want what the other cannot give. When this happens, don't fall into the trap of resignation. Instead, consider the possibility of asking for outside help. We are not islands. We all have the same basic issues, and we don't have to deal with them in isolation. Counseling and support groups are available for every aspect of personal relationships. Once you view your relationship as a form of nourishment, it becomes natural to seek out ways to improve and sustain it so both you and your partner can feel satisfied.

Physical Activity

People need to exercise. Our bodies thrive on movement and quickly degenerate without it. An emerging field of inactivity research suggests that sitting is actually lethal. Most people sit all day at a job, and researchers estimate that people who sit too much are easily shaving a few years off their lives.[3] For those people who work at a desk all day, be sure to get up every hour or so, and stretch, walk around your office, or even consider a standing desk. When it comes to working out, the challenge is to find the types of exercise you enjoy most, and then build them into your life. Physical activity can take simple and modest forms, like getting off the subway or bus one stop earlier and walking to your destination. It can be taking the stairs, instead of the elevator, to your office or apartment. It can be taking your dog for a walk or your children to the park. A 30-minute brisk walk every day may be all you need to keep yourself in shape. It's good to find something you can do every day without altering your schedule too much, especially if you are first starting to incorporate it into your routine. Making physical activity a simple daily habit greatly increases your chances of staying active.

Something interesting I've noticed is people's inclination to choose exercise that aggravates their current condition. In gyms, the bulky, aggressive people tend to lift weights, making them even bulkier and more aggressive. People who only take yoga classes may be grounded or strengthened by doing some weightlifting, just as a yoga class would lighten weightlifters. I am a big proponent of creating balance, and exercise is a great way to do that. Different forms of exercise will give you different types of energy, and by listening to your body you can find the movement that will work best for you.

After living at Kripalu Center for Yoga & Health, doing yoga every day, I realized I was all stretched out. I was practicing a very relaxing style of yoga, and I needed to get more grounded. So, I stopped practicing yoga and switched to weightlifting and running. It provided great balance and stability in my life. In this way, movement is a lot like food. Once you understand how different types of movement nourish your body, you can put together a menu of activities to keep yourself in balance. For example, if you have been feeling frail and unfocused, you could choose vigorous exercise to make you feel stable and powerful, such as kickboxing or running. On the other hand, if you feel tight and tense, you can choose gentler exercise to increase lightness and flexibility, such as swimming or yoga.

Consider what time of day is best for you to get physical activity. Just as some people think more clearly in the morning and others think more clearly at night, some people prefer to exercise first thing in the morning, while others prefer to exercise later in the day. There's no right or wrong; it's simply a matter of personal preference.

Different people require different types of exercise to stay healthy, and your exercise needs will change with time. Stay open to all of the options. You can go rock climbing, paragliding, surfing, in-line skating, or canoeing, or you can take up Pilates, karate, or ballroom dancing. You can find team sports like baseball or volleyball, which have the added benefit of human interaction. Maybe exercising outside in nature is more pleasurable for you. If you are a quiet person who likes a lot of alone time, consider buying a small trampoline or a set of hand weights so you can move in the comfort of your home. Your options are endless. Be experimental, and find a routine you can nourish yourself with on a regular basis.

Career

In today's society, most of us spend eight to 10 hours a day at work and very little time with our loved ones. While we are choosy about who we relate with intimately, we spend years doing work we can't stand and that may be completely opposed to our personal values. Think about it for a moment. We have 24 hours each day. We sleep for eight hours, work for at least eight hours, and have six to eight hours left for other activities. More than half of our waking hours are spent working—and even more if we include commuting. Work is a huge part of our daily routine, yet how many of us really enjoy it? How many of us complain constantly about what we do but feel powerless to change it? This feeling of helplessness is not a nourishing lifestyle.

A great example of this connection between job satisfaction and health is weight gain. I've known many people who were struggling with their weight, wanting to lose those last 10 pounds. They had tried many diets, and some were even very healthy eaters. But the weight would simply not come off. What they had in common was being unhappy at their jobs. And when they finally found work they liked, the extra weight came right off.

We don't realize the extent to which our lives would improve if we were doing work we loved. We have little to no understanding of our ability to walk away from a particular job or career and begin a new one. In the flexible, fast-moving job market of today's business-oriented society, we can easily have three, four, or five careers in a lifetime. Most of our parents and grandparents didn't have such choices. They knew one craft, one skill, and that was all they did. They were dedicated to the company, and the company was dedicated to them. But the modern business environment is different. Each of us has the power to try working for different companies, reinventing our careers, and seeking out jobs that we find personally and financially satisfying.

We all know someone who has made a satisfying job change—a banker who quit Wall Street to open a bakery, a plumber who retrained as an IT consultant, an editor who started her own publishing company, or a salesman who became a stay-at-home dad. Although the modern work world is challenging, it is also a world of opportunity. We have the luxury of creating work that nourishes us and gets us excited about each day. I encourage you to think about your current job—some of your likes and dislikes of what you do each day. Finding work you love is essential to living a healthy, balanced life.

Entrepreneurial pursuits are on the rise. Worldwide, more people than ever are starting their own businesses. More than 60% of adults see entrepreneurship as a good career choice, and more than half of working-age people feel they could start a business, according to research from The Global Entrepreneurship Monitor.[4] Women entrepreneurs are thriving—with more than 200 million starting or running new businesses in 83 economies throughout the world.[5] I'm not surprised, as it's easier than ever to start a business. Launching an online business has very few startup costs, and connecting with new customers through social media and blogging is a great way to begin. One interesting trend in the U.S. is the rise of senior entrepreneurship. About 25 million Americans ages 44 to 70 are interested in starting their own business or non-profit venture, according to research by Encore.org.[6]

Finding the Work You Love

"Finding the work you love, loving the work you find" is a well-known exercise in the field of job reeducation.

For the first part, "Finding the work you love," take a sheet of paper, and list all of the things you love to do, including your hobbies, activities you enjoy in your leisure hours, and subjects you read about with great curiosity. This list may include food, massage, exercise, coaching, fashion—almost anything. Take your time; make sure the list is exhaustive. Somewhere in this list lies the key to your new career.

Now review your list. If you could spend eight hours a day thinking about or working with some of these subject areas, which ones would you pick? Circle your top five. Use these as indicators of the kind of work you might find enjoyable. For each item, list as many job titles as you can think of that relate to a subject area. You might need to do some research. Look up jobs in that field. Call someone you know who works in that area. Find out all you can about it.

Once you've listed possible jobs, circle three that are the most appealing to you. You may be strongly drawn to jobs in several areas. In that case, brainstorm how you can blend these together into one career that you would love.

You now have in your hands a key to a new, exciting career. When you have identified and selected your strongest interests, start taking steps to make your new job a reality. It may take some time and effort, but the benefits to your health and quality of life will be enormous. Keep in mind that what you need from a job may change with time. You can always use your creativity and intelligence to create a new situation.

Loving the Work You Find

The other half of this exercise is "loving the work you find." Sometimes it is simply not optimal to go out and create a new career. Or perhaps you like your career, just not your current work environment. This exercise can help you increase the pleasure and nourishment you derive from your current job.

Take a piece of paper, and make a list of everything you like about your work. On the back of the piece of paper, make a list of everything you don't like. Think about the content of your work, the structure of your day, your colleagues, your salary, your work environment, opportunities for advancement, any successes or disappointments you have experienced, and how deeply you feel about the importance of the work. What is working, and what is not working?

Now imagine you have a job offer from another company. This other job may pay you more, be in a better location, or offer more exciting projects. Imagine going to your supervisor's office to give notice. Imagine that when you come out of your supervisor's office you have decided to stay with your current company. Why? What did your supervisor offer you? A raise? A nicer office? A more flexible schedule? A new project? Circle these items on your list.

By making adjustments in these few key areas, you could make your job more exciting and rewarding. Your job could become a positive influence in your life instead of a drain. By using good communication skills, you can enlist the support of your coworkers and supervisor to try to make these improvements. Ask for a raise or for flextime, redecorate your office, or request to join a new project. It is up to you to ask for what you need. You may be surprised by how easily you get it.

For example, I think many of my students enroll at my school because they want to work in holistic health instead of their current jobs. They start seeing clients, enjoy the process, graduate, develop momentum to break through to a new career, and go to their bosses to give notice. I can't tell you how frequently they walk out with a pay raise. Usually when this happens, they realize they actually enjoy the stability of their full-time job and choose to do coaching after work or on the weekends as a part-time supplementary career. Sometimes all you need is a pay increase to have renewed appreciation for your job. If you are a responsible, intelligent, and hard-working employee, there's a good chance you'll get paid for it.

One of my students was working for a large brokerage firm for many years, and her working hours were just under the requirement for full-time employment because this allowed the company to avoid paying for her benefits and insurance. She was fed up with the way they were treating her, and after months of thinking it through, she decided to quit. She walked into the office and announced she was leaving in two weeks. They immediately gave her the extra hours, switched her to full-time staff, and bumped up her pay, saying they'd been thinking of giving her new responsibilities and more money anyway. She decided to stay on.

"I wished I'd done it two years earlier," she confided in me. Whatever it is you need to make your job a more positive place to be, I encourage you to go after it. Feeling happy and productive in the place you spend most of your time will dramatically increase your sense of well-being.

The Meaning of Work

Although it's important to be fairly compensated for our work, too often we equate work with a paycheck. We may think of our jobs only as a means to earn money. Having money to take care of yourself and your family is obviously very important, but it's a limited view of work. For example, some people go to work to make the world a better place. They may be involved in a project that improves the lives of a few people, hundreds of people, or the whole planet. For others, work is a form of creativity and self-expression; whether in a corporate office or an artist studio, work is a place to hatch new ideas and to put their personal stamp on the world. Few things are more rewarding in life than meaningful and exciting work. You feel confident and stimulated. Time stops, and the outside world fades away. You are totally absorbed and energized by it. Doesn't it make sense to work on something you are passionate about?

Maybe you are interested in finding work that you can dedicate yourself to, but you haven't come across something that seems worthy of your time. I encourage you to try out new hobbies or interests. Join a club, volunteer with an organization, or start a study group with a few close friends. As you explore your interests, you will discover whether you really enjoy this new area, and, if you do, you will make contact with people who could help you start a new career.

Another way to identify meaningful work is to notice what you already spend your time on. Many of my students have been doing health coaching for years without knowing it. They have been coaching their friends, family members, or coworkers about their diets and lifestyles—they just haven't been paid for it. This is a good clue that they will be happy making health coaching their career. Our school helps them take their natural talents and make a career out of it. Once they build confidence and learn the basic skills, they find they are much happier working hard for their own businesses rather than working for someone else.

There is no one right answer about what work means or how to find happiness in your career. Maybe you love working hard in a corporate environment. Maybe you need a less conventional, more flexible relationship with work. Everyone is different. Be honest about what works for you. Remember that we all need to nourish ourselves is finding work we love and being paid fairly for it.

Spirituality

Plato said, "The greatest mistake in the treatment of diseases is that there are physicians for the body and physicians for the soul, although the two cannot be separated." Spiritual nutrition can feed us on a very deep level and dramatically diminish cravings for the superficial desires of life. We all search for meaning in our lives, and feeling at one with the world can help satisfy that longing. Cancer researcher Kelly Turner, Ph.D., writes about the healing power of a daily spiritual practice in her book, *Radical Remission*. In it, she discusses nine of the top factors she found in people who have healed from serious cancer cases without medical intervention, including those who make time for spirituality. Research has also found that people with spiritual beliefs adapt more quickly to health issues than those who don't.[7]

I encourage you to develop and deepen your spiritual practice, whatever that might be. Some people follow their traditional religion of birth. Others explore Eastern religion or New Age spirituality or evolve an integrative approach. I was raised in an orthodox Jewish family, which valued ritual, tradition, and the sacredness of daily life. We celebrated the holidays, fasted, and traveled to Israel. I was taught "tikun olam," which translates to "repair of the world." It's the idea of trying to make the world a better place, and I felt very connected to this value. It felt good to be one of the "chosen" people. However, it all kind of fell apart when I went to a Catholic college, and I found out *they* thought they were the chosen people, too. So, I decided to let it all go and find a path for myself that made sense to me, which took many, many years to evolve.

For me, spirituality means seeing myself as a microscopic part of the cosmos. I believe that whatever force makes the day turn into night, night turn into day, and winter become spring and fall become winter, whatever keeps all of the stars and planets going around perfectly in their orbits, creates new buds in spring and moves old leaves to drop away in autumn, can surely look after this one little life of mine. So, I take steps to keep myself in harmony with the order of the universe. I try to eat naturally grown foods, spend time outside, rise when it is light, sleep when it is dark, and adjust my activity level according to the season of the year. By doing this, I tend to increasingly be in the right place at the right time, doing the right thing, just like all of the other major elements in the universe.

Harmonizing with nature is my spiritual practice. For you it may be something different—daily meditation, attending religious services, reading inspirational texts, or walking in the woods. Whatever it is, I encourage you to commit to and deepen your practice. Developing spiritual openness and sensitivity can add depth and meaning to your life in a way that nourishes you on a profound level.

Synchronicity

Carl Jung popularized the term "synchronicity," indicating the subtle interaction between individual will and universal law (or God's will or the movement of the cosmos, depending on your perspective). A spiritual practice can help a person become more attuned to synchronicity—to read the signs, to see the way the wind is blowing, to feel the direction in which life wants to go, and then use his or her creativity and intelligence to help it happen in the best possible manner. Once we develop a knack for noticing and welcoming synchronicity, life becomes more interesting and rewarding. We start to meet the right people at the right time to lead us to the next station in life.

It's easy to embrace synchronicity when things are going well, but there are times when events seem to conspire against us. Some days, the computer system decides to crash at the very moment I am about to complete an important document, and then I get stuck in a huge traffic jam when I'm in a hurry to get somewhere. Three or four things all seem to conspire against me, preventing me from doing whatever I think I need to do. At such frustrating moments, all kinds of interpretations can pop into my mind, including the self-defeating attitude that life is against me.

Life is never against me or anyone else. In these situations, the most effective strategy is to pause for a few minutes and reflect on the balance between the apparent antagonism of life that is disrupting our plans and how much or how urgently we want to achieve our goals. Maybe, upon reflection, it's to our advantage that the goals are delayed a little. Maybe we're trying to push events faster than they can go out of fear that things won't turn out the way we want. Take a break. Step back. Reflect. Might there be a reason that life is intervening at this moment?

At the same time, paying attention to synchronicity doesn't mean we should give up on our efforts and goals. It doesn't mean that every time something goes wrong we are on the wrong path. We shouldn't let the negative or challenging influences in life justify procrastination or allow us to abandon our goals in favor of temporary pleasures and distractions.

A spiritually healthy life is lived in delicate balance between these two extremes: will and letting go, goal orientation and spontaneous impulse, personal desire and the cosmic plan. We need to learn how to walk a middle path, to be sensitive to the natural flow of events while not throwing away our own determined idea of where we want to go.

Some helpful tools are available, if you desire to become more attuned to synchronicity. These tools include the Chinese masterpiece *The I Ching*, or *Book of Changes*, astrology, numerology, and tarot cards. They can all help you learn to read the signs and signals of life, but don't take these tools too seriously; otherwise, you may wind up relying on them to make simple, ordinary decisions.

If you want to explore the same phenomenon without such tools, try creating a record of all of the moments in your life when you felt synchronicity was happening to you: the people you met at pivotal moments by coincidence, the chances you took on a gut feeling, the decisions that somehow happened by themselves, the dreams you had that eventually happened during waking moments. When you have finished, see if you can apply this understanding to your daily life now, paying more attention to little synchronistic happenings, like when the phone rings and it's the right person at the right time. You'll soon get the hang of it.

Awareness

Almost all forms of spiritual practice come down to one thing: The more we bring our individual lives into alignment with the whole of existence, the more we feel nourished and at peace. Awareness practices can help connect that alignment. They are designed to quiet the busy mind, relax the body, and bring a sense of attunement with existence. Prayer, meditation, and ritual meals are all common awareness practices found in many religions and spiritual traditions.

Jon Kabat-Zinn, known for bringing mindfulness practices, especially Mindfulness-Based Stress Reduction (MBSR), into the mainstream, defines mindfulness as "awareness that arises through paying attention, on purpose, in the present moment, non-judgmentally." How can you become more aware of each moment without criticizing it? You can start by simply noticing your surroundings and what is on your mind.

I encourage you to incorporate simple practices (check out the exercises at end of this chapter) into your life on a regular basis. As you deepen your connection to the greater processes of life, you may find yourself coping with stress and emotions more easily, relating more lovingly with others, and finding more joy in life.

Exercises

1. The Circle of Life

Discover which primary foods you are missing and how to infuse joy and satisfaction into your life. Refer to the Circle of Life graphic at the beginning of this chapter.

Step 1: Place a dot on the line to indicate your level of satisfaction in each area. A dot toward the center indicates dissatisfaction, and a dot toward the periphery indicates satisfaction. For example, if your social life is abundant, place a dot on the line somewhere toward the outside of the circle.

Step 2: Connect the dots to see your Circle of Life.

Step 3: You will now have a clear visual of any imbalances in primary food and a starting point for determining where you may wish to spend more time and energy to create balance and joy in your life.

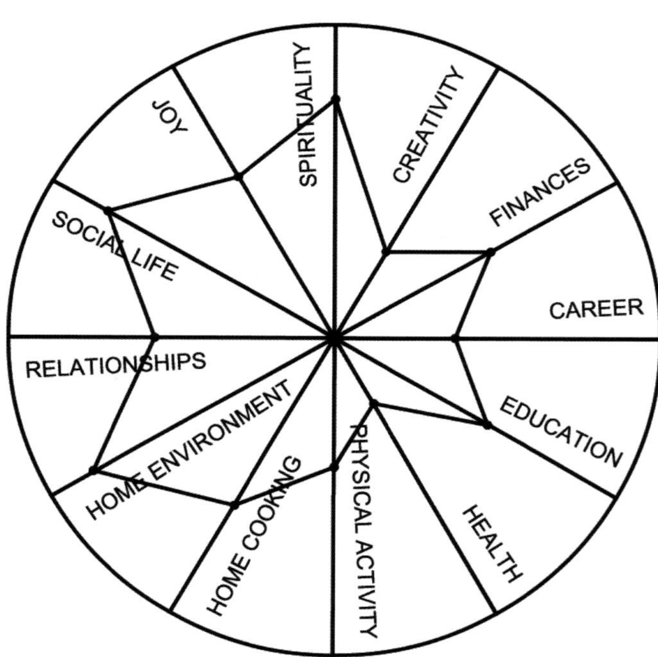

2. Practice Awareness

Sit in a relaxed, comfortable position. Breathe through your nose, and notice how the air is slightly cooler going in and slightly warmer going out. Place one hand over your heart and one hand over your belly. Feel your heart beating, and thank your heart for being there for you all day every day, pumping your blood and keeping you alive. Feel your belly, noticing the rise on the inhale and the fall on the exhale. Thank your belly for digesting all of the food you eat. Sit silently, with your eyes closed, and allow yourself to be with yourself. When you feel ready, take a deep inhale and exhale, open your eyes, rise, and move back into your day.

3. Three Deep Breaths

Upon waking, take three deep breaths—in through the nose and out through the mouth. Notice how this simple act of bringing attention to your breath can help you find the present moment. Use this exercise anytime throughout the day.

Chapter 8

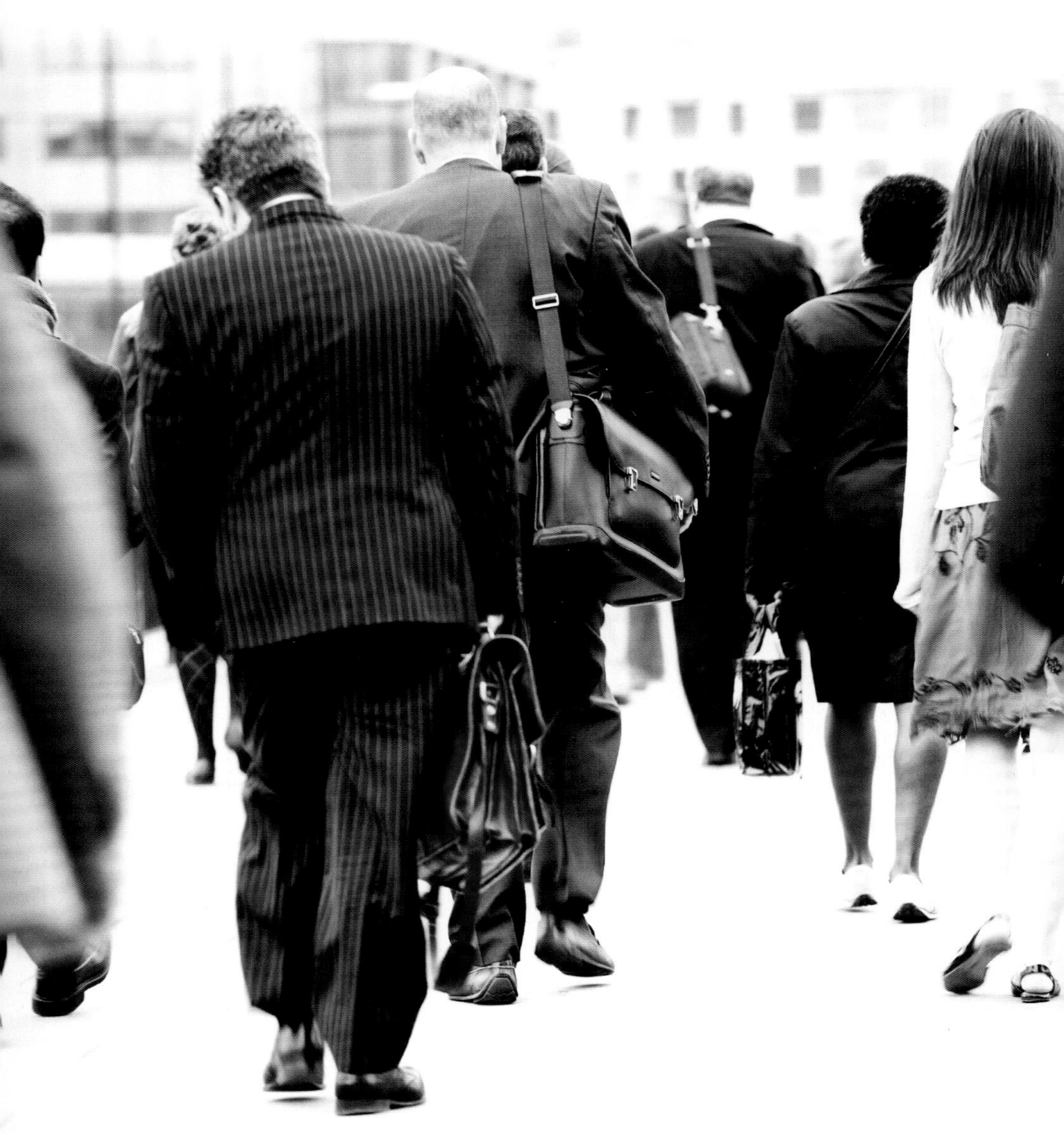

Escape the Matrix

People tell you the world looks a certain way. Parents tell you how to think. Schools tell you how to think. TV. Religion. And then at a certain point, if you're lucky, you realize you can make up your own mind. Nobody sets the rules but you. You can design your own life.

—Carrie-Anne Moss

We may live a large portion of life never questioning what we've been taught. We go along with this sort of matrix mentality, unaware of what other realities are possible for our lives. Escaping the matrix and reclaiming our own individuality and lifestyle is the task at hand. It is extremely challenging and rewarding. And when you start to wake up and look around, you will find many other intelligent people on the same path.

What is the matrix? As Morpheus said in the 1999 sci-fi movie, "The matrix is everywhere." We are completely surrounded and enveloped by it. It's the accepted beliefs and false concepts about the world that drain our life force. It's a kind of mental, emotional, and spiritual programming. It's more than the corporate agenda; it's from the government, the church, big business. It's the insistence that we all should get married, have children, join a church, and buy stuff. You can feel it at work or at the grocery store. You may feel it from your family and friends, too.

It creates our collective beliefs about food, fashion, and most aspects of life. It's the constant drum that calls us to produce, process, sell, and buy. It's the voice in our heads that tells us not to rock the boat, not to take risks. It's the treadmill many of us feel beneath our feet, on which we can never move forward. The matrix is what's familiar and even comfortable to most people, yet the beliefs and practices it demands disrupt our happiness and our authenticity. The matrix dictates to us its rules about our food, our health, our relationships, our spirituality, and how we should live.

Think about what the matrix looks like. It's slender women who are young forever, virile men who are wealthy and powerful. It's an endless parade of things to buy, to play with, to wear, and to consume. The matrix has us running on stress, in survival mode, and it always tells us we're not enough and we need more. The matrix says we never look good enough. It insists that we are really alone in this world. It tells us not to trust others. And it hypnotizes us into forgetting our true essence and greatness.

We may show our independence by making cynical, sophisticated remarks about aspects of the culture that surrounds us, about TV commercials or certain products, but in the end, it is nearly impossible not to succumb to the overwhelming forces that bombard us every day with these messages. Millions of dollars are spent every day to persuade us to do things and to buy things that we would never otherwise buy.

We allow clothing companies to brand us, abandoning our individuality and covering ourselves with logo-emblazoned sneakers, pants, shirts, purses, and jackets. Then we parade ourselves in front of each other, trying to gauge who has been branded best. We equate these brands with lifestyles. They represent youthfulness, luxury, or fun. These brands even fill needs, like the need to belong or to feel respected.

The matrix is an extremely powerful set of attitudes, beliefs, and thoughts that are relentlessly imposed on the public, every day, through many media channels. And the business-oriented motives that drive it are escalating and causing damage to the mental and physical health of millions of people and the planet.

Corporations have developed their own self-interested economic laws and dynamics because their survival depends on it. A fundamental economic law is that the corporation must always do what is best for the corporation, which is to maximize profits, outperform competitors, expand, grow, and keep shareholders happy with high-performance stocks and regular dividend payouts. The health and welfare of the consumer is irrelevant.

U.S. Measured-Ad Spending by Category

RANK IN 2015	CATEGORY	2015 (in millions)	2014 (in millions)	% CHG
1	Automotive	$13,829	$14,312	-3.4%
2	Retail	$12,965	$14,086	-8.0%
3	Medicine and remedies	$9,522	$8,357	13.9%
4	Telecommunications, internet services, and ISP	$8,613	$8,547	0.8%
5	General services	$8,458	$8,268	2.3%

Table includes 17 measured media; excludes free-standing inserts, Internet display, and paid search
Source: Kantar Media, Ad Age Datacenter Analysis of Kantar Media Data

Escaping the cultural matrix of needing to look, dress, and eat a certain way means mustering the courage to step away from outside influences, to look inside and ask yourself, "Who am I, and what do I really want from my life?" As an example, look at the U.S. One of the most fundamental concepts embedded in the American psyche is freedom. Americans like to think we are the freest people in the world, and, in a way, we are.

But I see two types of freedom: freedom from and freedom for. Where "freedom from" is concerned, we are doing well. Through our democratic institutions, particularly the U.S. Constitution and the Bill of Rights, we have achieved a great deal of freedom from religious persecution, from monarchy, from undemocratic political systems like communism, fascism, and military dictatorships. But what is "freedom for?" Freedom for what? To work our butts off all day and then sit in front of a TV, a computer, or video games until it's time for bed? To stuff our mouths with processed food until our pants burst or our bodies deteriorate? To chase after the latest products that will make us feel complete? Isn't there something more to life? Our "freedom for" habits have spilled over to the rest of the Western world. I urge everyone to consider what freedom means to you.

Meanwhile, other places exist without this matrix mentality. Costa Rica, a small country in Central America, consistently ranks as one of the happiest countries in the world. People living there have higher rates of overall well-being than those of many other nations, including the U.S. and the U.K., and they live longer than people who reside in the U.S. Despite having a lot less stuff than people in Western countries, Costa Ricans are generally happy. They even have a saying, "Pura Vida," or pure life, which is synonymous with "enjoy your life." Researchers speculate that the happiness there is related to strong social and family connections, along with a culture that takes pride in people expressing themselves and being happy with who they are.

Hungry? Why Wait?

One of the most insidious features of the matrix is that it tells us that life is about instant gratification. And if life is about getting what we want as fast as possible, then so is eating. In fact, our nutrition woes today can be summed up in a one-liner from a Snickers commercial: "Hungry? Why wait?" Introduced to the market in 1930, global sales of Snickers reached $3.5 billion in 2012, and it's the world's best-selling candy bar due to savvy marketing techniques based on giving people what they think they want—fast, convenient, colorfully packaged food.[1]

As the slogan implies, there's no need to wait until the next meal, no need to cook food or wait for other family members to get home to sit down together for a meal. Just grab the nearest tasty thing, and pop it in your mouth. Modern marketing and distribution have ensured that when we feel hungry, many products are lining the shelves of the local stores or stacked in the office vending machine. Almost all these foods are loaded with calories, fat, refined sugar, processed salt, and artificial chemicals, making them foods that are not really fit for human consumption. Just look at the ingredients listed on the Snickers wrapper. They are as follows: milk chocolate (sugar, cocoa butter, chocolate, lactose, skim milk, soy lecithin, artificial flavor), peanuts, corn syrup, sugar, skim milk, butter, milk fat, partially hydrogenated soybean oil, salt, egg whites, and artificial flavor. I have nothing against Snickers bars, but I'm using Snickers as an example of the way people are being seduced into buying foods that, when eaten regularly over time, increase weight and decrease health.

It seems the less healthy a food is, the more money companies spend on its marketing. Advertising is a multibillion-dollar industry charged with stimulating the buying impulses of the biggest consumer society on the face of the earth. We are constantly bombarded with ads encouraging us to eat and drink more. From the billboard on the side of the bus to the back cover of a stranger's magazine on the subway, from commercials slotted between songs on the radio to the pop-up ads on our social media and Internet searches, we are inundated by commercial messages every day.

New research also shows that binge-watching TV, one of the most popular pastimes in many countries around the world, makes you eat more and may even be associated with higher rates of depression. No surprise there! Marathon TV-watching sessions encourage mindless snacking, especially with frequent exposure to unhealthy food and beverage marketing. When you are distracted while eating, you don't pay attention to the food right in front of you. This mindless eating will often cause you to miss satiety cues that let you know you are full.

For children, it's even worse. They're bombarded with junk food ads for high-sugar and high-fat foods like Pop-Tarts, cereal bars, and many types of processed cookies, cakes, and snacks. Is this really what we want to teach young people today? Good nutrition is crucial in the formative years, but our kids are eating junk, especially in the school system, and it shows. In the U.S., childhood obesity rates have doubled for children and quadrupled for adolescents in the last 30 years.[2] Worldwide, the numbers are equally staggering, as the number of overweight and obese young children (up to 5 years old) went from 32 million in 1990 to 42 million in 2013, according to the World Health Organization.

Scientists predict our children will be the first generation in history to live shorter lives than their parents. The number of 30-second TV commercials seen in a year by an average child is 20,000, and the top-ranking advertiser for child-oriented advertising on television is the junk food, fast food industry.[3]

Most parents would be shocked to see ads for cigarettes or alcohol accompany children's television. They should be equally upset by junk-food advertising, especially as childhood obesity rates continue to skyrocket.

It's no surprise that obese children are also more susceptible to food ads seen on TV, which makes them more likely to eat, according to a study published in the *Journal of Pediatrics*. The study's authors also found that companies spend more than $10 billion each year on food and beverage ads for children and that 98% of those products are high in fat, sugar, and salt.[4]

Small strides have been made with children's television networks like Walt Disney Co., Nickelodeon, and the Cartoon Network, who have begun reworking ads to meet federal guidelines for nutrition and restricting their characters from promoting unhealthy products.[5] Schools are also making slow improvements. In 2010, the U.S. Congress passed the Healthy, Hunger-Free Kids Act, which, in addition to improving the health of all school meals, also applies to competitive foods—the ones sold outside the school meal program, which include fast food items, sodas, and junk food in vending machines, etc. But in April 2013, public health lawyer Michele Simon, wrote that the "USDA's narrow focus on nutrients, such as grams of fat and sugar, will still result in highly processed junk food with only slightly improved nutritional profiles." I would say we still have a long way to go to help kids escape the junk food matrix.

I'd like to make it clear that I am not against fast, convenient food. I think it's a great idea. But I long for the day when the colorful packages on our supermarket shelves and at fast food restaurants offer good, wholesome, nutritious foods that keep us healthy. It is possible, and we are seeing some changes. We need enough people to keep demanding it. Then the companies whose existence depends on knowing what we want and supplying it will switch to healthy products in order to guarantee their own survival. It's really up to us.

I've said it before, and it's important to remember that what we're dealing with today is something totally new. Nothing like this massive consumer society of ours has ever happened in the history of humanity, and it's very possible nothing like it will ever happen again. This message may seem simplistic. Even if you're mindful of your exposure to advertisements, the ads keep coming. They keep entering your brain, and their influence is powerful and escalating. How can one be vigilant enough to filter out the useless messages the matrix communicates?

Think of how its influence affects your own moods and feelings. Compare the way you feel after spending a few hours in the park versus watching a few hours of TV. Or think of a time when you were chasing things outside yourself to fulfill you. Consider your relationship to food after spending the morning at a local farmers' market talking to the people who grew the food versus sticking a few quarters into a vending machine to satisfy an afternoon craving.

The Pressure to Be Thin

The idea of being thin enters our minds very early in life. Increasingly, young girls in particular say they want to be thinner. About half of girls in the United States between the ages of 11 and 13 see themselves as overweight.[6] Most of these girls own a Barbie doll, and Barbie has a body shape that is impossible to attain. If Barbie were a real woman, she would be about 6 feet tall with a bust measurement of 39 inches, a waist of 18 inches, and hips of 33 inches. Her weight would be about 110 pounds.[7] If women were really built like Barbie, they would not be able to walk, have a menstrual cycle, give birth, or breathe. If young girls see this doll as an image of what it is like to be a woman, what kind of message does that send to them about how they should look?

Despite the strides women have made in education, politics, and the workplace, many women still struggle immensely with body image and self-esteem. We still live in an overly masculine modern society. The world needs strong, powerful, nurturing women to balance this energy. But many women are limited and silenced by their insecurities because of the messages they have received throughout their lives about what it means to be female.

Read any women's fashion magazine, and you will see that the content and advertising are incessantly inflaming, and cashing in on, obsessions with measuring up to media-driven images. What is shown in mainstream magazines, however, is not reality. The magazines don't publish disclaimers announcing that the models work for hours with the world's best hair and makeup artists, that the clothes are tailored to fit their exact shape, or that professionals retouch the photos. Blemishes are removed, cellulite airbrushed, and any extra fat from the belly, thighs, and arms is erased.

Women see these ads and begin to believe they are supposed to roll out of bed being as beautiful as these models on the pages of the magazine. Men also see these ads and impose their unrealistic ideals onto women. And men also see these images and feel pressure to maintain rock hard abs or unrealistic muscle mass.

At least 30 million people in the U.S. alone deal with an eating disorder at some point in their lifetime, thanks in large part to these unrealistic expectations of body type. Eating disorders do not discriminate. Both men and women and people of all economic classes and ethnicities feel this pressure.

Supermodels represent the cutting edge of all that is supposed to be beautiful and desirable. But typical models are thinner and taller than 99.9% of women. The average model is 5'11" and weighs 117 pounds. In the U.S., the average woman is 5'4" and weighs 164 pounds. To keep their jobs, models must maintain as little body fat as possible. The human body, especially the female body, is simply not designed to operate without body fat. It's an inhuman concept. Small wonder that, on any given day, more than half of the women in this country are on a diet, trying to mold themselves into an artificially created cultural concept of what it means to be beautiful.

Advertising encourages all of us to substitute food for love, while glamorizing distorted images that seem unattainable to most people. The media is reluctant to examine the impact of advertising on the public's health because it depends on advertising for commercial viability and cannot afford to bite the hand that feeds it. As discussed in Chapter 1, governments are compromised by the power of corporate interests. Left to ourselves, we can just drift along with the collective cultural mindset and try to make the best of it, or we can choose to stand up for what we know is the truth, regardless of what the media pushes us to believe.

Superwoman Syndrome

Liberated from the confinement of traditional female roles, with increasing opportunities to explore areas once exclusively for men, modern women frequently end up leading chronically stressful lives as they struggle to balance all of their options. They want to be successful in business, have a dynamic love life, maybe children, a perfect figure with a flat belly, enjoy time with friends and family, travel around the world, or do whatever makes them happy. Phew! Just thinking about it makes me stressed out. I know many women who suffer from the Superwoman Syndrome, trying to maintain this stressful lifestyle, and then wondering why it's not making them happy.

I am a great believer in encouraging people to slow down. I understand why women want to explore all of the possibilities open to them, having been denied them for so long, and I admire those who manage to do so. But sooner or later anyone who maintains such a high-powered lifestyle, man or woman, is bound to see that an intelligent selection of priorities is required. Courage is needed to stand up and stay true to you. You can prioritize based on your needs rather than the traditional priorities or responsibilities attributed to women and take time for what really matters most to you.

Superman Syndrome

Men today have enormous pressure to be strong, to provide for their families, and to be there for their partners. In recent years, marketing geared toward men has dramatically expanded to include images of men with fit bodies who are also highly successful in their careers.

When I teach about gender roles at the school, I am always reminded of the pressure men feel to be successful in their professions. Just as women are seen as "sex objects" in our society, men are seen as "success objects." Somehow, men in our culture get the message that if they don't "bring home the bacon," and in large quantities, they are failures. The drive to be a success object often causes men to override their bodies. They don't listen to the wisdom of their bodies, to the gentle voice inside that would have them go slower and be more self-loving. After all, by our culture's standards, this isn't very manly.

In helping men overcome the pressure to be "perfect" by our society's standards—to have a fit body and a well-paying job and to be open, but not too sensitive—I encourage men to seek support. I urge them to create communities where they feel comfortable, free from the pressure to conform to other people's ideals of who or what they should be and where they can express their emotions openly, without judgment. Lastly, I support them in continuing to move forward.

Men in our culture are ready to learn that they don't need to sacrifice their bodies for success. Males are often expected to lay it all on the line, to sacrifice their health to toxic jobs, to push themselves with pride, and to take injuries or wounds "like a man." Yes, men can be strong, but they can also be vulnerable. Many men want to nourish themselves and care about their own health. They need encouragement and permission, not only from the women around them but also from their fellow men.

The Self-Improvement Superhighway

When we start making healthier choices and going against the matrix mentality, we sometimes bump into something I like to call the self-improvement superhighway. A superhighway is designed for high-speed traffic and to accelerate our ability to get from point A to point B. In our efforts to feel good and get healthy, we can encounter this idea of endless self-improvement—whether it's new foods to try, a better workout, or making changes in other areas of life. It's a subtle but persistent thought that we must be striving to advance ourselves. And it's really just the matrix in disguise telling us to read another book on productivity, do another cleanse, or buy a certain kind of yoga pants.

Even those of you with the best intentions can get caught up in the idea that you must always be fixing or improving your life in some way. Fixing yourself implies that you are broken, and thankfully that's not the case. No matter what your circumstances look like right now, you are more capable than you can imagine.

Change is a natural part of life. In fact, it's something we can count on! But always struggling to be better can end up feeling like a bit of a trap and that you never really arrive. So, take a moment to distinguish for yourself between natural growth and that empty feeling that goes with obsessing over your own self-improvement. Start by being in the here and now. Remember all of the good things in your life, and feel whatever you need to feel. I'm not saying you can't set goals or even track changes; just notice when you are feeling out of balance with all of it.

Self-improvement can become tiring and stressful. Ultimately, if we are stressing ourselves out about being healthy, it's counter-productive. I encourage you to make changes at a pace that feels comfortable for you. Remember your own bio-individuality, and don't try to compare your rate of growth to others'. You can apply the 90-10 rule to your ideas about self-improvement if that's helpful. It's great to be committed 90% of the time, but allow yourself to spend at least 10% of your time to having fun and enjoying your life—even if it looks completely different from what you expected.

The Individual

Even though I look at the big picture, my focus is always on the individual sitting in front of me and on listening carefully with an open mind to what she or he is saying. This perspective is from Zen Buddhism. It's called "beginner's mind," and it refers to the art of approaching something with an innocent attitude, in a fresh, receptive, and inquiring manner. This is a wonderful way to starve the matrix and let your beauty and truth shine through.

I look at the person in front of me—whether a student, client, or friend— as a *tabula rasa,* a clean slate, and I ask them, "How are you? What is your health concern?" A lot of evidence exists in the counseling and coaching worlds that a person will get themselves well just by speaking about their problems and receiving love without the listener making any recommendation. This approach takes time and runs counter to mainstream healthcare, in which the focus is to get the job done quickly by diagnosing symptoms, identifying diseases, and prescribing medications.

Looking back, I notice that many of my clients have recovered quickly without the need for medications or other interventions. I attribute this to my careful listening skills, my sincere appreciation for them, and my deeper knowledge that they need not suffer. Many of my clients and students could probably have worked out their problems on their own, without my help, if they were willing to put as much attention and intelligence into their own health care as they do into their professional lives. But this rarely happens.

Society, culture, and media all shift people away from caring for their own health, drawing the focus away from what's "inside here" to what's "out there." Fashion, the lives of celebrities, and gossip take precedence over our own physical health and well-being.

I like to remind my students to love and respect themselves and to take time to listen to the needs of their bodies, minds, and souls. I encourage people to notice the issues that are troubling them, and then invest time and energy into fixing them. Our method makes people focus on themselves and address the issues that are bothering them. Once this happens, the solution is usually quite obvious, and the person with the answers is usually the individual, not the professional. But having that person there, a trained listener who is devoted to helping them get better, is how people discover their answers.

Fitting Out

One of the more powerful ways we can free ourselves from the matrix is to learn to "fit out" rather than trying to always "fit in." We are all susceptible to the age-old social pressure to conform, be accepted, and keep up with the Joneses. Who cares about the Joneses? This need to fit in keeps us locked into the matrix, which pushes for a poor diet and fast foods. Its illusions push us to work harder, relying on addictive stimulants, like coffee, sugar, and cigarettes. We feel compelled to push forward with all our life force. Getting off this treadmill requires a willingness to stand on our own and disregard others' opinions.

I am personally sensitive to this tendency because, being raised in an Orthodox Jewish family, I grew up with a need to fit in, not attract unnecessary attention, and pretend I was just like everyone else. That's why it's easy for me to spot the same tendency in others. I have noticed that, when people shift to significantly different lifestyles, they sometimes try to hide it or play it down for similar reasons. So, as you're starting to make healthier food choices, quit drinking, or do whatever new things to nurture yourself, I encourage you to be open about it, and let people know what you're about.

Many IIN students do not fit into average society. In one way or another, they live on the periphery and don't want to attract too much attention, so they mimic the customs and habits of their families and neighbors, despite feeling like the black sheep of their families. They tell me, "I'm nothing like my brother or my sisters, my parents, or my next-door neighbors. I see myself as being quite different from the society around me." But they'll blend in with the crowd, chatting about the latest sporting event or social happening, and wear the same clothing, just to be acknowledged as part of the collective. Others may have an interest in healthier eating habits but feel that they don't want to interrupt their usual routines, whether it's lunch at a fast food restaurant with coworkers or food served at family events. Our eating habits—at home, at the office, or in a restaurant—are sure to reflect our willingness to compromise for the sake of social harmony. I suggest starting small. Experiment with bringing a healthier dish to a family function, or let your coworkers know about a new healthy restaurant that just opened.

Another area in which people, including myself, often compromise for the sake of appearances is in relationships. After three years of marriage, I felt mine wasn't working, but I stayed married for another three years because my parents were so happy that I had married a Jewish woman. I couldn't imagine disappointing them. This same pressure manifests in a thousand different ways in other parts of our lives. I often refer to sections of the newspaper to illustrate this topic. We have a section for wedding announcements with smiling, happy couples. But we don't have a divorce section with pictures of smiling women or men who have decided to take their own path. Are you caught in your own picture, trying to uphold something that's not working? Maybe it's a relationship, a job, or a way of eating.

People often struggle to maintain healthy habits once in a relationship as well. It's funny how people tend to take care of their health and personal development when they are single, but after a few years in a relationship, they become more comfortable and "let themselves go." Habits like going to the gym or taking a meditation course get replaced with movie nights or going out for pizza. Personal development coach Jim Rohn said it best when he said, "The greatest gift you can give to somebody is your own personal development." If you find yourself getting lost in the relationship or losing healthy habits, find creative solutions to maintain your health and personal path while also enjoying quality time with your partner. Maybe you go hiking together. Or take a workshop on your own, and make time to share what you learned with your partner. Examine how much self-care you need versus relationship comfort, and don't be afraid to speak up to your partner about it. If you're afraid taking time for yourself may impact the relationship, have a conversation to find out whether that's really true. Many times, people are afraid to talk openly about their struggle, but once they share what they need, their partner can become an amazing ally in helping them achieve health or personal goals.

I'd like you to pause for a moment and reflect on how much of your intelligence and creativity is being channeled into "fitting in." My own experience is that if you put the same amount of effort into "fitting out"—giving yourself permission to be spontaneous, natural, and authentic in the way you live and behave—you'll immediately become much happier and more content.

Escaping the matrix is a key step in creating true health and happiness. Start by noticing the places in your life where you feel inauthentic. Are there certain people you have difficulty expressing your true self around? In what circumstances do you try to fit into other people's expectations? Without self-judgment, begin to notice when and where this occurs, and start building the confidence to express your true self at all times, to embrace what makes you different from the norm. By loving yourself completely, you will reach a new height of health that no food could ever give you. And by expressing your authentic self, your life force will soar, your heart will open, and the world will never look the same.

Exercises

1. Turn Off the Media

I encourage you to experiment with turning off the media for a day, a week, or a month. Hide the TV, skip the magazines or newspapers, and avoid the Internet. Notice how your thoughts about the world and about yourself change without constant media messages. Notice that you have more time for the people you love or to face the fact that you are overly isolated.

2. Be Bad

Now that I've covered foods that can lead to health problems when over-consumed, I want to introduce you to the joy and freedom of throwing away the rules and being bad. Over the next week I invite you to do something bad every single day. When I say "bad," I mean something you feel you shouldn't do or feel is irresponsible. Obviously, I'm not asking you to rob a bank or hurt another human being. Perhaps you'll delete unread emails, play hooky from work, or tell someone what you really think. Start slowly. Gradually build your "being bad" muscles.

The purpose behind this exercise is to put you back in charge of your life. Many of us feel like being good is what makes us worthwhile. We put pleasing others above pleasing ourselves. Learning to put yourself first and find your voice is priceless. If people like you, great. If they don't, know that you are still a very good person. This way, you remain true to you. There's nothing more health promoting than that. Now write down three things you want to do this week to practice being bad.

Examples

1. Leave early from work to get a massage.
2. Order the expensive dessert at my favorite restaurant.
3. Schedule a playdate for me, instead of the kids.

3. Wish List

This is a tool for you to let go of societal ideals of what your life should look like and connect with your deepest desires for your future. Write down the elements that are most meaningful to your future, such as relationships, children, career, health, and spirituality. Write what you want to accomplish or obtain, the places you want to go, the people you'd like to meet or become closer with, or anything that your heart, mind, and soul truly desire.

Start listing your desires. Begin with the simple and obvious, and you will notice that more ideas come to you once you start writing. Allow yourself to go crazy—write down all that you desire. Use any language you're comfortable with, such as "I want . . ." or "I desire . . ." or "I intend . . ." Allow yourself to have fun with it.

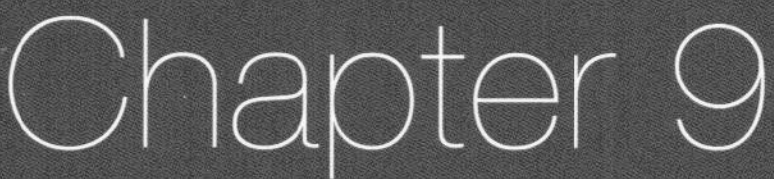

Chapter 9

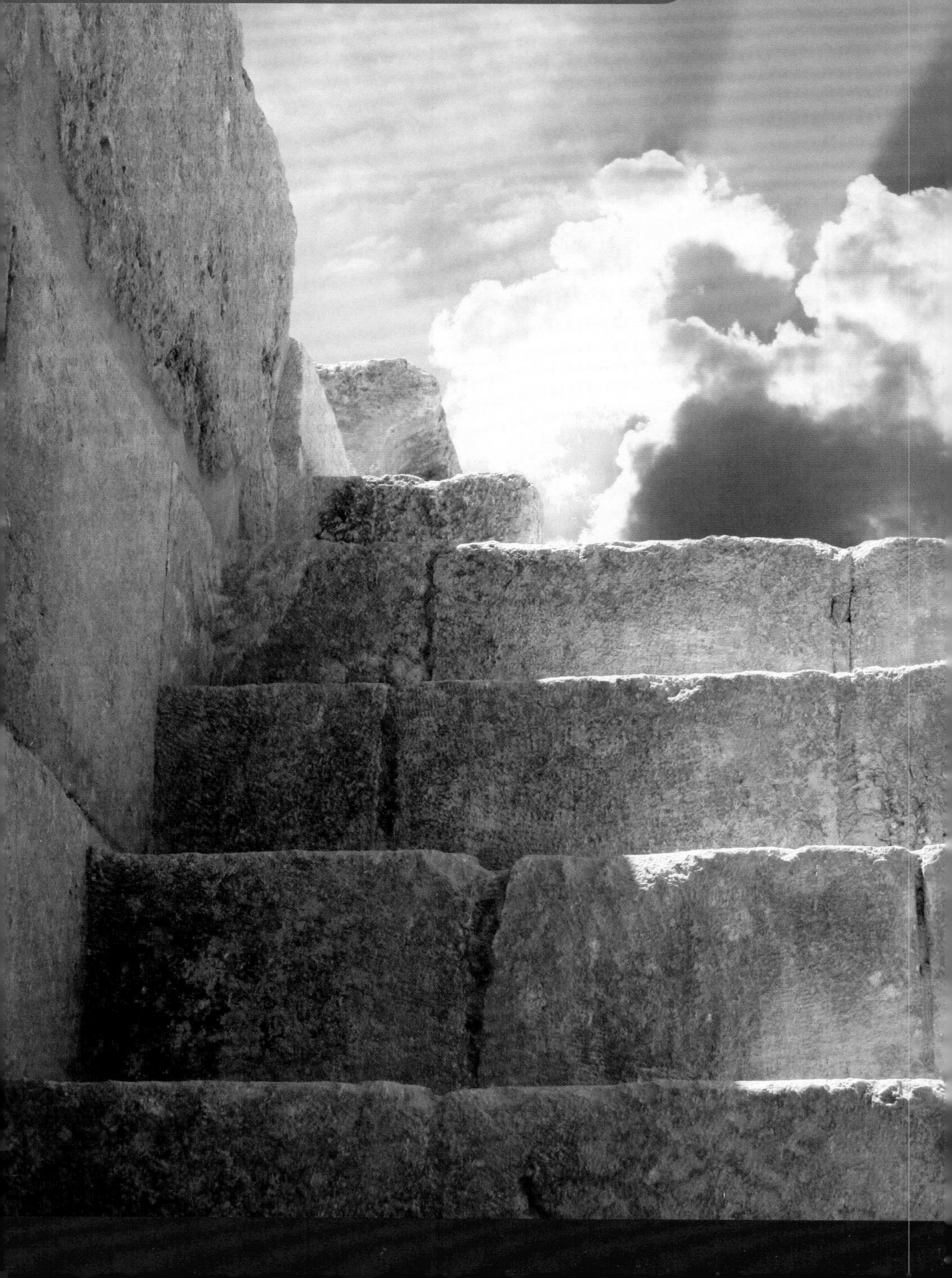

12 Steps to Better Health

To get through the hardest journey, we need take only one step at a time, but we must keep on stepping.

—Chinese Proverb

We've examined the politics surrounding the food industry and the difficulty of breaking out of contemporary cultural attitudes that influence our eating habits. We've looked at the innate wisdom of the body, learning to trust it and to understand the importance of the signals it sends to us in the form of cravings. We've examined dietary theories and looked at the pivotal issue of primary food. Now it's time to integrate this knowledge into one of the most laid-back health plans out there. No one way of eating will work for everyone, but you can take steps each day to improve your health. The steps in this chapter act as general principles and suggestions, not rigid rules. This approach has flexibility according to each individual's needs, recognizing that no two people are alike, and no two people have the same food preferences.

I don't expect you to make changes all at once. On the contrary, I have found that drastic, sudden shifts are difficult to maintain because they force people to repress their food cravings and embedded eating habits. The more habits are repressed, the more powerful they become, leading to internal stress that builds until people fall off the wagon and the diet fails. A gradual introduction of basic changes allows people to create a larger shift without as much effort or strife.

Even by choosing to follow just one step from this chapter, significant changes are likely. Think of it like climbing a ladder. You have to take it one rung at a time, or you might fall off. I'm offering many suggestions, but it's up to you to find the ones that fit. Most diet books recommend that you completely alter your current way of eating and follow their strict rules. I say choose the things that you most want to do, and leave the hardest ones for later. As you start doing the easier ones, your body's energy will kick in, and you will pick up momentum. You will find yourself doing the hardest things with greater ease because you're not starting from zero. If you like the idea of a hot towel scrub, do that. If it's appealing to eat more sweet vegetables, do that. Whichever suggestion you want to follow is the right one for you. One thing I can tell you is they all work. You don't need to follow the steps in any particular order. Pick one, and then go on to another when you are ready. Go at a pace that's suitable for you. You could tackle one new step a day, a week, or a month. This isn't a short-term diet; this is a long-term lifestyle. Trust your instincts, and know that each change you make has a tremendous impact on your present and your future.

I also wish to make one more recommendation. You don't have to do it all alone. Everyone has someone in their life who also wants to improve their health. Who is that for you? You can be supportive and hold each other accountable for making the small changes that lead to improved health. Friends make life a lot more fun, and you are more likely to keep up a healthy lifestyle when you surround yourself with people who are on a similar path.

Integrative Nutrition Plan: 12 Steps to Better Health

1. Drink more water
2. Practice cooking
3. Experiment with whole grains
4. Increase sweet vegetables
5. Increase leafy green vegetables
6. Experiment with protein
7. Eat fewer processed foods
8. Make a habit of nurturing your body
9. Have healthy relationships
10. Enjoy regular physical activity
11. Find work you love
12. Develop a spiritual practice

1. Drink More Water

The body is 75% water, so it makes sense that this essential fluid must be continually replenished. We can go for a month without food, but we can live only two or three days without water. Water is crucial to our survival. Many people are confused by how much water they should be drinking; they are always told to drink more. What is more? What is the correct quantity of water for your body? Some experts recommend eight glasses a day, but this raises the question, how big is one glass? Eight ounces? More? Less? The answer must come from your own experience. Much will depend on your size. A smaller person will need proportionately less water than a bigger person. It also depends on your level of physical activity, the climate in which you live, and your diet.

According to Traditional Chinese Medicine, drinking more water increases yin, making the body light and airy and expanding energy through the whole system. If you are too yang—too tight or contracted, suffering from stress, headaches, and bodily tension—you may want to try increasing your water intake to balance these symptoms. In addition, cravings for sweet (yin) foods may actually be signals of dehydration. Drinking water may reduce or eliminate the cravings.

The late Dr. Fereydoon Batmanghelidj, an Iranian-born physician, gained international attention with his claim that regularly drinking water can treat a vast array of illnesses. "You are not sick, you are thirsty," he asserted in his best-selling 1992 book *Your Body's Many Cries for Water*, which attributes most pain and sickness to chronic dehydration. Through years of reading and research, Dr. Batmanghelidj concluded that ordinary water prevents and cures depression, asthma, arthritis, back pain, migraines, high blood pressure, multiple sclerosis, and many other illnesses. He also opposed the use of costly drugs for treating illnesses, saying that you "don't treat thirst with medication."

Dr. Batmanghelidj was jailed as a political prisoner in Iran following the Islamic Revolution in 1979. Because he was a medical doctor, other prisoners came to him with medical problems. Having no access to medicine or drugs, in desperation he told an ulcer patient with severe abdominal pains to try drinking two glasses of water. To his surprise, the patient's pain receded within minutes. During three years in prison, he treated more than 3,000 fellow prisoners who suffered from peptic ulcers, viewing the prison environment as an "ideal stress laboratory." After his release in 1982, he came to the United States and continued to explore the role of water metabolism in the human body until he passed in 2004.

A large majority of people are dehydrated, which contributes significantly to a poor state of health. Regularly flushing out the kidneys and bladder with water ensures that waste products can be expelled before they reach toxic levels. Maintaining hydration can prevent premature aging, reduce pain and headaches, lessen hypertension, and promote weight loss. Some people say they can't drink water because they don't like the taste. I advise them to add a squeeze of lemon, a slice of cucumber, or anything that creates an appealing flavor.

People always ask me what kind of water I recommend. This issue has become increasingly complex. In the past few decades, bottled water has become one of the most popular beverages in the world. Global bottled water consumption is big business, and worldwide consumption reached almost 75 billion gallons in 2014.[1] That's a lot of plastic! It's fascinating to me that people, including holistically minded ones, drink water flown in from Fiji, Holland, and other parts of the world. Many times, the cost of the water is for the brand, and the water is not much different from what comes out of your tap. Federal standards for tap water in the United States are actually higher than those for bottled water.[2] Plastic water bottles are also a huge strain on the environment. The amount of fuel, not to mention plastic, used in these bottles is tremendous. I'm not saying everyone should drink only tap water, but drinking solely bottled water is simply not sustainable for our planet. When you're out and about, sometimes drinking bottled water is the only option. I recommend you try different kinds—look for options in glass bottles and even eco-friendly boxes.

Most tap water does contain chlorine, fluoride, and sometimes lead. So if you are going to drink tap water, I recommend getting some kind of filter system. A wide variety of filters are on the market, and they vary in price as well as quality. Most people are familiar with the pitcher filters or faucet filters, such as Brita, which are relatively inexpensive. You can also try a carbon water filter or a reverse osmosis filter, both of which are more expensive but are known for eliminating a higher amount of toxins. You can research the different kinds of filters online to find one suited to your needs and your budget. If after researching water filters you decide to invest in one, be sure to change the filter regularly.

Timing is also important in water intake. After waking up in the morning, it's good to drink one or two glasses of water to hydrate the body. Many people realize late in the day that they didn't get enough water, so they drink a lot right before bed. Good sleep is integral to health, and you don't want to disrupt it by waking up to go to the bathroom. Complete regeneration occurs only when we sleep deeply. If you notice that you are waking up at night to go to the bathroom, I suggest drinking most of your water in the morning and early afternoon.

Many health experts say water is the only liquid that can hydrate the body and that juice and tea don't count. As far as I'm concerned, caffeinated drinks, like coffee, soda, and black tea, don't count because they are dehydrating. Herbal tea, soup, and juice all help hydrate the body, although not as much as pure water.

Others recommend drinking warm water with lemon first thing in the morning, claiming it's good for cleansing the liver. If you try this, notice how your body reacts. It may bother your stomach or have a diuretic effect on some people. Experiment to find out what really works for your body. The same thing applies to ice water and hot water. A lot of people refuse ice in their water, thinking it's unhealthy because the water used is poor quality or the coldness disrupts digestion. These people may think nothing of drinking pints of hot tea, creating an overheated condition. The body, through its natural wisdom of seeking balance, will often compensate by craving something cooling, such as ice cream. Ice water can often help restore the imbalance caused by excessively drinking hot liquids without the side effects of sugar.

Remember to look at your whole day's intake when deciding how much water you need. Certain foods are more water dense than others. Cooked grains are two parts water, one part grain. Vegetables also have high water content. Steaming or boiling vegetables, as opposed to frying or baking them, further increases their water content. If you eat a dry breakfast cereal or a muffin, you will take in little to no water from these foods.

Considering the proven impact of water on human health, it amazes me that people remain so unaware and uneducated about this subject. They spend most of their lives dehydrated, needlessly suffering from low energy, cravings, and symptoms, not realizing they could feel much better by merely drinking more water. Also, most of the added sugar in our diet comes from sugar-sweetened beverages, so a simple switch to water can have huge health benefits for those who are looking to reduce their sugar intake.

2. Practice Cooking

It's a well-known paradox that only a skilled cook knows how to prepare a meal in just a few minutes. You would think expertise would bring complexity, but making a meal can actually be divided into two simple stages: preparation time and cooking time. Preparation time for rice is short—about a minute. Take it out of the bag, measure it, rinse it, and put it in the pot. The cooking time is longer, but this doesn't mean you need to hang around the kitchen, impatiently testing the rice every few minutes to see if it's ready. Just flip on a timer, and go about doing whatever else you need to do.

Vegetables, which are seriously lacking in most people's daily diets, are especially easy to prepare. Making a salad involves rinsing and chopping. Cooking vegetables takes a couple of minutes of prep time to rinse and chop and then a few minutes of cooking time to steam, sauté, or boil. Juicing is an instantaneous way to prepare vegetables; all you need is a juicer and a few minutes to clean it once you are done. Other easy ways to eat vegetables are buying bags of baby carrots or celery sticks or simply washing vegetables and eating them in their natural, crunchy state. Dip them in hummus, yogurt, or nut butters. The key is to have them available and ready for snacking. Learning the art of simple meal planning will help you get all the nutrients you need as well as release you from dependency on restaurant food, fast food, and other processed foods. We eat differently when we are feeding ourselves from when we are out and about. Restaurant food is usually very salty and highly flavored, as it's designed to be a taste sensation. It often comes in oversized big portions, more than enough for the average person. By buying and preparing our own food, we eat in accordance with our body's actual needs, and we are less likely to overeat or consume excess salt and flavoring. Cooking delicious, satisfying meals in a brief period of time is a skill worth learning. It's not difficult, but it takes practice. At first, you may burn the rice or overcook the kale, but that's okay. You may go through an initial period of trial and error. Give yourself permission to make mistakes. It's like starting a new office job. The first few weeks seem complicated because you have to figure out how the phone system works, how the photocopy machine works, where the bathroom is, and who's who in the office. In the beginning, it seems like a huge task, but a month later you are doing it without even thinking about it. You know it all by heart. Cooking is just like that.

For many people, the task of cooking seems daunting. They are puzzled and ask questions like, "How do plain, ordinary vegetables turn into such a delicious meal in a few minutes?" A chef is like an alchemist, turning simple ingredients into gold, transforming a caterpillar into a butterfly. But few cookbooks talk about the initial, most-challenging period. They don't mention that cooking a meal takes much longer when you are an inexperienced chef than when you have had some practice. It is a great gift to be able to cook with ease and confidence. It just takes some patience and practice. In a short time, you will be effortlessly washing, chopping, cooking, and nourishing yourself and others.

Creatively selecting combinations of foods is similar to a painter choosing colors from a palette. Cooking is the only art form that actually enters the bloodstream. You can look at a painting and find it inspirational or listen to a piece of music to create a mood, but homemade food has a much deeper effect because it goes into your body. A very intimate relationship exists between a meal and the person who consumes it.

3. Experiment with Whole Grains

Many fashionable diet theories advise people to avoid carbohydrates, naming them as a culprit in our obesity crisis. This advice is a huge and faulty generalization. By looking at the delicate, thin bodies of Japanese people, who consume high-carbohydrate diets composed of large amounts of rice and starchy vegetables, it's impossible to conclude that all carbs lead to weight gain. Still, the subject of whether to eat grains does stir up emotions for many. Some people live on brown rice and oatmeal; others do better with less grains, and some swear by getting off grains altogether. No food is inherently "good" or "bad," so I encourage you to experiment with whole grains and see which ones work best for you, if any.

Whole grains have been a central element of the human diet since we stopped hunting and gathering and settled into agrarian communities. Until very recently, people living in these communities on all continents had lean, strong bodies. In the Americas, corn was the staple grain, while rice predominated in India and Asia. In Africa, people had sorghum and millet. People in the Middle East enjoyed whole-wheat pita bread and couscous. In Europe, it was corn, millet, wheat, rice, pasta, and dark sourdough breads. Even beer, produced by grain fermentation, was considered healthy. In Scotland, it was oats. In Russia, they had buckwheat or kasha. For generations, very few people eating grain-based diets were overweight.

People are gaining weight today because they eat too much processed junk food containing refined carbohydrates. Remember refined carbohydrates, like sugar, are associated with weight gain, while complex carbohydrates are associated with healthier BMIs. People will eat all kinds of junk food, yet they avoid natural, whole grains, which might significantly benefit their health. Whole grains are some of the best sources of nutritional support, containing high levels of dietary fiber and B vitamins. Because the body absorbs them slowly (due to the fiber), grains provide long-lasting energy and help promote satiety. Whole grains can especially help people who struggle with maintaining a steady level of blood sugar. Whole grains release sugar into the bloodstream slowly, in contrast to the sudden rush and energy crash caused by refined sugary foods and sodas.

Sally Fallon Morell points out that people traditionally soaked or fermented their grains, often for a few days before cooking. Soaking grains, or fermenting them by soaking in hot water with vinegar, reduces the phytic acid and makes the grains easier to digest. All grains contain phytic acid in the outer layer of the bran. Phytic acid combines with certain minerals in the body, such as calcium, magnesium, copper, and iron, and can block absorption in the intestines, which may lead to digestive disorders, mineral deficiencies, and bone loss. Eight hours of soaking in warm water will significantly reduce the phytic acid and greatly improve the nutritional benefits of grains. Even an hour of soaking will help. If you have difficulty digesting grains, you may want to try soaking them overnight.

The most common grain in our culture is wheat. Some people may be sensitive to wheat and not know it. Wheat products are heavily subsidized, and the food industry incorporates it into almost all breakfast cereals, cookies, cakes, and crackers. Gluten, a protein found in wheat, barley, and rye, is difficult for some to digest. If you are sensitive to gluten, you can experience bloating, constipation, diarrhea, or gas after eating wheat and other glutinous grains. Other related problems are brain fog, chronic indigestion, and candida. In more severe cases, someone might have celiac disease, which causes an autoimmune reaction to gluten that damages absorption sites in the small intestine. If you are allergic, you may experience hives or have difficulty breathing, and need to remove all gluten from your diet. Sometimes the symptoms occur immediately after eating, but they can also take time to manifest. If you think you have a gluten sensitivity, experiment with removing or reducing wheat and gluten products from your diet for a couple of weeks, and see how you feel. During that time, stick with gluten-free grains, such as amaranth, brown rice, buckwheat, millet, quinoa, sorghum, and teff.

Creating Great Grains

- Measure the grain. Rinse. Remove any unwanted material.
- Optional: Soak for 1 to 8 hours, to eliminate phytic acid and make the grain more digestible. Drain the grain, and discard the soaking water.
- Add grain to recommended amount of water, and bring to a boil.
- A pinch of sea salt or piece of kombu may be added to all grains except amaranth, kamut, and spelt (it interferes with cooking time for these).
- Reduce heat, cover, and simmer for the recommended time.
- Check your grains halfway through and near the end of cooking to determine whether they are done or if more liquid is needed. If too much liquid has been added, remove the lid, and boil off excess. You can change the texture of grains like quinoa, millet, and buckwheat with different cooking methods. Bringing the liquid to a boil before adding the grain will keep grains separate, like rice. Boiling the grains and liquid together will create a softer, porridge-like consistency.
- Tip: To reheat cooked grains, simply add a bit more liquid, and reheat on low on the stove.

4. Increase Sweet Vegetables

Almost everyone craves sweets. Instead of depending on processed sugar, you can add more naturally sweet flavor to your daily diet and dramatically reduce sweet cravings. Certain vegetables have a deep, sweet flavor when cooked, like corn, carrots, onions, beets, winter squash (butternut, buttercup, delicata, hubbard, and kabocha), sweet potatoes, and yams. Some lesser-known vegetables that are semi-sweet are turnips, parsnips, and rutabagas. And there is another group of vegetables that don't taste sweet but have an effect on the body similar to that of sweet vegetables. These include red radishes, daikon radish, green cabbage, red cabbage, and burdock. Because many of these vegetables are root vegetables, they are energetically grounding, helping to balance out the spacy feeling people often experience after eating other sweets. Other delicious ways to incorporate sweet vegetables into your daily diet include eating raw carrots, baking sweet potato fries, roasting squash, making soup with corn and onions, or boiling beets to put on top of your salad.

Serving Up a Sweet Sensation

A simple way to cook sweet vegetables is to follow a recipe I call "Sweet Sensation." It has few ingredients, and preparation time is minimal.

- Use one to five of the sweet vegetables mentioned above.
- Chop the hard vegetables, like carrots and beets, into small pieces
- Cut the softer vegetables, like onions and cabbage, into large chunks
- Add enough water to a medium-sized pot to barely cover the vegetables. You may want to check the water level while cooking, and add more water if needed. Remember, vegetables on the bottom will get cooked more than the ones on the top. Cook to desired softness. The softer the vegetables get, the sweeter they become.
- Add any of the following ingredients: Spices, salt, and/or seaweed. You may also add tofu or beans for extra protein.
- When the vegetables are cooked to your satisfaction, empty the ingredients into a large bowl, flavor as desired, and eat. The leftover cooking water makes a delicious, sweet sauce and is a healing, soothing tonic to drink by itself.

5. Increase Leafy Green Vegetables

If vegetables are the scarcest food in the Western diet, leafy green vegetables are lacking most of all. Learning to cook and eat greens is essential for creating lasting health. The color green is associated with spring, a time of renewal, refreshment, and vital energy. In Asian medicine, green is related to the liver, emotional stability, and creativity. Nutritionally, greens are high in calcium, magnesium, iron, potassium, phosphorous, and vitamins A, C, and K. They are crammed with fiber, folate, chlorophyll, and many other micronutrients and phytochemicals.

Some of the benefits gained from eating dark leafy greens are:

- blood purification
- reduced cancer risk
- improved circulation
- immune strengthening
- promotion of healthy intestinal flora
- improved liver, gallbladder, and kidney function
- reduction of congestion, especially in lungs, and reduction of mucus

When most people hear "leafy green vegetables," they probably think of iceberg lettuce, but the ordinary, pale lettuce in restaurant salads doesn't have the power-packed goodness of other greens.

You can choose from a variety of greens. Broccoli is very popular among adults and children—each stem is like a tree trunk, giving you strong, grounded energy. But remember to be adventurous and try greens you've never seen before. Rotate between bok choy, napa cabbage, kale, collards, watercress, mustard greens, broccoli rabe, dandelion, and other leafy greens. Arugula, endive, chicory, lettuce, mesclun, and wild greens are generally eaten raw. Get into the habit of adding these green vegetables to your diet as often as possible. Nourishing yourself with greens will naturally crowd out less health-supportive foods. Try it for a month, and see how you feel.

Cooking Greens

Try a variety of preparation methods like steaming, boiling, sautéing in oil, water sautéing, waterless cooking, or chopped in salads. Boiling makes greens plump and relaxed. I recommend boiling for under a minute so that the nutrients in the greens do not get lost in the water. You can also drink the cooking water as a health-giving broth or a tea, if you're using organic greens. Raw salad is also a wonderful food. It's refreshing and cooling, and it supplies your body with live enzymes.

6. Experiment with Protein

Protein is the basic building block of the human structure, helping our bodies form muscles, skin, and hair. Because of our bio-individuality, protein requirements vary dramatically from person to person. I recommend experimenting with reducing or increasing your protein intake, trying different sources, animal and vegetable, and noticing the impact on your body. So many people today eat way too much protein. Some people need protein-rich foods more often because of their constitution or dietary needs like iron deficiency. Low protein can lead to low energy and a variety of cravings. On the other hand, many people feel lighter and clearer and notice a decrease in physical symptoms when they reduce animal protein in their diet. Disorders such as heart disease, cancer, obesity, and high blood pressure can all be linked to an excess of animal foods. People often find that reducing animal protein consumption helps clear up constipation, low energy, body odor, and sugar cravings.

Vegetarian and vegan people often attempt to get their protein needs met through beans and bean products. Some individuals may find beans difficult to digest, but little things like choosing smaller beans (like lentils), cooking with a piece of kombu, or cooking for slightly longer than normal may help to facilitate digestion as these foods are introduced into the diet. In Mexico and Central America, where beans are a fundamental part of the daily diet, the most frequent bean dish is refried beans. The beans are cooked then fried in oil or butter to ensure easier digestion. A similar situation exists in Japanese cuisine with soybeans. Rarely, if ever, do the Japanese eat soybeans unless the beans have first been fermented or aged. They convert the beans into foods like miso, soy sauce, tempeh, and natto. They also eat tofu in small amounts.

Soy is a popular, and sometimes controversial, ingredient derived from the soybean legume. It is a complete protein rich in calcium, iron, magnesium, fiber, and potassium. Soy is a typical replacement for dairy and/or meat in the diets of vegetarians and vegans. Although it may be considered a health food, not all soy products are created equal.

Soy products, both fermented and unfermented, range in their degree of processing, from soy flour and soy protein to more traditional foods like miso, tempeh, and tofu. Highly processed items to limit include soy cheese, soy yogurt, and imitation meats. Focus on traditional forms to maintain the soy's nutrient density, and keep in mind that nearly 95% of soy products come from GMO beans, so if you want to limit your consumption of these foods, opt for organic soy.

Some research shows that a certain chemical found in soy, called genistein, can potentially damage fertility, especially in men. Traditionally, in Zen monasteries, men would eat tofu to help reduce their sex drive so they could sustain a celibate lifestyle. So men, if you want to be celibate, tofu is a great food for you. However, if that is not your mission, you may want to avoid eating too much tofu. Soy isoflavones can also increase estrogen activity, and some research shows that consuming soy products during menopause can ease some of the negative symptoms that some women experience. But other research links increased estrogen activity to higher risks of developing breast cancer. In general, much research is still needed on the effects of soy. My basic advice is to eat soy in moderation and listen to your body.

For those who don't eat meat but who are okay with eating animal products, eggs may be a good source of protein. High-quality yogurt may also be a good option for those who are not lactose intolerant. I strongly encourage buying organic eggs and dairy that are free from hormones and antibiotics.

When it comes to animal-based sources of protein, I encourage you to seek out variety. Many Western diets rely on beef, but you can try other meats, such as duck, pheasant, buffalo, lamb, chicken, and fish, and rotate these in your diet to avoid the stagnancy and health concerns associated with excess beef consumption, including heart disease, high blood pressure, constipation, and high cholesterol. Quality of meat is really important, and organic is always the best option. Search for humane and more sustainable options whenever possible. As I mentioned before, we take in an animal's energy when we eat it. Wouldn't you rather take in the energy of an animal that was treated humanely throughout its lifetime?

When deciding how much animal food to eat with a meal, I urge you to follow the guidance of Dr. Barry Sears. He recommends eating a piece of meat "no bigger and no thicker than the palm of your hand." A proper serving is about 3 ounces per portion and a much healthier choice than having a huge slab of meat as a main course. Think quality not quantity.

Again, there is no right and wrong here. Food is not religion. No special heaven is reserved for vegetarians. So please find the fuel that is most suitable for your current needs. Finding the optimum protein intake is a key to a balanced, healthy life.

7. Eat Fewer Processed Foods

One of the biggest hurdles to having a healthy diet these days is avoiding the bounty of highly processed junk foods available. These foods are typically found in boxes, cans, bags, and bottles, i.e. soda, crackers, candy, and more. But notice I still said eat less, not eliminate completely. That's because not all processed foods are created equal. Remember, processing a food could be as simple as grinding coffee beans, shredding carrots, or buying spinach in a bag. These minimally processed foods are convenient and generally healthy. You may also find processed foods like canned tomatoes (cooking tomatoes actually makes the nutrients more available) or frozen veggies that are picked at their peak and stored for later use useful. But when it comes to a bag of chips with a long list of ingredients or refining a grain and removing its more nutritious parts, these are the foods to reduce as much as possible.

The problem with highly processed foods is that they have become too common for most people. One study[3] found that almost 58 percent of all calories consumed in the U.S. alone come from these ultra-processed foods. Highly refined foods can be a major contributor to inflammation, a precursor to many chronic disease states. Most people who reduce processed junk foods in their daily diet feel more energized. If someone is already sick, cutting back on these foods can help to support recovery and vitality.

I think where people struggle the most is with processed foods that seem healthy, such as salad dressing or canned vegetable soups, which can contain added sugars, preservatives, or unhealthy fats. You need to be a food detective and read labels to determine what works for you. My easy rule is that if the list is too long or has ingredients I don't recognize, I just put it down. The good news is that you can make your own salad dressing at home in less than five minutes by whisking together olive oil, lemon, mustard, and maybe some chopped garlic or shallots. A great way to practice cooking and avoid more highly processed foods in your diet is to make more of your own sauces, dressings, and snacks.

I would rather *add in* than take away from anyone's diet—a process I call crowding out. This concept is simple: Focus on *adding more good things* into your diet as opposed to reducing the not-so-good. By adding more real, whole foods without trying to change everything all at once, a natural cycle of abundance and curiosity sets in that gradually "crowds out" the junk foods. You'll find that your preferences change with time, and it will become much easier to have balance in your food choices. You can explore a diverse diet of different colors and textures, including vegetables and fruit, grains, different sources of protein, legumes, nuts, and seeds. It doesn't matter if you're an omnivore, vegetarian, macrobiotic, dairy-free, or any combination of them all. The most important thing you'll learn is how to truly listen to your body.

When you are surrounded by highly processed convenient foods, find strategies you can use to choose more whole food options. Will you practice making more of your own foods, give yourself more time at the store to read labels, or simply start by replacing highly processed foods with more minimally processed foods? The choice is yours.

8. Make a Habit of Nurturing Your Body

The tongue cleaner, hot water bottle, and hot towel scrub are three of my favorite daily tools to establish a loving relationship with the body. This relationship is a key component of overall health, and it's often overlooked by the medical community. Increasingly, I'm happy to see more people taking an interest in self-care. It's not just about eating healthy foods, but about deepening our connection with ourselves. Try some of these habits, or make up something new that works for you. The key is to find simple ways to consistently give back to your body for all it does for you each and every day.

The tongue cleaner, an inexpensive yet transformative tool, is a simple, thin, U-shaped piece of stainless steel with a blunted edge to remove gunk from the surface of the tongue. Dentists recommend the tongue cleaner more and more because it helps fight cavities by removing bacteria from the mouth. It also prevents bad breath, especially for people who eat a lot of dairy and build up mucus in the mouth, nose, and throat. The tongue cleaner comes from the tradition of Ayurveda, which says people who use them are better at public speaking, expressing themselves more thoughtfully, and speaking more sincerely and authoritatively. Some people ask if the same effect can be gained by brushing the tongue with a stiff toothbrush. Brushing the tongue moves the coating around and is helpful, but a tongue cleaner is more effective, since it clears out the deep deposits and generally keeps the area cleaner and more stimulated.[4]

The tongue cleaner also helps with cravings by cleaning the tongue of leftover food residue that could lead to cravings for those foods eaten previously. A clean tongue has fewer "food memories" on its surface. A tongue cleaner reverses the process of desensitizing your taste buds, which happens to everyone to some extent. It allows you to taste more subtle flavors in food so that you can eat vegetables, fruits, and whole grains with greater enjoyment. When old residue remains on the tongue, we aren't able to taste the natural flavors in whole foods. When you have a clean tongue, you will be better able to taste your food, and you won't need to eat as much, since you will have gained greater satisfaction from your meal.

A big advantage of using a tongue cleaner is that it enhances kissing by making the tongue sweeter, fresher, and more sensitive. If you are in a relationship,

I invite you to check this out with your partner. Make an agreement to scrape twice a day for one week, and feel the difference. The tongue cleaner takes just seconds to use, and it can easily be worked into your morning and nighttime rituals. You can purchase tongue cleaners at most health food stores or online.

It's an ancient and natural feeling for both men and women to seek some kind of warm coziness at night, and a hot water bottle can help create this feeling. It's also an easy and inexpensive way to heat up your bed before sleeping. For years, I've recommended people try using a warm compress on their bellies. The lower belly is the home of your Hara, the central balance point of your body, and, according to Asian philosophy, it is the center and source of your life energy. The Hara is the gate, the doorway to the universal energy surrounding us. Heat from a water bottle brings more energy and more blood circulation to the digestive organs in this area, which are really the engine of your body. It aids in digesting food and in unblocking energy that may be stuck after a heavy meal.

At bedtime, place an old-fashioned hot water bottle on your belly for about 15 to 20 minutes. Most hot water bottles today are plastic, so you'll want to put the bottle in a pillowcase or get a cover before placing it against your skin. On a psychological and emotional level, warmth on the belly may promote absorption and digestion of whatever feelings or mental input are left over from the day's events.

I get a lot of feedback from single people about how they dread getting into a cold, empty bed at the end of a busy day. After being introduced to the hot water bottle solution, some of them even start using two or three of them to create a soothing, comforting feeling that helps them relax and sleep better. It's a simple and effective way to feel nourished.

Women can also use a hot water bottle, similar to a heating pad, to help relieve the pain and tension associated with menstrual cramps. It conforms to your body, and you can use it at night and not worry about falling asleep with it. British scientists have proven that applying heat to your abdominal region actually deactivates pain at a molecular level, similar to the effect of taking over-the-counter painkillers.

The hot towel scrub is an incredible tool for relaxation, circulation, and detoxification. The skin is the body's largest organ of elimination. More dead cells, toxins, and waste products from the body get eliminated through the skin than through urinating and having a bowel movement. Stimulating the pores of your skin with a rubbing action allows them to eliminate better. The only thing separating you from your external environment is your skin. The hot towel scrub rejuvenates this living organ, creating a better two-way flow of sensory information between you and your environment. It's a great source of primary food because it creates a loving connection between you and your body. Also, the heat and friction may help to reduce the appearance of cellulite.

Here's how it works: Dip a washcloth into hot water, or hold it under running hot water, then wring it out, and rub your entire body with it for five to 10 minutes. There is no right direction in which to rub. Try head to toe, toe to head, toward the heart, away from the heart, whatever feels easy and natural for you. It's invigorating if you do it in the morning and relaxing if you do it in the evening after work or at night before you go to bed. It has a neutralizing and balancing effect on the mind.

Some people say it's similar to using a loofah or skin brush, but the added effect of using heat to open pores is very important. So, don't settle for brushing. Also, take the trouble not to do this in the shower. Instead, stand by a sink. It makes a difference because showering is such a routine, mechanical act. By the sink, you are looking in the mirror and seeing your body, and you are more present to the sensations the hot towel scrub is creating in you.

When I show a washcloth to my students and say, "This will change your life," they are naturally skeptical. But afterward, I get a lot of positive feedback, like "I can't believe how well this works!" and "I feel my skin opening up, vibrating," and "I've fallen in love with my body." If you use it for a few minutes every day, or even once a week, your body will thank you.

These simple tools really speak to improving the quality of each day. The tongue scraper, hot water bottle, and hot towel scrub are three of the fastest, easiest, and least expensive means of creating a loving relationship with your body and, in turn, a new level of health. You can also find other methods that work for you, like stretching your body in the morning, starting a meditation practice, or spending more time in nature. What nurturing habits appeal most to you?

9. Have Healthy Relationships

It's rare that I meet someone who feels entirely supported by his or her family, friends, coworkers, boss, and significant other. Sometimes the answer to getting the support you need may be as simple as asking for help from your loved ones or from a professional. Other times, the answer may lie in creating new relationships and letting go of the old ones that no longer serve you. Start by developing the relationship you have with yourself. When you find ways to nurture and love yourself, you will be better able to communicate your needs more effectively to others.

Figuring out what kind of love relationship works best for you is essential to your well-being. Love is food for the soul and nourishes the body, mind, and spirit. For some, a happy marriage early in life is their main goal. They are clear that they want to have children and build a firm structure for their whole life and for future generations. Others look for alternatives to marriage or wait until later in life to settle down with one person. Many people feel pressure from their families or society to get married and have children, while this is simply not the right path for some. It is important that you take time to determine what you want, and then work practically and positively toward it.

Some people love being alone, while others love being around lots of other people. Most people fall somewhere in the middle. I encourage you to find a type of love and intimacy that is appropriate and nourishing for you. Find the right balance of togetherness and aloneness, and know that these needs will change with time, just as dietary needs change and just as everything in life changes.

How can you make sure that the relationships in your life are nourishing your soul and keeping you healthy? Consider these tips.

Open Communication: In a healthy relationship, whether it is with your mom, best friend, or partner, you should have an open line of communication. If something is bothering you, talk to that person about it. If you are happy about something, call that person, and share your joy with them.

Mutual Support: A strong relationship lasts through the good and the bad. You should be able to lean on each other when you are going through hard times like a breakup or losing a job. If your friend is constantly coming to you with problems but seems to be absent from your life when you are going through a hard time, then it may be time to reevaluate the relationship.

Laughter and Fun: Celebrating in the good times is just as important for a healthy relationship as supporting each other through the tough times! Being able to spend time laughing and rejoicing with your loved ones will feed you in a way that food cannot.

We all need to discover what kinds of relationships work best for us, so take the time to look at your relationships and find people in your life who support you.

10. Enjoy Regular Physical Activity

A lot of people go to great lengths to make sure they are eating healthy food, but they don't bother to exercise regularly. Inactivity is more prevalent than ever, with 1 in 3 adults not active enough worldwide.[5] Movement aids digestion, assimilation, circulation, and respiration, and it is a crucial part of any healthy person's regimen. Many people don't like exercising. It's challenging for them to find an exercise routine they enjoy. Think about what you loved to do as a kid. Did you dance, bike, or hike? This is a good place to start when looking for a new exercise routine. Look for a gym or yoga studio near your home or on the way to the office where you can work out. It's important to find a location that's convenient and where the atmosphere is pleasant, comfortable, and welcoming. This will enhance your chances of going regularly.

Exercising can be an opportunity to reconnect with nature, perhaps by going to a large park if you are a city dweller. Research shows that exercising outside has mental benefits, too, including increased energy and feeling less tense.[6] Getting out to a rural environment—somewhere you can breathe clean, fresh air, hear the birds, and see the sky—on a regular basis can be very healing. We can live without food for months and without water for days. However, we cannot live without air for more than a few minutes, so it makes sense that air quality is essential to life quality.

11. Find Work You Love

Career can be one of the most dysfunctional areas of adult life. Many people resign themselves to doing tedious work in jobs, offices, and corporations that are not in alignment with who they are. They do this not for a day, a week, or a month but for years and even decades. Sometimes they are working in fields that are diametrically opposed to their own personal values. As a long-term lifestyle, this path is bound to affect their health. If you are one of these people, I encourage you to explore potential options to proactively improve or remedy the situation. Do you believe we are spiritual beings in a material world? If so, I think you'll agree that what we do all day, every day is central to why we are here.

Many people feel trapped in jobs because they have a retirement fund, 401(k) plan, or accrued benefits. They know they should leave, but they have a mortgage or bills to pay. And they just need to work a few more years before they can quit or retire. If this describes you, the challenge is to find a way to love the work you have. You can try making your office environment more attractive, identifying people at work who can be allies, and avoiding people who are irritating. Get an office with a nice view if you can. Use a comfortable chair that supports your back, and take stretch breaks every hour.

You can also try to identify what isn't working in your job on a personal level and find ways to address these issues. Maybe your deadlines are too quick, and you have problems with procrastination. Or maybe you have a hard time communicating with large groups because you are shy. Maybe you feel you are overqualified for your position and feel bored at work. Instead of putting all the blame on your work environment, see what you can learn from your current situation and how you can make changes. Research local seminars on organization, public speaking, or continued learning in your field. You may be surprised to find that when you make changes in yourself, your job may feel more fulfilling.

12. Develop a Spiritual Practice

Spirituality is what gives depth and meaning to life, creating the feeling of divine order and harmony that exists above and beyond human limitations. Spirituality, like food, comes in all forms. I don't recommend a specific path, but I encourage people to have a spiritual practice. For some, this means embracing their religion of birth, following the traditions of their ancestors, and seeking depth through prayer and with God. Others feel discontented with the past and explore new avenues, such as meditation, mindfulness, or the religion of their partner. Some people blend together different religions or spiritual practices that align most with their values, which I call "integrative religion." For people who are agnostic or atheist, being spiritual may mean going for a walk in the late evening and feeling the vastness of the night sky or walking by the ocean and enjoying the sense of infinite, endless space. It has been my experience that when people feel connected with the big picture, they get healthier faster. We all crave meaning and purpose in life, and developing a spiritual practice can help us feel connected and deeply committed to our lives.

If the idea of developing a spiritual practice sounds overwhelming, you might begin with ways to keep your spirit lifted. You may find doing random acts of kindness for others or unplugging for an hour at the end of the day could be the perfect avenue to experience this part of life. For others, you may schedule time to attend church, read inspirational texts, or attend a silent retreat. Ram Dass, author of the best-selling book *Be Here Now*,[7] says that when he wakes up each morning, he takes time to read a spiritual passage. He keeps books by his bed to help him remember to keep up this regular practice.

Sometimes the biggest challenge when it comes to something new is simply the act of beginning. Start small, and don't overcomplicate it. If you aren't sure what kind of practice you want to develop, make time to talk with others, or research various forms of spirituality on your own. You may feel like you don't have 30 minutes a day for a meditation practice, so start with a set time that feels doable for you. Remember, a seed doesn't struggle to become a plant; it just takes the right amount of nourishment. Find a practice that is enjoyable and feeds your soul.

Exercises

1. Your First Step

Choose one of the 12 steps to try for a week. What will your first step be? What are three things you can do to support yourself in making this happen over the next week? Great! Now go and do them. Check back in with yourself after one week. How did it go? What worked, and what didn't? Are you ready to add another step? If so, pick the next one that resonates with you. If not, focus on maintaining the first step until you are ready to add the next. Continue this process until you are doing all 12 steps. Go at your own pace. You will see and feel the difference in your body, mind, and spirit.

2. Daily Journaling

For more support on incorporating these steps into your daily life, check out the *Integrative Nutrition Daily Journal: Your guide to a happier, healthier life*. This book contains daily, weekly, and monthly exercises to keep you on track with your personal goals around health.

3. Create a Self-Care List

Make a list of at least 10 things you can do on a regular basis to help reduce stress and care for your body beyond food or exercise. You can start with some of the examples I gave in Step 8: *Make a habit of nurturing your body*. Keep the list in a safe place, and regularly check in on how it's going. If you notice your stress levels on high alert, make more time to nurture and give back to your body.

Chapter 10

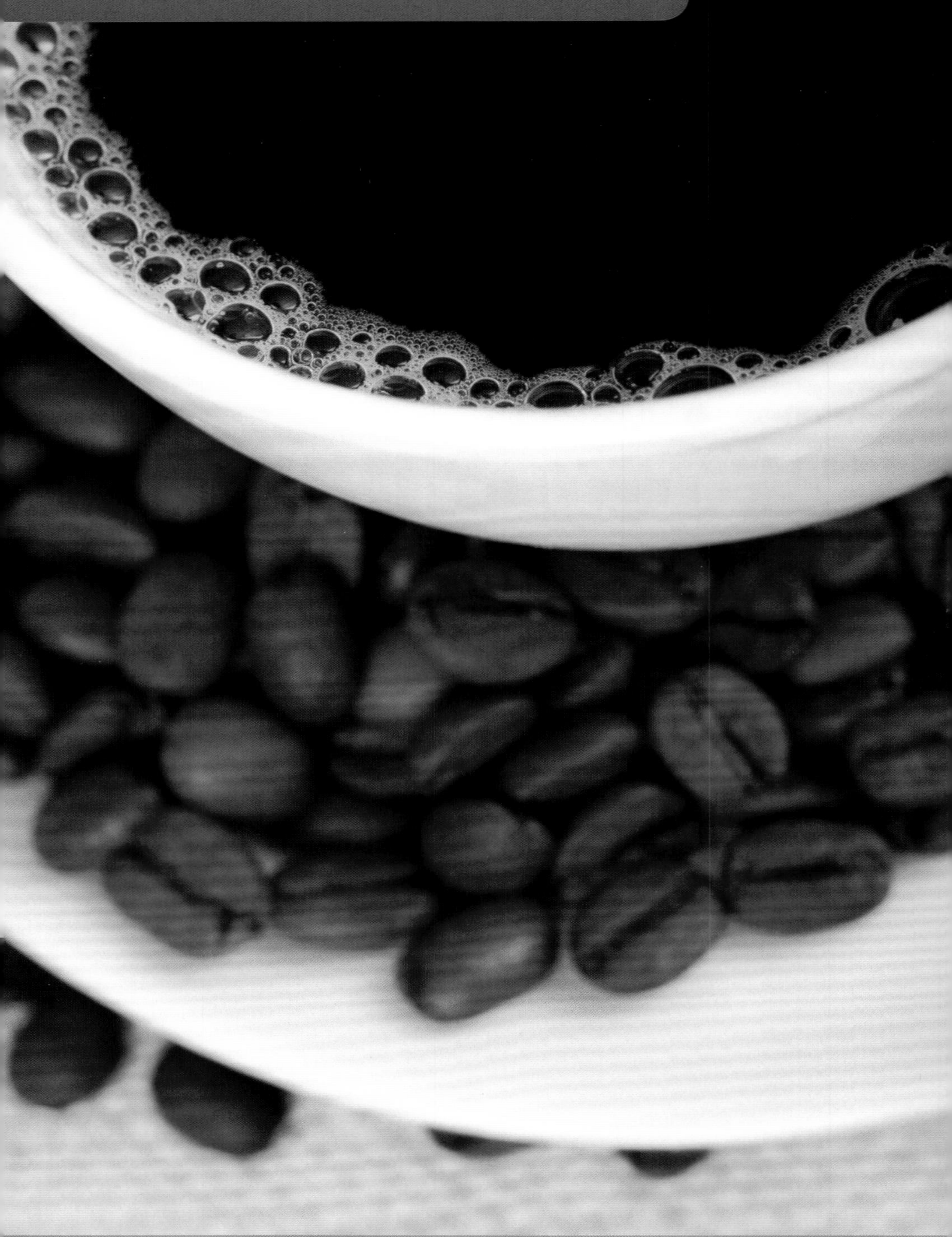

Dealing with Food Triggers

No foods are forbidden except when your body tells you so.

—Lima Ohsawa

By now you've grasped the fundamentals of maintaining a healthy diet. In spite of the enormous amount of confusing and contradictory information that regularly floods the world of nutrition, the basics are simple. Most people would be much better off consuming less processed junk food and increasing their consumption of water, experimenting with whole grains, and eating more vegetables, especially dark leafy greens.

I want to emphasize, however, that no food is innately bad. If you really want to have fried chicken, a burger, or ice cream, it's okay within the overall context of a healthy diet. I am not in favor of fanaticism or extreme food practices. As I've said before, it's not what you eat some of the time; it's what you eat most of the time that makes a difference.

Certain foods or drinks are considered "triggering," meaning they tend to set off some kind of negative reaction in the body or the mind. Not everyone is triggered by the same kinds of foods (because of bio-individuality), but, generally speaking, junk foods—the sugary, salty, and/or fatty ones—can mess with your brain's ability to regulate your appetite and cravings. Up until quite recently, the term addiction was only used for drugs that activate the brain's reward center, but now research shows that many of these pathways in the brain can be activated by food as well.

In some cases, foods are designed to make you crave more and more. Food industry scientists have revealed that they develop and test levels of sugar, salt, or fat in ultra-processed foods until they find what's called a "bliss point," or just the right amount to keep us eating more and more of it. Potato chip companies even capture this feeling using the slogan "Bet you can't have just one." It's true. These foods have been engineered to send signals to our brain to reward us each time we take another bite, leading to compulsive eating habits, and the effect can last for days.

These foods might make you feel out of sorts or act as a gateway to poor eating choices that can bring you out of balance. We tend to have these experiences when we've been "good" all week, then indulge in a trigger food and spend the weekend binging on other junk foods. Of course, everyone is different. Some people can keep one bar of chocolate in the house for weeks or months, slowly nibbling away at it. Other people may bring that same bar home and eat it that night. I invite you to notice and become aware of any imbalances with food in your life. It's so important to learn how to listen to your body and become your own health advocate.

Two helpful concepts when it comes to food triggers and other imbalances are moderation and mindfulness.

Moderation means having balance. If you enjoy eating something sweet once in a while, do it. Find the highest-quality ingredients. Prepare your food with love, and let it nourish you. As long as your overall diet includes a variety of wholesome, unprocessed foods, and you're not overdoing it on any particular food group, then you can indulge once in a while. If you follow the 90-10 rule and take good care of yourself, your body can handle a cookie or a glass of wine from time to time.

Mindfulness is being aware of what you're consuming on a deeper personal and environmental level. This means consuming more whole foods than packaged goods and taking time to slow down and enjoy the food you eat. Tune into how your body responds on a bio-individual level to each meal, and address health issues before they escalate.

This chapter looks specifically at some of the common trigger foods and drinks to give you a clearer understanding of how they may affect you, along with some of the history of how these foods became so popular. We'll start with the most challenging of all: sugar.

Sugar

It's no surprise that the United States is the largest consumer of sweeteners and one of the largest global sugar importers. Starting in 1689, when the first sugar refinery was built in New York City, colonists soon began to sweeten their breakfast porridge with refined sugar, and within 10 years individual consumption reached 4 pounds a year. By 2012, Americans consumed more than 130 pounds of sugar and sweeteners per year.[1] In contrast, Americans consumed an average of about 5.6 pounds of broccoli.[2]

While the U.S. might have the biggest sweet tooth in the world, you can certainly find pastries, candies, and other treats throughout the globe. Germany is the second most sugar-loving country, with the Netherlands and Ireland not far behind. The World Health Organization recommends that adults and children should limit daily added sugar intake to less than 10% of their total calories and that going below 5%, or about 6 teaspoons per day, is even better for your health. These recommendations are not for sugars naturally found in fruits, vegetables, or milk. Instead, they are talking about both table sugar and the "hidden" sugars found in many processed foods. For example, one tablespoon of ketchup has about 1 teaspoon of added sugars, and a single can of soda contains 10 teaspoons.

Humans love sweet things. Even before we started refining sugar, we sought out foods with sweet tastes. Sugar is a simple carbohydrate that occurs naturally in foods such as grains, beans, vegetables, and fruit. When unprocessed, these foods also contain a variety of vitamins, minerals, enzymes, and proteins. When brown rice or other whole grains are cooked, chewed, and digested, the natural carbohydrates break down uniformly into separate glucose molecules. These molecules enter the bloodstream, where they are burned smoothly and evenly, allowing your body to absorb all of the good stuff.

Refined table sugar, also called sucrose, is very different. Extracted from either sugarcane or beets, it lacks vitamins, minerals, and fiber, essentially only adding calories to the diet. These calories often end up displacing more nutritious calorie sources, so, instead of providing the body with nutrition, they may lead to deficiency. Refined sugar enters swiftly into the bloodstream and wreaks havoc on the blood sugar level, first pushing it sky-high, causing excitability, nervous tension, and hyperactivity, then dropping, causing fatigue, weariness, and exhaustion. Health conscious people are aware that their blood sugar levels fluctuate on a sugar-induced high, but they often don't realize the emotional roller-coaster ride that accompanies this high. We feel happy and energetic for a while and then suddenly, unexplainably, we may find ourselves arguing with a friend or lover.

Sugar qualifies as an addictive substance for two reasons:

1. Eating even a small amount creates a desire for more.
2. Suddenly quitting causes withdrawal symptoms, such as headaches, mood swings, cravings, and fatigue.

Today, sugar is found in many of the usual suspects, like cakes, cookies, and candy. But you will also find it "hidden" in baby food, cereals, peanut butter, bread, salad dressings, and tomato sauce. It is often disguised in fancy language, labeled as corn syrup, dextrose, maltose, glucose, or fructose. Even some so-called healthy foods contain sugar. Energy bars that are touted to give you lasting strength throughout the day can contain up to 20 grams of sugar.[3] Compare that to a chocolate-glazed cake donut, which can contain 14 grams of sugar. You may think your afternoon cup of coffee only has a little sugar, but a 16-ounce Frappuccino actually contains 50 grams of sugar—that's like eating three donuts!

Overconsumption of refined sweets and added sugars found in everyday foods has led to an explosion of type 2 diabetes and other health problems. Glucose is a type of sugar that provides energy to every cell in the body. Our bodies normally maintain blood glucose levels within a narrow range. A poor diet, especially one with an excess of refined sugars, can cause a gradual breakdown in our body's ability to manage blood glucose efficiently. When this happens, blood glucose levels may initially spike after a meal (hyperglycemia) and then crash to abnormally low levels several hours after the meal (hypoglycemia). This roller-coaster effect is implicated in the onset of type 2 diabetes. It may take years for pancreatic function to become so compromised that type 2 diabetes may occur, but the sooner you intervene, the better.

Worldwide, more than 420 million people have diabetes. Experts say that by 2040 this number will increase to more than 640 million people. The rates are increasing in every country each year, and it's estimated that about half of the people with diabetes are undiagnosed.[4]

When a person without diabetes eats something that creates glucose in the blood, the pancreas produces insulin in order to maintain blood sugar balance. Insulin acts as the gatekeeper, allowing the proper amount of glucose into the body's cells to be utilized as fuel.

In type 1 diabetes, which typically develops in childhood or early adulthood, the pancreas is unable to produce insulin. People with type 1 diabetes must rely on daily injections of insulin to keep their blood sugar from getting too high.

Type 2 diabetes usually develops much later in life, though recently it is on the rise among children and adolescents. In fact, type 2 diabetes was commonly referred to as "adult-onset" diabetes until the rates of children diagnosed with the condition became more common. With type 2 diabetes, the pancreas is still capable of producing insulin, but it may be producing less, with the insulin it is producing becoming less effective. One of the most alarming statistics in medicine right now is the rate at which people are diagnosed with this type of diabetes, which is far more prevalent than type 1. This news is especially heartbreaking when we know that reducing processed sugar and eating a healthy, balanced diet can help prevent the condition.

When people lose the ability to maintain a steady blood sugar level, the entire human organism is affected. A healthy body exists in a state of homeostasis, maintaining a steady balance within all systems that ensures smooth functioning for the whole organism. Take body temperature, for example. Somehow the body knows how to maintain a temperature of 98.6 degrees. If we get overheated, we perspire to cool down; if we get too cold, we shiver to warm up. Many systems in the body are designed to maintain this status. We know when to urinate so our bladders don't swell and explode. We know when to stay awake so we don't drift into slumber while driving and crash. The body maintains these interlinked systems by itself, for itself, without any need for conscious control. Maintenance of blood sugar is controlled by the hormonal system, which is interconnected with many other vital body control systems, including the sexual reproductive system, adrenal glands, thyroid, and pineal gland. The breakdown of blood sugar regulation can lead to the breakdown of other systems, until the entire organism is out of whack. Results from a large-scale epidemiological study published in 2013 showed that sugar has a direct, independent link to diabetes. California researchers looked at data on sugar availability and diabetes rates in 175 countries from the last decade. They found that increased sugar in the food supply was linked to increased rates of diabetes.[5] Elevated blood sugar is also associated with inflammation, which is the cause of many chronic disease states and also impacts our homeostatic functions.

Sugar Alternatives

One way to help reduce your intake of refined table sugar is to experiment with more natural sweeteners. Remember to use any sweetener with moderation.

Date Sugar

Date sugar consists of finely ground, dehydrated dates, utilizing this fruit's vitamin, mineral, and fiber content. If you like the taste of dates, this will definitely appeal to you. Date sugar can be used as a direct replacement for sugar, and it comes in a granulated form.

Honey

One of the oldest natural sweeteners, honey is sweeter than sugar. Depending on the plant source, honey can have a range of flavors, from dark and strongly flavored to light and mildly flavored. Raw honey contains small amounts of enzymes, minerals, and vitamins. Some vegans choose not to eat honey, as it is a byproduct of bees.

Maple Syrup

Maple syrup is made from boiled-down maple tree sap and contains many minerals. Forty gallons of sap are needed to make one gallon of maple syrup. It adds a pleasant flavor to foods, and it's great for baking. Be sure to buy 100% pure maple syrup and not maple-flavored corn syrup.

Maple Sugar

Maple sugar is created when the sap of the sugar maple is boiled for longer than is needed to create maple syrup. Once most of the water has evaporated, all that is left is the solid sugar. Maple sugar is about twice as sweet as standard granulated sugar but much less refined.

Molasses

Organic molasses is probably the most nutritious sweetener. It is derived from sugar cane or sugar beet, and is made by a process of clarifying and blending the extracted juices. The longer the juice is boiled, the less sweet, more nutritious, and darker it becomes. Molasses imparts a very distinct flavor to food. Blackstrap molasses, the most nutritious variety, is a good source of iron, calcium, magnesium, and potassium.

continues

Sugar Alternatives *(continued)*

Monk Fruit

Also known as lo han gu, this small green melon is native to Asia, where it was traditionally used to sweeten foods or drinks. The extract, made by crushing the fruit and collecting its juice, is up to 200 times sweeter than sugar, which means a little goes a long way. It typically comes in a concentrated powder, liquid, or granule form. Sweeteners made with monk fruit don't impact blood sugar levels, which makes it a good choice for those with diabetes. Just be sure to read labels to make sure the extract is not mixed with dextrose.

Stevia

Native South Americans have used this leafy herb for centuries. The extract from stevia is 100 to 300 times sweeter than white sugar. It can be used in cooking, baking, and beverages, does not affect blood sugar levels, and has zero calories. Stevia is available in a powder or liquid form, but be sure to get the green or brown liquids or powders, because the white and clear versions are highly refined.

Sucanat

Short for "Sugar Cane Natural," this brand-name product consists of evaporated organic cane juice made through a mechanical, rather than a chemical, process; thus, it is less refined, retaining many of sugarcane's original vitamins and minerals. It has a grainy texture and can be used in place of white sugar.

Coconut Sugar

This sugar is made when the sap of coconut palm trees is dried and granulated. It's a very low glycemic sweetener that is light brown in color and exhibits a rich, caramel-like flavor.

Yacon Sugar

This sweetener comes from a root vegetable in Peru that gets extracted to create a slightly sweet syrup. Yacon does not elevate blood glucose levels, making it a safe alternative to sugar, especially for diabetics and people with candida overgrowth. It contains prebiotic qualities that help promote calcium absorption and strengthen the immune system.

Remember, a small amount of sugar in the diet isn't the problem. The problem is the vicious, addictive cycle we have created by eating processed sugar, feeling the rush, crashing, and then taking in more sugar to begin the cycle again. If we are on a healthy, balanced diet, nourishing ourselves with milder forms of sweetness, we don't need a big sugar hit from a candy bar or soda to boost our energy levels. Unfortunately, more research shows that intense sweet flavors are as addictive as drugs like cocaine to our bodies. Sugar, and in particular high fructose corn syrup, are so overused in foods today that we are all left addicted and wanting more.[6]

When people look for alternatives to sugar, some find the $2 billion industry of artificial sweeteners, like saccharin (Sweet'N Low) and aspartame (Equal, NutraSweet). Although these products have been linked to serious health problems, such as cancer, public demand for sugar alternatives continues. Research shows that these substitutes actually cause weight gain by stimulating your appetite and your body's fat storage capabilities, even though they are touted as "diet" products.[7]

So, manufacturers continue to explore other options. Sucralose (brand name Splenda) has become a popular artificial sweetener. Splenda claims to be the perfect sugar substitute—as sweet as sugar with no calories, no surge in insulin, and no side effects or long-term health damage. Studies have found that Splenda is not so sweet. Studies show that it reduces beneficial bacteria in the gut, which impacts metabolism and leads to obesity and other health issues. Furthermore, Splenda is a synthetic compound made from sugar in a patented five-step process substituting three atoms of chlorine for three atoms of hydrogen-oxygen, converting sugar into a fructo-galactose molecule. This type of molecule does not occur in nature. So although sucralose tastes like sugar and sweetens like sugar, the body does not know how to assimilate it, which is why it has zero calories.

From a holistic point of view, it makes more sense to go with naturally occurring sweeteners, rather than artificial products. However, switching from white to brown sugar or coarse turbinado sugar is also not the answer. These alternatives contain 96% sucrose—not much of an improvement on the 99.9% sucrose content in refined white sugar. An easy way to reduce your overall intake is to just use less. If you are baking a recipe that calls for one cup of sugar, try using 1/2 cup. If you put three tablespoons of sugar in your coffee, try using two and then one until you are ready to try something more natural like coconut sugar. As you slowly decrease your sugar intake, you will notice your palate changing, and you will crave fewer sweets.

Italians have a saying, *la dolce vita*, which translates to "the sweet life." Let yourself live a sweeter life, and you may notice you will crave less sugar. Balanced primary foods can be much more satisfying than any sweet food.

Dairy

Of all of the triggering foods out there, dairy may be most linked to addictive behavior, according to scientists. Research, including questionnaires and brain scans, looked at why certain foods seem to be more addictive than others in the Yale Food Addiction Scale. Milkshakes and pizza came out on top! Of course, processed foods in general were the foods that gave people the most trouble, so chips and cake are in a similar boat. But when it comes to cheese, research has found that it stimulates the reward system in the brain. Casein, the protein part of dairy products, releases opiates called casomorphins when it breaks down in our digestive system. Some people can be quite sensitive to this reaction and crave more and more, thus creating the trigger.

But let's look back in time at our relationship with dairy. Female mammals in the wild nourish their babies with their own milk and stop after a relatively brief period of growth. After this time, young mammals never again show any interest in milk, nor do they have access to it. Humans are the only mammals who continue to consume milk into adulthood. The plain truth is we don't need dairy; sorry, cheese lovers.

I am not saying we should stop enjoying the wide range of dairy products available in modern society, but it is worth acknowledging that dairy is not an essential part of the human diet, and, in fact, most adults around the world do not consume it at all. Many of them can't because they are lactose intolerant, which means they lack the digestive enzyme needed to digest dairy. Many people also have dairy sensitivity that may contribute to health issues like congestion, asthma, skin conditions, and more. A brief break from consuming dairy often leads to surprising improvements in many of these health conditions.

Calcium Content in Dairy and Non-Dairy Foods*

Dairy	
Whole Milk	113 mg
Whole Yogurt, Plain	121 mg
Cheddar Cheese	710 mg
Non-Dairy	
Sesame Seeds	975 mg
Sardines	618 mg
Almonds	269 mg
Collard Greens	232 mg
Soybeans	197 mg
Dandelion Greens	187 mg
Dried Figs	162 mg
Amaranth	159 mg
Kale	150 mg
Fresh Parsley	138 mg
Mustard Greens	115 mg
Beet Greens	117 mg
Pistachio Nuts	105 mg
Spinach	99 mg
Sunflower Seed Butter	64 mg
Leeks	59 mg
Swiss Chard	51 mg
Buckwheat flour	41 mg
Broccoli	47 mg
Brussels Sprouts	42 mg
Wild Rice	21 mg

*Calcium content of foods based on 100-gram or 3.5-ounce portions.

Source: USDA, Agricultural Resource Service, National Nutrient Database Reference Release 28 in 2017

Modern methods of dairy processing are cause for concern. The typical cow produces milk for about 300 days after giving birth.[8] In an attempt to keep daily production levels high throughout this time, the industry began widespread use of bovine growth hormone, or BST, a controversial, genetically engineered growth hormone that is injected into cows to increase milk production. The manufacturers of BST claim the hormone has no adverse side effects on animals or humans, but many experts disagree. Canada and the European Union have banned its use.

In order to maximize milk production, dairy cows are kept pregnant most of their lives on both commercial and organic farms. During pregnancy, female cows' hormones, like estrogen and progesterone, go sky-high, and these hormones are present in their milk. There is both concern and evidence that high hormone content in dairy products is linked to high rates of breast cancer among women in America. I suggest women who regularly consume significant amounts of dairy products consider seeking alternatives, like the ones listed in the Dairy-Free Options section, or at least take care to improve the quality and reduce the quantity of dairy they are eating.

If you eat dairy, I strongly encourage eating organic. The organic cow's natural diet contains no added hormones, chemicals, or antibiotics. Studies show that organic milk contains higher levels of omega-3 fatty acids, vitamins A and E, and antioxidants.[9] On organic dairy farms, cows are raised on open pastures, fed grass, and not given extra hormones. While organic milk costs more than regular milk, I contend that it is worth it. Just make sure you are educated about its source.

Contrary to popular belief, dairy does not prevent osteoporosis or bone fracture by boosting calcium intake. In fact, numerous studies have demonstrated that countries with the highest intake of dairy, such as the United States, Sweden, and Holland, have the highest incidence of osteoporosis and fractures, while countries with the lowest dairy intake, such as Japan and South Africa, have the lowest rates of osteoporosis and fractures.[10] Harvard University's landmark Nurses' Health Study followed 78,000 women during a 12-year period and found that those who consumed the most dairy broke more bones than those who rarely consumed dairy. Healthy bones need calcium, magnesium, phosphorus, boron, copper, manganese, zinc, and many vitamins. An excess of calcium without these other vitamins and minerals actually increases the likelihood of fracture.

Vegetable foods high in calcium, such as collards, bok choy, and sea vegetables, also contain an abundance of magnesium and other minerals. Eating plenty of green vegetables, whole grains and sea vegetables can provide all of the essential calcium needed for the human body, without the added negative side effects of dairy.

For some people, dairy is an emotional issue. It's a food that provokes a lot of feelings and attachment, possibly stemming from early memories of breast-feeding. When I point out the hazards of high dairy consumption at school, many students adamantly refuse to give it up. If you have an emotional response to the idea of reducing or eliminating dairy, it may be helpful to examine the source of these emotions. Perhaps dairy is providing you with nourishment outside of the protein, fat, and minerals, nourishment that is not about secondary food nutrition. If so, try to think of other ways you can get this nourishment.

If dairy is not a triggering food for you, then enjoy it at the amount that feels right for your body. One of the plus sides of cheese is that it's a fermented food, and research suggests that the bacteria in cheese can be beneficial for your gut and help maintain your metabolism.

Dairy-Free Options

If you are choosing to reduce or eliminate dairy, these dairy-free options have you covered. It's all about bio-individuality!

Soy

Made from the liquid extract of whole soybeans, soy milk is a popular alternative to milk and has been produced in Asian countries for centuries. Plain, unfortified soy milk is a great source of protein, B vitamins, and iron, but it does have a strong aftertaste. This alternative is the most processed of the dairy-free options. It's not suitable for infants or anyone with soy allergies.

continues

Dairy-Free Options *(continued)*

Rice

Rice milk is made from blending brown rice and water. It contains more carbohydrates than cow's milk and has a lighter taste and texture. Commercial varieties usually add some type of sweetener and fortify the milk with calcium, iron, and B vitamins. Rice milk is the base for a popular Latin American drink called horchata, which is made with a blend of cinnamon, vanilla, and sugar.

Almond

Almond milk is made from ground almonds. It contains no lactose or cholesterol but is high in natural fats. Commercial varieties usually contain added vitamins, vanilla, and sweeteners, but unsweetened varieties are also available. You can also make nut milks with other nuts, including hazelnuts, walnuts, and Brazil nuts.

Oat

Oat milk has a creamy taste that comes from blending cooked oats and water. It's naturally high in fiber and low in protein.

Coconut

Coconut milk is a naturally sweet, white liquid made from the meat of a mature coconut. This milk is very rich, due to its high oil content. You typically find it canned, usually in the Asian foods section of a grocery store, since it's used as a base for many Thai curries. You can also use it for desserts and making creamy sauces.

Hemp

Made from soaking and grinding hemp seeds with water, this milk is quite creamy. Hemp seeds have an amazing amount of healthy fats, with a 3:1 ratio of omega-6 to omega-3, along with magnesium, calcium, fiber, and amino acids, making this drink a great source of vegan protein.

Meat

While meat is not necessarily a trigger food, excessive meat eating has been implicated in many types of chronic disease. Advertising and high-protein diet books emphasize the need to eat more and more meat for many reasons. Red meat is full of saturated fat and has no fiber and no phytochemicals, and any kind of mass-produced, factory farmed, commercially grown meat, whether it is beef, pork, or chicken, is loaded with hormones and antibiotics that are designed to generate the maximum amount of meat per animal, which means the maximum amount of profit for the producers. When you eat the meat, you eat the hormones and antibiotics. These animals are also subject to life in unnatural, confined environments and fed processed diets.

Commercially raised chickens spend their lives in tiny cages, crammed in with thousands of other birds, which leads to major stress and disease outbreaks. These chickens contain excessive levels of antibiotics, steroids, and growth hormones, all of which are fed to them in an attempt to keep them healthy and fat while confined in these unnatural conditions. Moreover, the fat levels of commercially raised chickens are more than three times the level of their free-range relatives. Organic, free-range varieties may cost two or three times as much as commercial chickens, but the price is worth it. Remember, too, that animals raised in factory farms suffer, and this suffering is passed on to those who consume their meat. I've already discussed how humans take on the qualities of animals we consume through cross-species transference, and we also take on their pain caused by being reared in cruel conditions.

Meat is something people either choose to include or omit from their diets. Some vegetarians and vegans are adamant in their belief that eating animals is inhumane. Other people feel as strongly about their need to eat meat to feel healthy. I believe people should choose whatever protein source feels comfortable for them. I pray for the day when all people can thrive on a vegetarian diet. But through my years of experience, I have seen many vegetarian-leaning people become healthier by incorporating small amounts of organic meat into their diet. I have also seen many heavy meat eaters become healthier after reducing the amount of meat in their diet. Meat is a very bio-individual food, and with this food group we need to focus on choosing quality rather than quantity.

Deconstructing Meat Labels

Organic

According to the USDA, the organic label means "produced without excluded methods, (e.g., genetic engineering, ionizing radiation, or sewage sludge)," produced per the National List of Allowed and Prohibited Substances (National List)," and "overseen by a USDA National Organic Program-authorized certifying agent, following all USDA organic regulations."

Natural

The terms natural and organic are not interchangeable. Only food labeled "organic" has been certified as meeting USDA organic standards. The USDA defines a natural product as "a product containing no artificial ingredient or added color that is not more than minimally processed. Minimal processing means that the product was processed in a manner that does not fundamentally alter the product. The label must include a statement explaining the meaning of the term natural (such as 'no artificial ingredients; minimally processed')."

Free Range

This term implies that animals are raised in an open air or free-roaming environment. The USDA defines "free range" as "producers must demonstrate to the Agency that the poultry has been allowed access to the outside."

Grassfed

The American Grassfed Association defines "grass-fed" cattle, bison, goats, and sheep as those that have eaten nothing but their mother's milk and fresh grass or grass-type hay from birth to harvest, or in other words for their entire life. Further, they are also raised with no confinement and no antibiotics or hormones and must be born and raised in the U.S. Pigs and poultry are "grass-fed" if they have had grass as a significant part of their diets. The USDA is reviewing its guidelines on grass fed marketing claims.

Pasture Raised

This term can be found on labels of meat, milk, and eggs to describe animals that were raised in open fields in an ecologically friendly manner. Some people consider this designation a step above organic. Always get to know your farmers or sources whenever possible, as this term is not regulated.

Marine Stewardship Council

This label found on seafood products aims to promote sustainable fishing practices. The council is an independent global nonprofit created to "ensure that the catch of marine resources is at the level compatible with long-term sustainable yield, while maintaining the marine environment's bio-diversity, productivity, and ecological processes." They work with various fisheries to maintain these standards and label fish accordingly.

Certified Humane

Humane Farm Animal Care (HFAC) is a nonprofit certification organization dedicated to improving the lives of farm animals in food production from birth through slaughter. The Certified Humane® Raised and Handled® label on meat, chicken, pork, eggs, or dairy products means that the food comes from farms where Humane Farm Animal Care's objective standards for the humane treatment of farm animals are implemented.

A funny thing happens to students at my school. Some who come in as heavy meat eaters may graduate with a more vegetarian-type diet, and some who enroll as vegans or vegetarians may leave as fish or meat eaters. When presented with the opportunity to experiment with food in a nonjudgmental, supportive community, people are able to find balance in their individual needs for protein.

Bearing this in mind, I generally recommend people limit meat consumption to a few times a week and supplement their diets with other protein sources, such as eggs, beans, and whole grains. If you are a regular meat eater, choose organic meats whenever possible. Many stores and restaurants now offer meat from small, local farms that has been raised in humane ways without the use of chemicals and antibiotics.

Caffeine

One of the most popular mood-altering substances throughout the world is caffeine, found in the coffee, tea, soda, or energy drinks that many people consume throughout their day. Caffeine is, essentially, an adrenaline delivery system that jolts the body's central nervous system to help enhance alertness, concentration, and mental and physical performance. In the short term, this jolting action wakes us up and gets us going. In the long term, the constant and unnatural stimulation of our nerves creates stress levels that damage the resilience of the immune system, which protects against disease. So many people rely on caffeine to keep up with the pace of modern life, and coffee itself helps to create the nervous energy of this pace.

Drinking coffee isn't just a matter of personal taste. It has become a cultural habit and a form of comfort. It's warm. It's foamy, and it tastes good with sugar, chocolate powder, or cinnamon on top. It's an enjoyable social moment, a ritual, and a symbol of dynamic, busy, working people.

Some like to talk about the aroma and the flavor of various coffee brands, just as they enthuse about certain vintage wines, and it's true to a point. But if you're knocking back a bottle of cabernet a day, it's not just the taste that's attracting you. It's the same with coffee. If you're drinking large quantities throughout day, you most likely have an addiction.

While a morning cup of coffee or a mug of black tea might be fine, you want to be sure that you are not using caffeine as a crutch to make up for lack of adequate sleep or the need to hustle through your day regardless of your energy levels. In the long term, this behavior is not mindful of what your body really needs.

Alternatives to Coffee

If you find yourself craving something warm in the morning, but you're experimenting with reducing your caffeine intake, consider the following options instead.

Dandy Blend

This instant dandelion beverage is an herbal coffee substitute made from dandelion, chicory, and sugar beet. Rich in minerals, this alternative provides extra energy without caffeine. Dandelion is known for its detoxifying properties.

Green Tea

Known for its popularity in Japan and powerful antioxidant qualities, green tea has been shown to reduce the risk of certain types of cancer and lower LDL cholesterol. Green, black, and oolong teas all come from the leaves of the same plant. What sets green tea apart from black teas is the way it is processed. The leaves are steamed rather than fermented, as they are for black teas and oolong teas. This steaming process is said to enhance its disease-fighting qualities. Green tea has about 30 mg of caffeine per 8-ounce cup. Many people describe its taste as earthy.

Oolong Tea

Oolong tea originated in the Fujian province of China. This tea is semi-oxidized, providing a milder flavor than black or green tea. Oolong is known for having digestive and detoxifying properties. The caffeine level is between the levels of black and green tea.

Pero

This caffeine-free instant-coffee substitute is from Switzerland and is made from malted barley, chicory, and rye.

continues

Alternatives to Coffee *(continued)*

Teechino

A blend of roasted herbs, grains, fruits, and nuts make up this caffeine-free coffee alternative. It brews similarly to coffee, can be used in a coffee machine, and has a similar aroma and taste to coffee. It has high levels of potassium, which helps to balance acidity. It offers a natural energy boost from the nutrients, not from the stimulants.

White Tea

White tea comes from the same plant as green, black, and oolong, but the difference is in the leaves. They are picked earlier in the season, when the leaves are young and the buds are covered with white hairs, giving this tea its name. White tea has gone through a minimal amount of processing and is not fermented. This tea has a light, sweet taste and has a small amount of caffeine, about 15 mg per serving.

Yerba Mate

Yerba mate is a species of holly, native to South America. It is prepared by steeping dried leaves in hot water rather than boiling hot water, as you would for coffee or tea. The flavor is bitter, herbal, earthy, and somewhat similar to green tea. The stimulants in yerba mate are called xanthines, which are similar to caffeine, although many people report fewer side effects. It also contains potassium, magnesium, and manganese.

In moderation, coffee does have health benefits, as it's a significant source of antioxidants, especially for people who consume an ultra-processed diet. Additionally, coffee consumption is associated with lower risk of total mortality and lower rates of Parkinson's and Alzheimer's disease, and it may even help protect against diseases like MS. It certainly affects each person differently. Some people can drink a cup of coffee or caffeinated tea at 9:30 p.m. and be asleep by 10 p.m., while others may be awake most of the night from one or two cups of caffeine in the afternoon. Quality can play a role in your overall health. A cup of unsweetened green tea or an organic coffee is quite different from a large sugary soda or an energy drink with a cocktail of mystery additives.

If you are interested in giving up caffeine, go slowly. Caffeine withdrawal is not fun, and people often report headaches and mood swings. I recommend quitting by reducing the number of cups of coffee (or energy drinks) you drink each day or by diluting full-strength coffee with decaf. Drinking water and healthy snacking throughout the day can help to crowd out coffee, boosting your energy through nutrition rather than adrenaline rushes. Rediscover the delights of drinking tea. Green and white teas contain much lower amounts of caffeine and can be great ways to get over the withdrawal headaches.

I encourage you to explore the role that caffeine plays in your life and see what works best for you. Can you enjoy a cup of coffee or tea mindfully? If you gave it up for a few days, would you feel okay or like you were sleepwalking through life? Heavy caffeine drinkers, consider what your life would be like with less. Think about your natural state as a person without all that speed. Maybe you would get to bed earlier, take more time to get places, or take a closer look at what foods really help energize you. Have you ever driven a car, ridden your bike, or walked through the same block in your neighborhood? Wasn't each experience completely different depending on your speed of travel? I often compare slowing down in life to riding a bike or walking instead of driving around town. In each action, we become more connected to our surroundings, and we take time to see with a new perspective. If you can't imagine a life without caffeine, simply find the highest quality available, and drink it in moderation.

Unhealthy Fats

Starting in 1975, government recommendations, food advertisers, medical doctors, and nutrition experts advocated a diet low in fat. What this fad failed to address was the difference between low-quality fats contained in junk foods and naturally occurring high-quality fats that can be beneficial to health. In the early 1990s a low-fat craze swept the U.S. Every cookie, cracker, and cake variety came in a low-fat version. Yet Americans continued to get fat. We became a nation of fat fearers, believing that eating fat made us fat. The truth is that our bodies need fat, and knowing what kinds of fats to consume and what kinds to avoid is not complicated.

Your body needs fat to nourish your heart, brain, nerves, hormones, and every cell. Fat is good for the health of your hair, skin, and nails too. Your body's fat storage is not necessarily related to the fat you consume. You could be overweight and still undernourished, especially if you are eating highly processed foods. Many people on low-fat diets feel hungry all the time and, as a consequence, overeat. Did you ever set out to have a few low-fat or fat-free cookies and end up eating the whole box? That's because there is nothing in them that makes you feel satiated. The brain doesn't get the "stop eating" message. You actually need the fat to feel full. Fat also makes food taste good. It carries flavors and smells more than carbohydrates or protein do. Cooks combine spices with a fat or oil, such as butter or olive oil, for this very reason. They know it makes their food taste great.

The four basic types of fat found in food are *saturated*, *monounsaturated*, *polyunsaturated*, and *trans fats*. All fats, or lipids, are composed of fatty acids, which are chains of carbon atoms with hydrogen atoms filling the bonds. The chemical composition of the fatty acid chains determines the type of fat. *Saturated fats* are found mainly in animal foods and tropical oils, like coconut and palm oils. The fatty acid chain is highly stable and straight-shaped, so these fats are solid or semi-solid at room temperature. *Monounsaturated fats* have a double bond, making them more flexible, so they tend to be liquid at room temperature and solid when refrigerated. Examples of monounsaturated fats include olive, sesame, and avocado oils. *Polyunsaturated fats* are considered essential because the body cannot make them and must rely on food sources to get them. The two polyunsaturated fatty acids found most frequently in food are omega-6 and omega-3. These fats have two or more double bonds, which makes them more reactive and unstable, especially at high temperatures. They also remain liquid even when refrigerated and can form free radicals when they are heated during extraction and processing or when used for cooking. These free radicals can initiate disease. Examples include corn, soy, safflower, and sunflower oils. So, although some of these oils seem healthy, they quickly become unhealthy when heated to high temperatures.

Trans fats are found in many processed junk foods, frozen foods, margarines, French fries, donuts, and other baked goods. On labels, these fats are listed as hydrogenated and partially hydrogenated oils. Trans fats are artificially produced by combining hydrogen with polyunsaturated oils in a process called hydrogenation. Consuming hydrogenated oil can interfere with your body's natural processes, leading to many health problems, including increased risk of coronary death. Thankfully, trans fats will be phased out of the U.S. food supply by 2018, joining European countries like Denmark, Austria, Switzerland, and Iceland, who have already banned them.

To beat the overall fat-fearing mentality, work on substituting good fats for bad fats. Choosing healthy portions of good fats can actually help you lose weight, increase your energy, boost your immunity, and optimize digestion. Coconut oil is one example of a good fat source that can help you lose weight, because the body converts it quickly to energy. It also contains lauric acid, a medium-chain fatty acid found in only one other naturally occurring place: human breast milk. Coconut oil is also more stable than other oils and can stand up to heat, which makes it a great choice for cooking. Other natural sources of good fats include avocados, olive oil, raw nuts, sesame and hemp seeds, and cold-water fatty fish, such as salmon, mackerel, and tuna.

Salt

Salt is not inherently bad. Throughout history, people have used salt to season and preserve their food. A good-quality sea salt can contain up to 92 minerals and can be considered a dietary supplement. Salt is composed of two minerals, sodium and chloride, and the average table salt contains about 40% sodium and 60% chloride. One teaspoon of salt contains about 2,300 mg of sodium. Sodium acts as an electrolyte and assists in regulating cell function, while chloride supports potassium absorption and helps regulate body fluids. We need salt in our diet every single day, but quantity really matters. The health problems associated with salt are from over-consuming the refined, processed, white sparkly salt found in ultra-processed foods.

The World Health Organization now recommends that adults consume less than a teaspoon of salt per day.[11] Yet most people consume more than twice the recommended amount. Most medical experts agree that diets high in sodium are a major cause of high blood pressure as well as pre-hypertension, both of which significantly increase the risk of having a heart attack or stroke. Today, raised blood pressure (hypertension) causes about 7.5 million deaths or about 12.8% of all deaths, according to WHO.[12] While excessive salt intake is not the only reason for these alarming statistics, it is a significant contributing factor. High blood pressure is the leading cause of preventable death in China, causing more than 1 million deaths each year.

Restaurant foods, fast foods, and processed, packaged junk foods contribute to the majority of sodium in our diets. Just one serving (half a cup) of canned chicken noodle soup has 890 mg of sodium, and one regular slice of cheese pizza contains 570 mg. If you have a full cup of canned soup, you've already reached your recommended daily sodium intake, and you're almost halfway there with two slices of cheese pizza.

Public health advocates claim that if we could reduce the sodium in processed and restaurant foods by half, we could save thousands of lives. My solution is simpler and more immediate: Master the art of home cooking. The next chapter will discuss how to get started on or improve your current routine. I strongly recommend using a high-quality sea salt for home cooking. For the most part, people today use processed, sparkling white salt that is stripped of the trace elements and minerals in high-quality sea salt. Food companies also put additives, such as sugar and potassium iodide, into refined salt. Potassium iodide is added to reduce iodine deficiency and thyroid disease, but it's actually been linked to the increased incidence of hyperthyroidism. All of this processing takes place to make salt less expensive and a prettier color, as natural sea salt has a brownish tint.

Using high-quality sea salt in limited quantities is a more nutritious and tastier way to get minerals and satisfy your body's cravings for salty flavor. Watch out for highly processed sea salts, which usually list magnesium carbonate as an ingredient. Look for sea salts that are free of coloring, additives, chemicals, or bleaching. They should have a reddish or brown tint.

Chocolate

I don't think I've ever met a person who doesn't like chocolate. Whether dark or light, sweet or bitter, chocolate has a widespread appeal in our culture.

Europeans account for almost half of the chocolate eaters in the world.[13] Americans consume more than 8 pounds of chocolate per person each year. The Swiss consume the most chocolate worldwide at close to 20 pounds per person. Part of why we love chocolate is that it helps release serotonin in the brain, which produces feelings of pleasure. This natural feel-good high may help explain why some people get such intense chocolate cravings. Its melting point is also slightly below our body temperatures, so it really does melt in our mouths. In a world that is becoming increasingly contracted and stressful, chocolate gives people a sense of expansiveness, comfort, and relaxation. In some ways, it's a really good food for people who are trying to gain weight. I have helped clients who were looking to gain weight add more chocolate to their diet with much success.

Chocolate encompasses a number of raw and processed foods that originate from the seed of the tropical cacao tree. The beans have an intense bitter taste. Cacao is high in iron, calcium, potassium, and antioxidants. It can also provide protection against health conditions like heart disease and high blood pressure. The Mayan, Aztec, and Olmec civilizations in Mexico and Central America first took these beans and mixed them with chili powder, honey, or vanilla to make a drink, creating chocolate. They considered chocolate a divine food. In Steve Gagné's book *Energetics of Food*, he writes that both the Mayans and Aztecs referred to cacao as a "food of the gods." Other research shows medicinal uses for chocolate, using it primarily as a means to deliver medicine. Cacao flowers were also used to treat fatigue, and cacao paste was used to treat poor appetite.

Of course, commercially produced chocolate does not contain many of these natural nutrients, nor does it have the same spiritual connection, although some people do create daily rituals around Hershey's or Godiva. One of the reasons chocolate gets a bad rap is because most chocolate sold in supermarkets has high amounts of added sugar, fat, and preservatives.

If you would like to experiment with chocolate in your diet, I recommend finding an organic brand with a high percentage of cacao—70% or more. Typically, the darker the chocolate, the fewer additives and sweeteners. Consuming raw cacao nibs as well as raw chocolate products found in health food stores or specialty shops is great options to reap the health benefits.

The issue of whether chocolate is good or bad really comes back to bio-individuality. Remember, one person's food is another person's poison. Some people are so addicted to chocolate that they may need to reduce or eliminate this food. For others, indulging in a small amount of high-quality organic dark chocolate every now and again can really be an enjoyable part of life.

Exercises

1. Become Friendlier with Your Food

Review the ingredient list of any food you eat this week. If it's a carrot, your job is simple: It has one ingredient. If it's a cookie, the list will be longer. Don't try to eat perfectly, but just bring more awareness to the foods you eat. What do you notice? Can you practice moderation and mindfulness with your meals and snacks? Do any ingredients seem to trigger you?

2. Try Reducing "Trigger" Foods

Consider the triggering foods within your own life. What role do they play in your diet? If you were to reduce one, which one would you reduce?

Why did you choose this food?

For one week, gently decrease your consumption of this one food and write down the results.

What is difficult about reducing this food?

What is easy about reducing this food?

Does your body feel different? Healthier? More energized?

How did reducing this food impact your cravings for other foods?

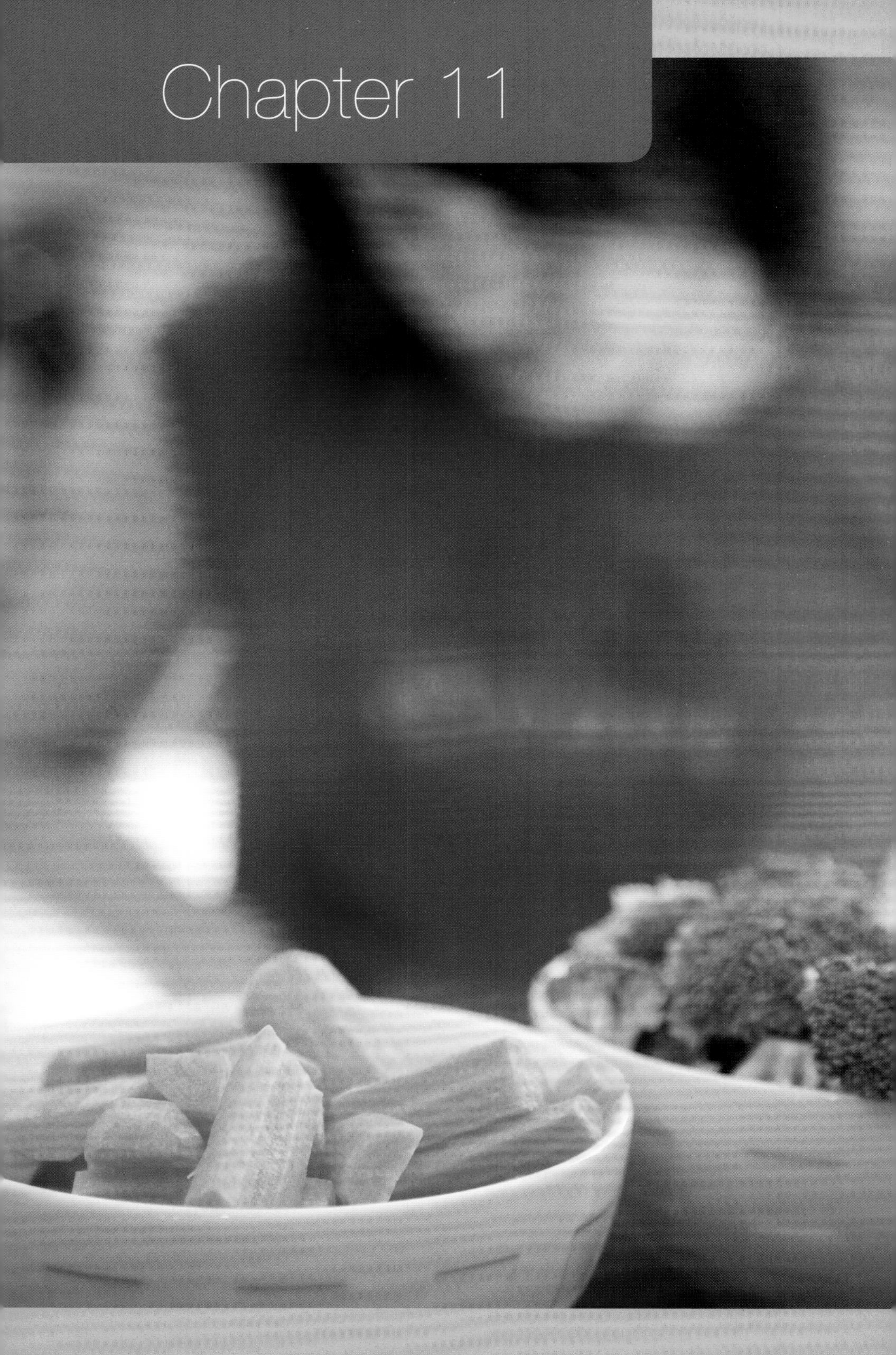

Chapter 11

Cook Like Your Life Depends on It

You don't have to cook fancy or complicated masterpieces—just good food from fresh ingredients.

—Julia Child

I tell people to cook like their life depends on it, because it does. The food we take into our mouth goes into our stomach, where it gets digested and eventually assimilated into the bloodstream. The nutrients we take create our cells, our tissues, our organs, our skin, our hair, our brains, and even our thoughts and feelings. We are, at our most basic level, walking food. Learning to cook high-quality foods for yourself and those you love changes everything. The three most important aspects of cooking are that the food be homemade, fresh, and made with love.

For me, there's nothing like when I am home and in my own kitchen. I get up, make some quinoa and vegetables and a cup of tea. When I'm home it's, "La-di-da. Maybe I'll add some ginger." It's so peaceful and so nurturing. It's strange to me that restaurant food has become so popular, minimizing the beauty and the value of home-cooked food. With restaurant food, people get caught up in the décor, the atmosphere, and even the menu. The food itself is often very flamboyant with lots of salt and flavoring. I love eating out on occasion, but the environment can be hectic. If I were at home and 30 people were moving around and talking in my kitchen, I would freak out. I understand that modern schedules can get busy and it may feel challenging to find time to shop, prepare, and cook all your own food. So, going out to eat feels like a timesaver. But once you master the basics of cooking, you may find that cooking at home actually saves you both time and money. It can be simple and easy, and for many people, it will transform your life in unexpected ways. What could be better than homemade vegetables and making food on your own time?

Homemade

Cooking nourishes our bodies on a variety of levels. When we put our own energy into the food, we ultimately put that energy back into ourselves. When we cook, we have control over the quality and quantity of ingredients we are eating. Our body's natural intelligence will fine-tune our cooking style to create meals that are just what we need. When we are in a restaurant, we relinquish that control. We do not know where the food came from, how much salt or spices were added, what kind of oil was used, the cleanliness of the kitchen, or the energy state of the people who touched our food along the way. By cooking our own food, we are in control of each of these factors and can adjust them to our needs.

As we have evolved from living together in tribal societies to living together in our extended families and nuclear families, meals have mostly been eaten together in groups. Not long ago, dinner was at 6 p.m. every night with few exceptions. Mom made the meal, and the rest of the family members would all come home from work or school and sit around the table together. The food would be served and everyone would eat while talking about the various events of the day. This ritual bonded people and helped foster familial relationships.

Today, everything has changed. People increasingly eat most of their meals out, in restaurants, delis, or fast food chains, or snacking along the way. Home is often like a hotel, serving only as a place for people to sleep at night. Parents, teenagers, and children wake up at different times, go in different directions, eat separately, and have little communication throughout the day. It's rare that everyone gets to have a home-cooked meal together. This schedule can create distance in family relationships, and the lack of quality, home-cooked food leads to a deficiency of primary nourishment. Of course, I recognize that everyone is doing the best they can, and I'm not suggesting we go back in time to traditional roles. Instead, we need to find creative solutions so that everyone can eat more nutritious food.

When families are dealing with two careers, longer working hours, and children with multiple extracurricular activities, it is unrealistic and unfair for the responsibilities of feeding the entire family to fall on just one person.

Everyone can participate in shopping, preparing, cooking, and cleaning. Just as sitting and eating together strengthens family bonds, so too can preparing a delicious meal together. Children can wash and peel vegetables, set and clear the table, and when they get older even help chop and cook. A good policy in the kitchen is that whoever cooks is free from doing the dishes. If you live alone, cooking doesn't have to be complicated. Find ways to prepare simple food at home so you are not reliant on takeout every night. Each household will be different, so please find a routine and system that works for yours.

Freshly Made

Food that is fresh affects us differently than food that's been sitting out for days. Think about the times you've been in a restaurant and a waiter passed by who was carrying a hissing tray of freshly cooked food, piled on a hot plate. The platter has so much energy that the whole restaurant turns around to see what is happening. We take in that same kind of energy when we eat food that's just been made.

Getting produce from the farm to the table is a complicated business. In Chapter 3, I talked about food miles, or the distance food travels to get to your plate. Many fruits and vegetables don't arrive in the store until weeks after they were harvested, then they sit on the store shelf for a few days and spend a few more days in the fridge at home. For many restaurants there's a similar delay, and food sourcing has become a big issue. Many restaurants have moved to work more closely with local farms to create farm-to-table or farm-to-fork restaurants. These restaurants locally source produce, meats, and seafood and put a bigger emphasis on fresh, slowly cooked foods, prepared simply. Some even grow herbs and produce in the backyard or on the roof of their restaurants. When you don't have time to make your own food, I recommend finding a farm-to-table restaurant to enjoy fresh, simple food.

Because of practical convenience, we often eat food that has been canned, sitting in a freezer, or made hours or days earlier. Sometimes we have to utilize these conveniences, and I'm not against it. In fact, I'm a big advocate of cooking once and eating two or even three times. Canned and flash frozen vegetables can be quite fresh since they're often packaged just after being harvested, and many stores now carry organic varieties. These foods are also a great transition for people looking to add more vegetables into their diets and are often more budget-friendly.

In countries where fresh food is valued, many people go shopping and cook vegetables on the same day. Most modern consumers, especially Americans, prefer the convenience of shopping only once a week. Wherever you live, I would like to point you in the direction of your local farmers. It wasn't that long ago that all food was grown locally. In the U.S. 97% of the more than 2 million farms are family-owned businesses. Many farmers now sell their products directly to the public through farmers' markets, food co-ops, CSAs, farm stands, and more. At farmers' markets the food is grown nearby, probably in the same county or at least in the same region or state. It's more alive, and this aliveness will transfer to your body.

Another way to have regular access to fresh, local food is to join a Community Supported Agriculture group. A CSA is when a group of people pledges to support a nearby farm in an economic partnership. The farm share model began in the 1960s in Europe and Japan in response to the rise of imported foods and urbanization of farmland.[1] Typically, members of the farm or garden pledge in advance to cover the anticipated costs of the farm operation and farmer's salary. In return, they receive shares of the farm's harvest throughout the growing season and the satisfaction of reconnecting to the land and participating directly in food production. Members also share in the risks of farming, including poor harvests from unfavorable weather or pests. Through this partnership, farmers receive better prices for their crops and gain some financial security. More than 12,500 CSA farms are in America today.[2]

Just as we have all kinds of vitamins in our food—vitamin A, vitamin B, or vitamin C—we still have a few undiscovered vitamins in the modern nutrition landscape and one of them is vitamin H, which is home-cooked meals. The foods you prepare at home and the foods that you eat in the restaurant have a whole different feel, even if you use similar ingredients.

Made with Love

After many years of personal observation, I've noticed that food prepared at home by a loving person has a different nutritional effect than the exact same food prepared in a restaurant. When we eat home-cooked meals, there's love in the food and care in its preparation, which creates a higher quality of energy. Invisible forces are at work, and they have an alchemical effect on the food itself. It tastes different. It feels different in the body. It affects us differently.

Foods made by someone you love contain another vital nutrient, which I call vitamin L, for love. Food that is cooked by someone who loves you, who is happy to be cooking and nourishing you, can be some of the best-tasting food in the world. The energy of love is passed into the food and nourishes you in ways that go beyond micronutrients.

Have you ever been in a restaurant kitchen? It has a lot of crazy energy. Having been in the restaurant business, I know there are huge discrepancies between what goes on in the front and the back. In the front, everyone is nicey, nicey. "Oh Mr. Rosenthal, good to see you," they say. In the back, people are throwing knives. Do you really think that energy doesn't affect the energy of your food? The people preparing most restaurant food are underpaid kitchen workers, living on minimum wage. I may be wrong, but I'm guessing most of these people are not in love with their jobs. This fact alone is bound to make the quality of the food we eat at restaurants very different from that of home-cooked food. In addition to the hectic energy, restaurant managers and cooks are pressured into reducing costs, maximizing profits, and getting food out on a very tight timeline. Their priority is to sell food, not to promote your health. Of course, in today's demanding world, we all need to eat out sometimes, and we all want to eat out and enjoy a new atmosphere. Just remember that eating out every night of the week can have an impact on your health.

It's a myth that preparing food is a complicated thing or that it has to look like Martha Stewart prepared it. When I'm at home, I use three to four ingredients, but when guests eat my food, they're like, "Oh my God. What's in this? It's so good."

Rituals can increase your awareness around cooking at home. You might simply wash your hands, put on an apron, or take a moment to close your eyes, take a breath in, and set an intention for the meal you are about to create. You may also want to light a candle or put on some gentle music—anything that helps you be more present.

The last few minutes of cooking are usually the most stressful. Everything has to be done at the same time: final flavoring, transferring from cooking pot to serving dish, getting the dining area ready. It's helpful to have a ritual at the end of cooking too, before you dash to the table, sit down, and start eating. Here are a couple of suggestions to re-center:

1. Pour yourself a glass of water and drink it slowly, to help you calm down and rehydrate. Cooks tend to become very tight—contracted and single-focused—and this simple act of drinking water helps ease you into a mellow, relaxed state of mind.
2. Serve yourself a small portion first and take a moment to smell the food and appreciate your gift of love through food.

When serving the food you've just cooked, please resist the temptation to apologize for imperfections. This habit will only focus your guests' attention on the limitations that you mention, rather than on their appreciation for your efforts. Instead, you want them to think, "Wow! Someone actually took the time to prepare a meal for me." If you are proud of your food, your family will enjoy it and appreciate you more, and it will help them remember the value of a homemade, freshly made, and lovingly made meal.

Cooking with the Seasons

In many parts of the world when we buy food at the supermarket, we are not buying what's really in season. In the U.S. we find mangoes and bananas in the middle of winter and winter squash in the middle of summer. When I pick up an apple at the store during the fall, I'm always amazed at how much better it tastes than in the winter. By following the natural harvest of fruits and vegetables, we can strengthen our connection to our surroundings. Cooking with locally grown produce is a great way to honor the natural environment in which you live. It helps you feel more at home where you are, and supports your body in adapting to changes in season. Of course, seasons are different throughout the world, but start to notice how you feel during each season and what kind of foods make you feel the best. For me, I know when it's warm, I'm drawn to more fruit and raw foods. When the weather starts to cool, I look for more hardy vegetables and whole grains. In the coldest months, I eat more protein and fat to help my body stay warm, and as the weather warms again, I eat more greens to help lighten my body. Eating foods out of season can lead to imbalance, making you more susceptible to colds, flu, and other illnesses.

You can also adjust your cooking methods for the time of year. During the colder months, put more heat into your food and cook your food longer. Try roasting, baking, using a Crock-Pot, and making stews to keep warm. When springtime comes, allow your food preparation to become a little simpler. You can start to incorporate more raw foods, quick sautés, and steamed dishes. Or notice how your body naturally craves more fruit, salad, and lighter foods during warmer months.

You may also want to consider how your lifestyle reflects seasonal changes. In the spring months, people feel refreshed, get their gardens going, start new projects, or spend more time with friends. When it's warm, people enjoy outdoor sports, play at the beach, go on vacation, and engage in other high-energy activities, which are appropriate for the season. With fall, children return to school and people get into a kind of organizing mode. People tend to become very busy in September and October, running around, getting ready for winter. I notice during the fall that many animals also scurry around in preparation for winter. Until recently, humans did the same thing, scurrying to see if we had enough food or wood to keep us warm. No one has alerted our DNA that we now have heating in our homes or that we can drive to the store anytime we need food; we are preprogrammed to act this way. We still tap into our ancestral, cellular memories of the harvest season.

All that preparation comes to a head with an extended holiday season that lasts from the end of October through the beginning of January. Come Halloween, children scour the neighborhood and gather as much candy as they possibly can. Next come the holidays, and our actions fall out of pace as we engage in the extreme sports of holiday shopping, partying, and eating. At Thanksgiving, Americans nationwide congregate and overeat. The next day everyone complains about how stuffed they are and goes shopping. Then we're into December, with office parties, family get-togethers, and social events that usually involve lots of food and drinking. This season leads to Christmas and more overeating, with a final blowout on New Year's Eve that entails even more eating and drinking. Other countries have your version of this cycle at this time of the year and others.

In North America, all this partying is happening when the normal, natural rhythms of life—colder weather, darker evenings, the end of the growing season—indicate this is the right time to turn inward. Humans are mammals, and mammals have a tendency to hibernate during the winter. They are not really sleeping; they are in a kind of battery-saving mode, a state not unlike meditation. But, oddly, Americans do the opposite. Instead of going inward, slowing down and replenishing our energy for springtime, society is set up to keep us burning the candle at both ends. Then, in January and February, people feel exhausted and depressed, and the country has a widespread outbreak of colds and flu. People's exhausted immune systems cannot cope with the demands of winter, combined with the inappropriate food consumption mentioned above.

Doctors have given a special name to the exhaustion and depression experienced during colder, darker months. They call it Seasonal Affective Disorder, or SAD, and attribute it to people not getting enough sunlight. If you have been diagnosed with SAD, I encourage you to go more slowly, respecting the seasons and eating and drinking more moderately. I also recommend finding ways to get more sunlight into your life at this time.

If you want to go to holiday parties, enjoy yourself, but be moderate with food and alcohol, and strive to get enough down time. Remember to keep up your own cooking with seasonal, locally grown ingredients and share with others during this season. If the majority of your food is healthy and homemade, the occasional party or indulgence won't affect you. In addition, your immune system will become stronger and you'll avoid getting sick in the wintertime.

Simplicity

One of the main reasons people don't cook is because they think they don't have the time. It looks too complicated, and they don't know where to start. From the very beginning, they feel overwhelmed. They may open a cookbook and see a recipe for lasagna that looks delicious but calls for a lot of ingredients and hours of labor. So they lose their initial enthusiasm, close the book, and forget cooking. Don't confuse taste with function. If you want a fancy, tasty meal, go out to a restaurant. You don't need to be a gourmet chef at home; you need to be able to feed yourself and those you love in a nourishing, convenient way.

Occasionally, you may enjoy making a complex recipe, but for daily diet, you probably want to have simple, down-to-earth meals that can be prepared quickly and easily. It takes about five minutes to prepare a piece of fish or meat, another five minutes to prepare greens, and less than 20 minutes of cooking time to get your meal on the table. If you decide to make a more complicated meal, prepare some ingredients, like grains and vegetables, freshly, and complement them with canned or frozen foods. With a little planning, you can soak beans overnight and reduce their cooking time for the next meal. Or if you're crunched for time, use organic canned beans. Cooking simple meals on a regular basis will lead you step by step to a simpler, more relaxed and enjoyable lifestyle.

Home cooking also saves you money. Many people unconsciously spend a lot of their income on eating out. People eat most of their meals in cafes, snack bars, and restaurants, and these outings can run about $30 a day or more—that's almost $1,000 a month. Although organic produce and meats are more expensive, I think you'll find they are still cheaper than eating out. Look for local produce markets with reasonable prices and shop for seasonal fruits and vegetables, which naturally have lower prices. Get familiar with your local health food store and the bulk foods section, where you can find many staples, including rice, pasta, beans, nuts, and even herbs. The bulk section not only saves money, but also reduces the amount of packaging waste.

Joshua's Keys to Healthy Cooking

Commercial Produce Is Okay

As I mentioned above, make sure you can get the freshest food possible, even if that means commercial produce. I know that organic options may not always be available, but fresh fruits and vegetables are healthful ingredients that will nourish you much more than ultra-processed foods.

Canned and Frozen Foods Are Also Okay

When using these foods, see if you can take a semi-homemade approach by mixing them with some fresh ingredients too. Remember, frozen foods are usually picked fresh and then frozen quickly, so they retain a lot of nutrition. Canned foods should be the last choice, as they're typically higher in added salt or sugar.

Organic Is Much Better

When you have the budget and access for organics, go for it! These foods will taste even better in your cooking. Organic is good for your body and it's good for the environment, too. Pesticides, herbicides, and fungicides not only kill the bugs, but they also pollute the soil and the water supply. So try to eat clean food without chemicals whenever you can.

Local Is Even Better

Local foods are always in season and many times available through your local farmers. When you know the people growing your food, you have an even deeper relationship with each meal. And sometimes local could be as close as your windowsill, if you choose to grow your own herbs or veggies.

Fresh Is Best

A good tip to remember when you're shopping at the grocery store is to stay in the outer perimeter of the building and try not to spend too much time in the inner aisles, where you will find most of the packaged food and the highly refined foods. Put your focus on fresh ingredients and whole foods.

Use a Timer

Just because a recipe takes 40 minutes to cook doesn't mean it takes 40 minutes of your time. Using timers helps you know what's due to be taken off the stove and frees you for other activities. People think if they make their own food, they have to follow a recipe and be in the kitchen for an hour or more. This thinking creates a negative attitude toward cooking. Maybe we don't really have much else to do, but the idea of waiting around the kitchen seems torturous. Timers allow people to eat in a healthy way without big demands on their schedules.

Keep It Simple

Rather than spending hours in the kitchen prepping elaborate meals, keep it simple. Save gourmet foods or complicated recipes as special treats, and instead cook with five ingredients or fewer. Part of keeping it simple can be prepping foods when you get home from the market so you can easily grab and go throughout the week. One great tip is to chop veggies and store them in glass containers with a little bit of water. You can also prep a big batch of greens for the week and use them as sides, as salads, or in smoothies.

Cook Once, Eat Twice

You don't have to start from scratch at each meal. I'm a big fan of cooking once and eating twice to increase the amount of homemade food in the diet without spending too much time in the kitchen. I always try to incorporate something fresh into my leftovers, by heating them with a little water, olive oil, and some fresh herbs, or sautéing carrots and onions and adding them to the dish. This gives my old food new energy and new flavor.

Whenever you cook, make extra. Take grains as an example. You can cook your favorite grain in the morning and use some for a hot breakfast cereal, perhaps adding some sweet flavor, like fresh fruit or raisins, and something satiating like tahini or nut butter. Then you can add some different flavor to the leftover grains, or put them into a soup and take it to work for lunch. In the evening, you can add vegetables and protein, and stir-fry the remainder with oil to give it some extra sizzle. You can also put leftover food into the fridge in small containers for a great, healthy, wholesome snack in between meals or freeze food for future meals. Cooking once and eating two or three times makes you feel like your investments of money on groceries and time in the kitchen were well worth it.

Vary Cooking Styles

It's easy to get stuck in a cooking rut. Don't be afraid to switch it up! Many different styles of healthy cooking exist, such as baking, grilling, steaming, quick boiling, stir-frying with oil, water sautéing… and the list goes on. If these words feel overwhelming to you, as they did for me when I first got started, you may find it helpful to invest in a good cookbook for beginners. You can also watch free YouTube videos on cooking methods that are unfamiliar to you.

Vary Flavoring and Condiments

One of the keys to an easy life in the kitchen is to cook food in a simple way, and then use condiments, spices, and other dressings at the table. Make a wide variety of flavorings available so everyone can personalize the meal to their own taste. Your best companion in this regard is a condiment tray or lazy Susan, a circular dish that sits in the middle of the table on a swivel and rotates with the touch of your hand. Stock it with your favorite condiments. Some love garlic, some love ginger and spices, others prefer more salt, less salt, more oil, or less oil. A lazy Susan can hold all of these, plus other standards like nut butters, sesame oil, tamari, and salad dressings. People love to personalize their food, and this method makes it much easier for the cook. A list of readily available condiments is at the end of this chapter.

Experiment

When you go grocery shopping, make it more fun by checking out other people's carts to see what they're buying. Try new recipes and explore new cooking methods. Don't be afraid to talk with the person stocking the veggies or the fishmonger to get ideas for new recipes or methods of cooking. Choose a new fruit or vegetable you've never had before and challenge yourself to use it! The more you experiment with new foods, the more fun cooking will be for you, and the more comfortable you'll feel in the kitchen.

Mistakes Are Okay

Try to keep your cooking simple. In the beginning, let yourself experiment and make mistakes. It's okay to burn the rice. Remember, everything in life has a learning curve. In the beginning, it will take time and may seem difficult, and you'll likely burn some foods and maybe some pots. But as you stay with it, cooking will become easier, more enjoyable, and hugely rewarding. Once you become confident, you will have a lifetime of delicious, home-cooked food for yourself, your family, and your friends, save thousands of dollars, and increase health, vitality, and family relationships.

Skip Self-Criticism

Don't fall into the trap of pointing out the flaws in your cooking or criticizing your efforts. Allow people to thank you, and ask for tips if something doesn't work out the way you'd hoped. At the end of the day, you are your worst critic! So whether you are new to cooking or you feel like a pro, remember that everyone has to start somewhere. Be kind to yourself and know that you will continue to gain confidence and enjoy your time in the kitchen as you continue to cook.

Notice the Effects of Your Cooking

Cooking for yourself is the best way to understand how you are affected by food. Since you know what you are putting into the meal, you can understand the food's effects on your body more directly. Maybe you feel sleepy after a meal and want to take a nap, or maybe you feel more active and have the urge to go somewhere and do something in order to generate energy to digest the meal. You will know if your cooking was too much for your body to handle, or if you feel unsatisfied and need more—an extra flavor perhaps or one more ingredient. I encourage you to explore, experiment, and learn to distinguish the foods and quantities that support your health from those that do not.

Healthy Restaurant Eating

Regardless of how hungry we are, we often find ourselves at restaurants ordering and eating large quantities of rich and heavy foods that we would never have at home. Most people don't realize it, but professional menus are designed to draw your eye to the most expensive food, or foods that are most profitable for the establishment. You need to sharpen your awareness to know clearly what you really want to eat, what you habitually eat if you don't stop to think about it, and what the restaurant owners would like you to eat.

When eating out, pause for a moment, keeping the menu closed, and take a moment to check in with yourself. What do you feel like eating right now? How hungry are you? What foods are right for your bio-individual nature? The restaurant menu is not designed to answer such questions. It makes food sound so tantalizing, you start thinking, "Oh my God, fudge brownie with drizzled chocolate and a few added twists of sugar-crystallized tangerine topped with whipped cream. That sounds incredible!" Your mouth is watering so much that you develop complete amnesia and forget your intention to be aware about what you are eating.

One way to avoid a few common pitfalls of eating out is to not read the menu. If you are out with friends, enjoying a social connection, it ensures you don't suddenly cut off from each other and bury yourselves in the menus, destroying the convivial atmosphere. It also invites a direct dialogue with the waiter, as you inquire, "What do you recommend that has some vegetables and some protein, either fish or chicken?" When the waiter comes up with a couple of recommendations, you can ask, "What does it come with?"

Keep in mind that restaurants have a lot of vegetables in the kitchen that are not necessarily on the menu. Ask the waiter what vegetables are available and if the kitchen can make a side dish of steamed, sautéed vegetables in olive oil and garlic, or any way you prefer. This kind of request will help you get accustomed to building vegetables into all your meals.

Be Flexible

Although I strongly encourage home cooking, I am not saying we must cook all our food or never eat out. It is important to have balance and a flexible attitude. Sometimes, it is healthier to go to a restaurant rather than stress out about preparing a meal. During busy times, I encourage eating at restaurants with healthy options and enjoying the food without guilt. Also, when dining at someone else's house, eating what has been prepared for all the guests can be extremely nourishing and healing, even if it is something we wouldn't usually eat on our own. It can be healthier to just have that piece of pizza, fried chicken, or ice cream cake, and not be singled out as the "healthy" one who always rejects other people's food. Remember the 90-10 rule?

Being too rigid in your diet can be isolating. Sometimes we just want to go out, eat whatever we want, and have a great time. And sometimes this flexibility can be healthier than staying home alone and eating high-quality healthy foods and chewing well. People can become overly obsessed with eating the "right" food, something known as *Orthorexia nervosa*. This condition can impede other important elements of life, including relationships, creativity, and just feeling part of a community. Either we avoid others because we don't want to see what they are eating, or they avoid us because they know we will disapprove of their undisciplined eating habits. Can you find a balance and not get stuck in either-or thinking? We want to relate with people as a friend, not as a preacher, and projecting our own food concerns onto others is a great way to lose friends fast. Let others eat as they wish, and learn to accept and enjoy their company, regardless of how many spoonfuls of sugar they stir into their coffee.

Exercises

1. Condiment List

Go to the store and choose a few new condiments to purchase. Keep them on the table at mealtimes so everyone can flavor and personalize the food to their liking. Getting a lazy Susan to keep on your table and store your condiments in is an option. Here are some condiments to try, plus you can add your own favorites.

Basic Spices
basil
black pepper in a grinder
cinnamon
cumin
curry powder
garlic
ginger
gomasio
oregano
sea salt
thyme
turmeric

Nuts and Seeds
chia
flax
nut butters: peanut, cashew, almond
nuts: pine, brazil, cashews, walnuts, almonds, pistachios
pumpkin seeds
sesame seeds
sunflower seeds
tahini

Sweeteners
honey
maple syrup
stevia

Oils, Vinegars, and Sauces
apple cider vinegar
balsamic vinegar
Bragg's amino acids
coconut oil
extra virgin olive oil
hot sauces
hot sesame oil
salad dressings
tamari soy sauce
toasted sesame oil
umeboshi vinegar

Sea Vegetables
dulse flakes
nori flakes

Other
chutneys
coconut milk
fresh limes or lemons
grated daikon radish
ketchup
mustard
nutritional yeast
sauerkraut or pickled vegetables
sliced cucumbers or scallions
sliced red cabbage
sprouts: alfalfa, sunflower, mung

2. Try a New Recipe

Now that you've read all about the benefits of cooking homemade, freshly made, lovingly made food, it's time to try a new recipe. The back of this book has many to choose from, so pick one and cook it for your family or friends. Be sure to get fresh ingredients and to cook with love, thinking about how the food will nourish both you and those closest to you.

Chapter 12

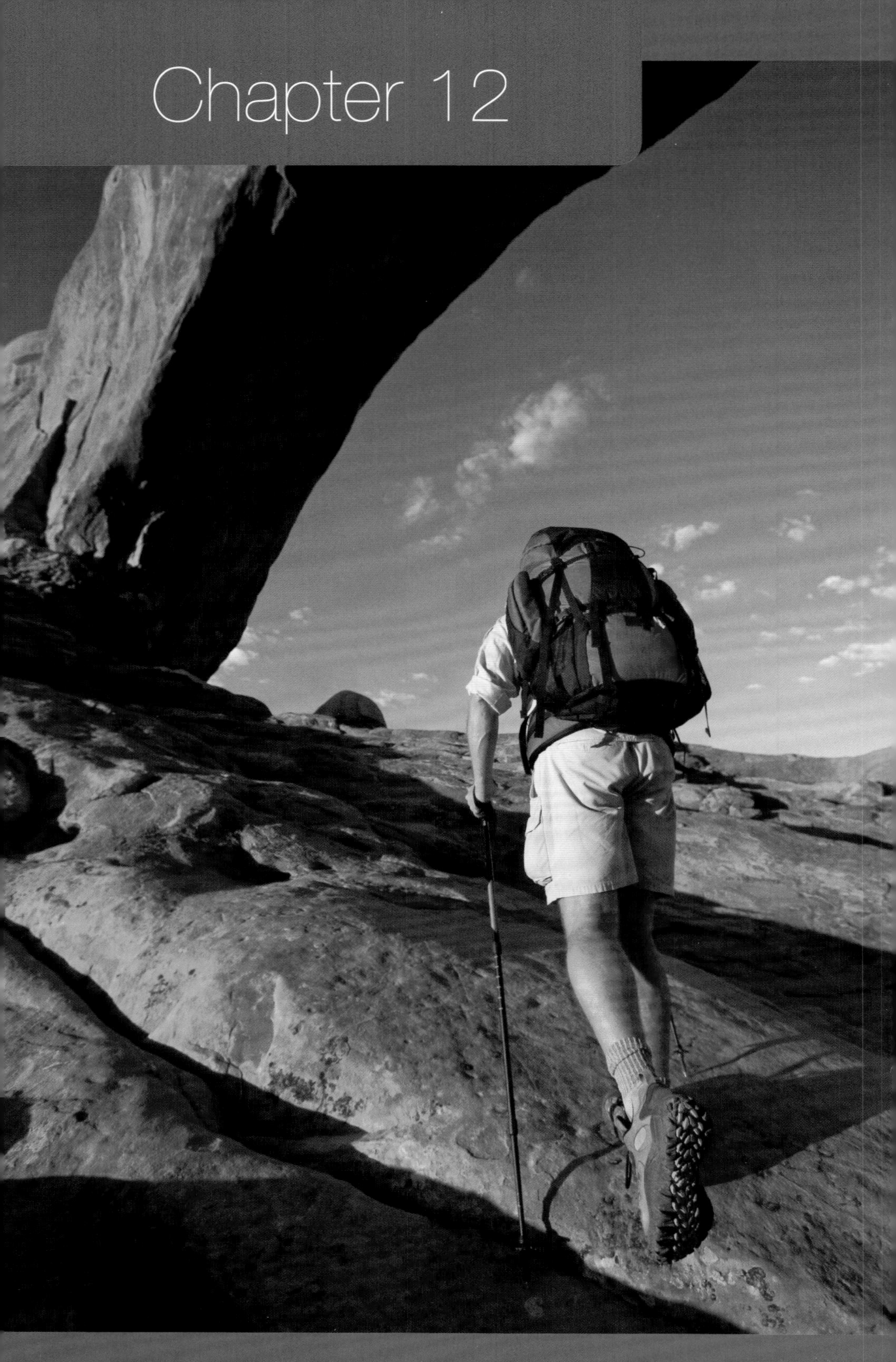

Why Be Healthy?

You see things; and you say 'Why?' But I dream things that never were; and I say 'Why not?'

—George Bernard Shaw

Health is a vehicle, not a destination. Excellent health is about more than just feeling good. Normally, when you are feeling low, dealing with a medical problem, or trying to lose weight, you think of health as something to achieve. Of course, good physical health is an important goal, but if you simply stop there, you will miss out on so much more. Robust health allows us to be active in the world and achieve more than we can when we are tired or sick. Your health is your most valuable asset.

You may have picked up this book hoping to learn the secrets of the perfect diet, but as you now know, nutrition is more than what is on your plate—so many factors contribute to your health and happiness. Taking a holistic approach to life considers the whole person and the relationship between body, mind, and spirit. You get to explore what brings you to balance and helps you thrive.

Ask yourself, "Why be healthy?" Imagine waking up every morning excited for your day. Envision what your life would look like as your best self. What would happen if you experienced high-level wellness most of the time? How would you use this gift to enhance your life and the lives of those around you? Sadly, most people are missing it. They eat processed junk food, don't move their bodies, and don't think about their health until they are diagnosed with illness. They deal with health concerns such as headaches, constipation, sugar crashes, and low energy as recurring parts of their lives. They are caught up in a matrix mentality concerned with keeping up, fitting in, and looking good. When you switch to a nutritious diet and healthy lifestyle, you begin dancing to the beat of a different drummer.

Each of us comes to Earth with a different agenda. As we get older, we continually make choices that individuate us from others and keep us on track with our destinies. And for some of us, the path is focused on personal growth and development, which frequently leads to a curiosity about food, diet, and lifestyle. In my experience, nutritious eaters tend to be smarter, clearer, and more in touch with themselves and the natural rhythms of life than people who eat highly refined foods. Trying to fit in has little value. Rather than pretending that you are like everyone else, you might as well take a deep breath, be authentic, and be yourself. As a health-conscious person, you have added potential to step out and create change in the world.

The first step is to shift away from a fitting-in mentality. By continuing to expend large amounts of your energy and intelligence just to fit in, you'll have less strength to focus on the more important aspects of yourself and your life. You may even create health problems for yourself, if you are not expressing yourself honestly. You are hiding your inner light, concealing your unique beauty, and shying away from your deeper destiny. I believe you have the capability to become an element for change. Think about people throughout history who have had a profound impact on society. Mahatma Gandhi, Nelson Mandela, Martin Luther King Jr., Mother Teresa, and Amelia Earhart come to my mind. Unconcerned with the status quo, they pushed their own potential and expanded the realities of the their times by "fitting out." They remind me of a German expression, "zeitgeist," which means the spirit of the time. In 1491, the zeitgeist was that the world was flat, and it took extraordinary courage for anyone to think outside that box and propose a different way of seeing the world—but that's exactly what happened. I see the people who are eating real, whole foods today in the same way as those who believed the world was round—they have a better capacity to see a healthy future not fueled by artificial junk food.

Authentic Self-Expression

As your diet and lifestyle improve, you will feel a greater sense of balance, and through this process become more fully present. You will probably notice your breath more fully, feel the breeze on your face, and really listen to what other people are saying. You will be more fresh and alert to new situations with access to a wider choice of behaviors at any given moment. This consciousness makes you more likely to steer away from foods and people that are detrimental to your health.

Our personalities are not fixed or rigid. The more we slow down and understand ourselves, the more flexible and present we become. Authentic self-expression means being the person we truly are at this point in time. Too many people live life based on events that happened a long time ago: a difficult relationship with a parent, a humiliating situation at school, or a challenging relationship that ended in an unsatisfying way. Many others live life as though they are constantly in preparation for something in the future, blind to the beauty of the present moment. It's time to snap out of this mentality. The past is over. The future never arrives. All you have is the present. The present is a gift, yours to treasure every moment, every day, in every way. You may have had a difficult childhood, challenges with your parents, and all kinds of things that happened to you that never should have happened. But that was then and this is now. Today, you are an adult who has a wonderful life. I urge you to let go of the past, forgive it, and know that, in some way, whatever happened was meant to happen. It is exactly those events that have made you who you are today.

Don't forget that authentic self-expression can apply to both primary and secondary foods. You don't need to hide what new foods you are eating, and you don't have to dial down your energy to make others feel better. It may feel hard at first to let go of certain friendships that drain you or to make the time to get to the gym, but I urge you to pay just as much attention to your primary foods and treat them with the same importance as eating greens. People might tell you it's selfish, but there's nothing wrong with prioritizing you. Think of it like when you are on an airplane. You have to put your oxygen mask on first before you can help others. When you start to prioritize the elements of your primary food circle, including career, relationships, exercise, and spirituality, you will enjoy an even higher level of health. I believe that ultimately, we are spiritual beings in a material world, so the more congruity we have with who we are and how we represent ourselves, the more likely we are to achieve the outcome that we came here in this lifetime to achieve.

Unpredictable Futures

I want to tell you the story of the frog in the grasshopper jar. It goes like this:

> A man had a grasshopper, which he kept in a glass jar so that he could admire it. A grasshopper, being a grasshopper, will jump. One day the grasshopper jumped and escaped from the glass jar. The man discovered that the grasshopper had gone missing and went looking for it. Fortunately, he found the grasshopper and placed it back in the glass jar. However, the man wanted to make sure the grasshopper wouldn't escape this time. So he placed a glass lid on the glass jar. When the grasshopper awoke the next morning, he saw that the sun was shining and the sky was blue. The grasshopper, being a grasshopper, jumped again. This time, the glass lid greeted the grasshopper. He didn't know what hit him. He jumped and jumped and jumped. The man was annoyed by the grasshopper's antics, so he lowered the glass lid to try to prevent the grasshopper from jumping. The next morning the cycle began again. This time the lid was so low that the grasshopper could only move forward and back, so he gave up and stopped jumping. When he woke again, he didn't jump. He didn't even try. He didn't notice that the man had removed the glass lid the night before. Freedom was staring him in the face and he didn't attempt to make it his.

Many people behave like the grasshopper, afraid to jump. They are so accustomed to their own views of life that they don't bother to try other ways of being. There are so many ways to live life and countless opportunities for each of us every single day.

Everyone has a predictable future, a future that would automatically occur by continuing to fit in, following the rules and moving along in the expected way. I had a predictable future. I was raised in an Orthodox Jewish household in Canada. I could have stayed there, followed my parents' religious belief system, and worked as a lawyer in a corporate setting, but that wasn't what my heart was telling me to do. Instead, I decided to travel and explore other life paths, which eventually brought me into the health food industry. I moved to New York and began health coaching. I had a passion for helping people and wanted to put my skills and education to use. I couldn't believe I was there, in my jeans, working with people to get well. When I decided to start a nutrition school that would cover all dietary theories, some people thought I was crazy. I was trying something that no one had done before. For years, I slept on friends' couches or in the school's offices, while I was building something I truly believed was possible. If I can do it, so can you.

Food has a powerful effect on our future. Avoiding junk food reduces brain fog and allows you to see opportunities that others can't. It's like when the grasshopper discovers the glass jar has no lid; suddenly a world of new options opens and all types of unimaginable things become possible. Nutritious eaters have a freedom and openness that most people can't fully understand. They are more able to step away from predictable, undesired futures and take advantage of the limitless openings of life. These people often move in unexpected directions. Family and friends sometimes find their choices odd, unwise, or threatening, but when all is said and done, these are some of the happiest, healthiest, most alive people in the world. They have the capacity and curiosity to start fresh, to explore more creative careers, begin new relationships, relocate to another area, or travel to distant lands. It's your life, and doors of opportunity are opening and closing at every moment. It's okay to take risks. The world is a safe place. It's a powerful experience to know you are strong enough and clear enough to survive and thrive through major life changes.

In Western thinking, we sometimes think, "I've got to make it happen for myself." We push and push to achieve success. Eastern philosophy says everything is going to work out for itself. In India, they have a saying, "Let go and let God." I think we have to find balance between these two ideologies and pay attention to both parts of the equation. You want to be aware of barriers and obstructions to progress and be willful about the future. But with one eye on barriers to progress, you must keep the other on how to surrender to them. One perspective is very yin and the other is very yang. Another saying from an Arabian proverb goes, "Trust in God, but tie up your camel." In other words, have faith that the world is working in your favor, and don't lose sight of the little commonsense things. You still have to wash your dishes, pay rent, or have difficult conversations, at times. But you don't have to get stuck in the mundane parts of life, either. In my experience, when we care for ourselves by eating well and listening to our authentic desires, we naturally move in the direction of our dreams, and even have the experience of surpassing them.

The more you live in balance, respecting nature and yourself, the more likely you will be in the right place at the right time, all the time. When you have that balance, you're one with nature and more connected to the system. You'll see synchronicity incessantly. You'll start planning a vacation to Spain and the next day you'll meet someone who just got back and offers tons of appealing advice. You'll be looking for a new job and run into an old family friend who just so happens to have an opening in your field. You'll meet a significant other who complements you beautifully; you'll find a career aligned with your personal values. People will call you lucky and you may think it's simply coincidence, but the truth is that you are aligning yourself with the natural order of everything. How are all those planets in the right place at the right time? How do the leaves all turn color in the fall and the birds know to fly south? Human beings are part of the same order. What looks after all these aspects of life will look after us too, the more we are in harmony with nature.

Building Your Future

As you learn to nurture yourself, space opens up for you to create your future. Whatever you dream is possible. The universe wants you to fulfill your dreams and achieve all your desires. The difficult part is getting clear about what you want and then having the faith and perseverance to make it happen. It's common to question your right to have what you can possibly dream of. But I'm here to tell you that the sky's the limit. Give yourself permission to make your dreams happen. Allow yourself to put time and energy into understanding what you would like your life to look like and feel like. What do you want to accomplish in your life? Where would you like to go? Who would you like to be with? The clearer your intentions, the more you can build your future according to your hopes and dreams. What do you really want to get done in this lifetime? You are free to create whatever you want in this world.

Stephen Hawking, the British theoretical physicist and author of *A Brief History of Time*, has a theory that the past and the future is a continuum, which means the future has already happened. When I first heard this concept, it completely fascinated me and really changed my life. When I ask my students who their fourth grade teacher was, they are able to trace back relatively quickly to remember that person. But when I ask them what they want their lives to look like in a year, I get that deer-in-the-headlights look. We have the ability to see the future too. It's a muscle that you have to train, just as you would for any sport. You can start by writing weekly, monthly, and annual goals. When you get clear about these goals, lo and behold, you see the future, because you're creating it.

Whether your goal is to have more energy, heal a health concern, or just to be the best version of your true self each day, relish every moment of that journey. Being healthy is about moving beyond a limited philosophy of nutrition and creating your own larger vision for your health and happiness. In my experience, people who adopt a well-balanced diet and lifestyle and avoid junk foods develop a higher degree of creativity, flexibility, and aliveness.

Spiritual Beings

As you begin to eat more intelligently, you stop medicating yourself by unconsciously using extreme foods as mood-altering drugs. When you stop eating extreme foods that bounce you around on a pinball diet, you naturally become more still. With this stillness, you are bound to disentangle yourself from the mundane attitudes that you received from the school system, society, and the media. This stillness offers benefits to your body as well. Your body will not have to work as hard to maintain homeostasis. Your blood sugar, temperature, and heartbeat will all operate at optimum levels. When our bodies slow down, we slow down. When we slow down, we increasingly come to experience "nothing to do and nowhere to go"—the sensation that life is just perfectly okay the way it is.

Despite this exquisite experience, you may find yourself noticing that most people are operating from a confused state, constantly looking for things outside of themselves to fill the void. You'll notice people who have everything and yet complain constantly. You'll notice people who feel that nothing is ever enough. You may fall into self-doubt and try to blend in, throwing yourself back into constant rushing and grasping for external sources of gratification— such as material goods, more money, or superficial relationships with others—since that's what everyone else is doing. Materialistic things can only get you so far. Yes, a better house or a better car can make life more enjoyable to a point, but it's not happiness. Nothing outside of yourself can ever truly fulfill you. Contentment and true joy come from within and are available to us at any moment.

I do understand the pleasure of being engaged by a strong mission. After all, I've invested a great deal of time in the development of IIN, so I'm well aware of the gratification that comes from using one's creative energies to contribute to the world. Remember, though, that you are a spiritual being in a material world. Spirit is your essential reality, and nothing you achieve or possess on a material level is ever going to fulfill you for long.

Please don't be in a hurry to dismiss or disturb the clear spaces when they come. When the tranquility hits, try to notice and resist the temptation to overeat, argue, seek distractions, or busy yourself for the sake of being busy. Allow yourself to live in this relaxed, unoccupied dimension of your being. Give it space. You are a human being, not a human doing. Enjoy the luxury of non-doing. It is an essential part of nature.

This Is Your Life

My father has a bumper sticker on his car that says, "This is your life, not a dress rehearsal." Now is the time to take action toward accomplishing whatever dreams, ideas, or aspirations may be lingering in the back of your mind. One of the easiest and most effective ways of making change in your life is to change what you eat. The foods you put into your mouth, together with primary food, create the fuel for your body, mind, and spirit. Health and happiness are inextricably linked. The better you feed yourself, the better you feel and the bigger impact you will have on the world.

Don't let yourself get stuck. A lot of holistic people are trying to get themselves healthier, but they're already healthier than 90% of the population. I propose that while working on getting yourself to a higher level, why not also work on getting the rest of the world to move up? By sharing what you already know with others, you may achieve a higher level of health than if you go to another yoga class or eat more broccoli. Get involved with your community, your kids' schools, your church, or your family. As Martin

Luther King, Jr. said, "Life's most persistent and urgent question is, 'What are you doing for others?'"

The surest path to success is by taking action. You do not need to know all the steps, just take the first one. Together, we can create a new future for our health and for humanity.

It is my genuine hope and desire that we can all make a difference by bringing the message of Integrative Nutrition into the mainstream. Imagine this world educated on whole foods and holistic practices that help to support our health and wellness. What we eat breaks down in our bodies and changes our whole way of thinking. It's hard to find something as significant as that. The future of nutrition is a world where primary foods and secondary foods are balanced and aligned for all. So, the question really isn't, "Are you healthy enough?" The question is, "What are you going to do with your health?"

Exercises

1. Write It Down!

Writing down your goals makes them real. It creates clarity. When you can see where you're going in writing, opportunities present themselves and help us get to the next step. Do this as often as needed—every day, every week, every month, and every year.

2. Identify Your Passions

What lights you up? What did you love as a kid, before you felt any pressure to do something well? Recall past successes. Reread your own résumé or ask a friend to share something they love about you.

3. Future Building

What do you really want to get done in this lifetime? You are free to create whatever you want in this world. The more specific you are, the easier it is to plan. Your hopes and dreams must be thought through and planned to make them happen. You may want to do this in a journal. You are not going to show this list to anyone, so just write freely and without judgment.

Write down all the things you need to get done or want to get done by:

1. the end of the day tomorrow
2. the end of the week
3. the end of this month
4. the end of next month
5. the end of the year

Now remember: This is your life. Make it happen!

Chapter 13

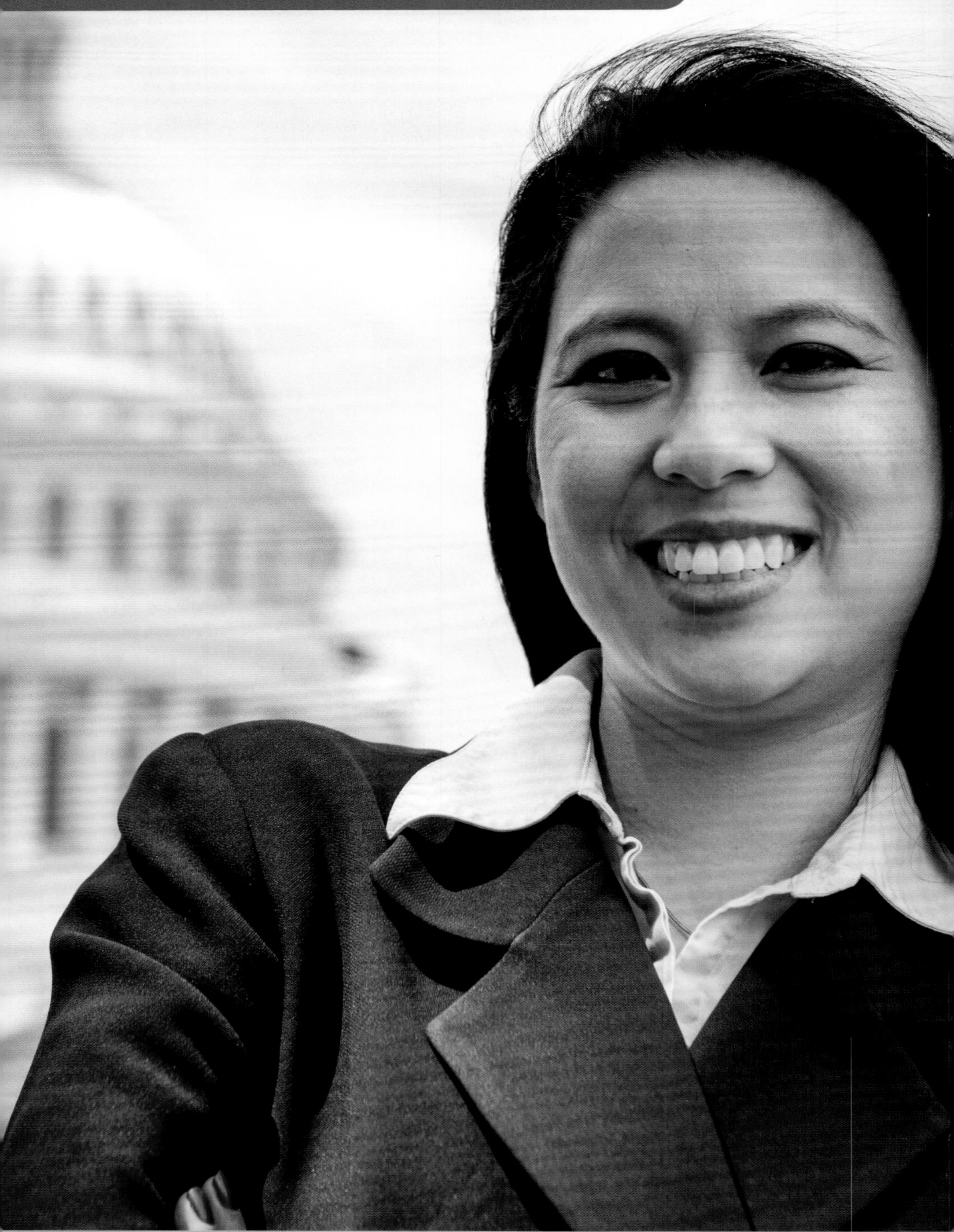

The Health Coaching Revolution

Never forget, no matter how overwhelming life's challenges and problems seem to be, that one person can make a difference in the world. In fact, it is always because of one person that all the changes that matter in the world come about. So be that one person.

—R. Buckminster Fuller

Now that you know the basics of the Integrative Nutrition philosophy, you are ready to become your own health advocate. But the biggest challenge is still in front of you. How do you take this knowledge and apply it your life? And even more importantly, how do you stay motivated?

Joanne Beccarelli was a fit, lean, athletic person before her 40s. But after years of working in the corporate business world, raising children, and living an overscheduled life, she had picked up more than a few unhealthy habits. She was an emotional eater who was more than 100 pounds overweight and on multiple medications.

She looked for help in traditional medicine, but the same advice kept coming back, "eat less and exercise more." Diets weren't helping.

"I let myself get lost," she said. "Not just my body but my whole being. Emotional and mental strains spilled over into food and physical ailments, and vice versa."

While attending IIN's Health Coach Training Program, she radically changed her food habits—steadily losing the weight and getting off prescription medications. She started to find more balance in her primary foods. Once she discovered what worked for her, she felt compelled to help others and launch her own health coaching practice. Today, she works with people one-on-one and in groups that are looking for help with weight loss and maintenance, immunity building, help with migraines, and more. She also teaches healthy cooking classes.

Joanne's story is like that of many IIN grads. She was looking for something more than a list of "eat this, not that." She learned how to navigate all of the contradictory nutrition information out there and found what worked best for her body—bio-individuality at its best. By making small changes at her own pace, she created a sustainable healthy lifestyle that she loves.

Just as athletes work with trainers, and students have tutors, people today more than ever before need Health Coaches. Someone who is trained in the art of listening who can help identify your struggles and help you figure out how to make healthy changes.

Ami Valpone spent a decade struggling with various health issues, from Lyme disease to colitis to leaky gut and more. She sought help from functional medicine and integrative doctors, and also wanted to learn more about how to truly be healthy. In 2009, she attended IIN.

"I was dealing with chronic illness and wanted to find a way to heal myself with food and mind-body practices," Ami said. "I took the classes while I was working a corporate job years ago, before I started my own business."

Not only did she heal, but also she says she really learned how to listen to her body and not be so concerned with what everyone else was doing or eating. Today, she's an Integrative Nutrition Health Coach, personal chef, professional recipe developer, and author, running a successful blog that helps others who are struggling and looking for balance with their health.

"I'm beyond grateful for IIN and the life that I live now," she said. "I love my clients, and I love waking up every morning to do what I do."

When people discover the school, hear about primary foods, learn about bio-individuality, and meet others who feel passionate about health and wellness, they become inspired. It's a ripple effect that really motivates me to keep going. And the stories I see and hear about through my students continue to reinforce my belief that everyone can do this. People can make simple changes that can dramatically improve their health.

Here's another story from an international student that truly touched me and really shows just how impactful one person can be in their community.

Dear Joshua and the Integrative Nutrition Team,

I am a British mother to three young children, and I reside in Dubai, United Arab Emirates, UAE.

My journey has been a truly fascinating one and I feel extremely grateful and proud. I had initially signed up to Integrative Nutrition in 2012 for my own health reasons, and since then so much has transpired that I have indeed started a movement here in the UAE! My company promotes ALL aspects of wellness and is aimed at children. We offer turnkey solutions to schools as well as providing awareness to our cosmopolitan community at large.

By the end of this year we will be offering accredited training courses on Mindfulness in Schools and Edible Education in Schools (gardening in some of the most extreme weather on earth can be an issue) on top of this we have food education, cookery, yoga, and edible educational lesson plans all downloadable from our membership website. We are also launching next week, a children's weekend cookery box to be delivered to the families' doorsteps with recipes and ingredients to encourage home cooking with fresh ingredients for children.

With the obesity rate and the anxiety/depression rate rapidly growing here in the UAE, I could no longer ignore the statistics. We have an ongoing pilot study of which the first phase of statistics will be presented to the city's school leadership and government at the end of this month, which is just amazing in itself, and as a result we are now beginning to work alongside the government in creating a healthier and happier community.

My training has allowed me to talk confidently in front of 900+ people (including very esteemed guests), and I feel so passionately in the need for change. I was awarded a jury seat on the Happy and Healthy Schools Awards, a government initiative. I was also given the role of facilitator for the Dubai Saturday Club, a separate government-funded free club, offering teens a chance to do something for good. Truly, my list could go on. Your ripple effect has certainly initiated a huge change here in the UAE.

With heartfelt thanks,

Justine Bain

What Is a Health Coach?

Have you ever wondered why we get a friendlier welcome when we go to a coffee shop than we when we go to a hospital or the doctor's office? Sure, you're not visiting your doctor to buy a warm beverage, but that time together is usually important, especially if you are dealing with a health issue. The average wait time in a doctor's office is about 20 minutes, and most doctors spend between 13 and 16 minutes with patients.

Traditional health professionals are on the frontlines of helping those in need, but they don't always have the time or resources to help patients build healthy habits. We have a huge demand for a new kind of health advocate and to help fill a void in our current healthcare system.

Enter Health Coaches.

Health Coaches work with clients to make shifts from unhealthy habits to sustainable habits for long-lasting health. A Health Coach is defined as "a guide and supportive mentor who empowers clients to take responsibility for their health and achievement of their personal wellness goals."

In practical terms, a Health Coach can tailor a personal wellness program to meet the needs of a client instead of prescribing one particular diet or way of exercising. They can educate and support clients to achieve their health goals through lifestyle and behavior adjustments by meeting regularly to discuss it all.

With more doctors and medical professionals seeing the value of nutrition, movement, and other lifestyle factors in overall health, more of them have begun to work with Health Coaches in their practices to serve their patients.

Health Coaches don't diagnose, prescribe medications, or take responsibility for bringing about wellness changes in a client's life. Instead, they can help patients stay accountable to recommendations that their doctors and health professionals provide.

Dr. Frank Lipman, a functional medicine doctor based in New York City and an Integrative Nutrition visiting teacher, practices what he calls "good medicine," focusing on healing and preventing the root cause of sickness. He has said that most of what people need support with is food-based recommendations, and he has a team of Health Coaches who work one-on-one with his patients to help him.

"Diet is the largest lever for health changes," Dr. Lipman said in an article. He encourages his patients to try cleanses, eat more leafy greens, include supplements, and make dietary changes, like reducing or eliminating dairy, gluten, or other inflammatory foods. "But telling my patients to take their turmeric and watch their sugar doesn't mean they do it. Compliance is a problem, even though my patients tend to be very motivated. With Health Coaches, it's so much better because they have time to work with patients, meet for regular sessions, stay in touch via email, and create a relationship."

Imagine if you had someone to talk with once a week (or once a month) who knew your health story, could really listen to your progress or struggles, and offer one or two simple next steps to keep you moving forward. More and more patients are looking for a partner in their health journey, and Health Coaches can provide that support.

They work not only at doctor's offices or in private practices, but also in corporate wellness, spas, gyms, wellness centers, and more. Even big health insurance companies like Humana and Aetna employ Health Coaches to help people set goals and create personalized action plans for health issues like weight management, stress management, smoking cessation, or improved eating habits.

In fact, the Department of Labor estimates a 21% increase—faster than all other occupations—for health and wellness professionals focused on preventive health. Right now only 2% of our healthcare dollars in the U.S. alone are focused on preventing disease. What would happen if we were able to double or triple that spending?

When Integrative Nutrition started as a small school in the early '90s, the wellness movement was just starting to take off in many ways, and chronic diseases were on the rise. I felt a deep sense of responsibility to do work that could make a difference and create a world where people would be happier and healthier than ever before—not, as my friend and IIN guest teacher Joe Cross said in the title of his documentary film, "fat, sick, and nearly dead."

Decades later, Health Coaches have made tremendous strides in improving global wellness and raising awareness that *food changes everything*. It's no small feat that our graduates have helped thousands of people throughout the world transform their health, prevent disease, and live more balanced lives. They've also played a role in school food programs, educating the public through media, and influencing government policy.

Integrative Nutrition is much more than a school; it's a movement. Students and graduates of all ages and backgrounds are revolutionizing the healthcare system by helping others take control of their health.

I believe that Health Coaches are the future of healthcare, and I'm not alone.

The *Wall Street Journal* recently reported that there is "a broader shift within the healthcare industry toward keeping people well instead of simply treating them when they're sick." And that, "although wellness coaching is a relatively new field, some recent research suggests that it does work—at least in the short term."

A Mayo Clinic study with 100 participants who worked with a Health Coach found that the majority of people improved their health—losing weight, creating better nutrition habits, and increasing physical activity in a 12-week program.

Another small study found that health coaching "improves the management of chronic diseases" and "produces positive effects on patients' physiological, behavioral, and psychological conditions and on their social life."

Ongoing research at the Department of Family and Community Medicine at the University of California, San Francisco, is looking at exactly how Health Coaches support and work with patients.

Researchers assembled focus groups (in Spanish and English) and conducted individual interviews with patients, their friends and family, Health Coaches, and clinicians at six public health primary care clinics.

The scientists found seven themes that help describe more fully how Health Coaches and patients work together—shared characteristics, availability, trust, education, personal support, decision-making support, and bridging the gap between the patient and clinician.

Shared characteristics can include language, culture, sex, and similar experiences or values. According to the study, these shared traits help the patient feel more understood by their coach. One coach reported that her patients saw her as a peer, and that was comforting for them. Availability was another factor to help create a deeper bond and offer more connection between the coach and client. Along with that was trust. "A trusting relationship enabled patients to be honest, ask questions, and express doubts or disagreements, which allowed the Health Coach to be more effective," study authors said.

When it comes to education, Health Coaches can share basic information about health conditions and assess their readiness for change. Personal support is about listening as well as providing hope, encouragement, and motivation. A Health Coach can help with decisions, too. One coach described how she works with patients, saying, "I'm not here to tell you what to do. I'm here to offer you options." Finally, a coach can also act as a liaison between patient and clinician. One doctor told researchers, "If I haven't explained something well or can't do follow-up or can't reinforce a message, I'm hoping the Health Coach can do that."

One of the most important findings from the research was that everyone involved, from patient to doctor to Health Coach, perceived the coach as a bridge between the patient and their primary care provider rather than as a barrier.

Other studies continue to look at health coaching, with researchers conducting randomized clinical trials (RCTs) to keep investigating its merits.

The Ithaca Coaching Project is one of the first large-scale RCTs to examine health coaching for primary prevention and to help provide data describing the effectiveness of coaching on behavior changes and health outcomes. They are currently recruiting, and I look forward to seeing more research in the field.

Four Benefits of a Healthy Lifestyle

Why would you want to improve your health beyond the obvious reasons? Some people simply accept the mindset, "Well, I gotta die of something, right?" This response may get the occasional chuckle, but there are more benefits to being healthy than a prolonged life.

1. Reduced Medical Expenses
A healthy lifestyle means fewer visits to the doctor. If you are overweight or obese, then you are subject to other diseases that can increase your medical expenses rather quickly. If you engage in a healthy lifestyle, you'll have a better chance of warding off harmful diseases.

2. Increased Energy
Sure, you can experience a sugar rush from candy and desserts, but you've surely felt the energy crash that inevitably follows. Saturated fats tend to drain your energy levels, and if your diet consists of many sugars and saturated fats, then not only will you experience significant weight gain, but your energy will slowly decrease. When you base your diet and lifestyle on nutritious choices, you'll experience more energy and vitality than ever before—which gives you more energy for quality time with family and friends.

3. Less Stress
It's no secret that regular exercise can be therapeutic and reduce stress, but healthy foods (such as foods high in vitamin C and magnesium) can help moderate your cortisol levels, which is the stress hormone. When you're stressed or in a chronic state, your body quickly breaks down protein. If you have sufficient protein in your diet you can help the body maintain those cortisol levels as well.

4. Improved Self-Confidence
When you change your habits and lifestyle to become more health-oriented, you start to feel good, too. It's easy to be hard on yourself when you constantly feel tired or out of shape. Start today on your path to a healthy lifestyle, and watch your self-confidence grow as a result.

Bottom line: If you've failed to meet your health goals in the past due to impossible diets, or if you're looking to learn how you can make the necessary lifestyle changes to improve your overall wellness, then seek out an Integrative Nutrition Health Coach.

Making a Difference

IIN students and grads are changing the world. I don't think very many schools can say they have a community as unique, diverse, and passionate as ours. I am very proud and humbled to be associated with these amazing people, and we now have 100,000 students and graduates in more than 155 countries. I want to share with you some of the stories of the real-life Integrative Nutrition Health Coaches out in the world today working to make a difference.

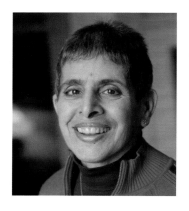

After finding herself facing a burnout situation, **Christine Boutross** *decided to change her career in education and ultimately her life. She pursued her passion for health by becoming a certified personal trainer. However, she still felt that something was missing…and that missing link turned out to be Integrative Nutrition. By the end of her journey with IIN, she had already built a significant client base, and her personal training business had exploded. Today, she successfully runs her business as a Health Coach alongside being a personal trainer.*

"My mission as a Health Coach is to inspire and educate busy professionals who want to make changes in their lifestyle through nutrition and fitness so they can live a happier, healthier life. It's wonderful to not only see my clients make these small changes, but to know that these changes have had an impact on their everyday lives."

Christine has continually taken her coaching practice to the next level since graduating from IIN in 2007. She first become certified by the International Association of Health Coaches (IAHC) and, more recently, board certified through the International Consortium of Health and Wellness Coaches (ICHWC). Additionally, she continuously gives back to the Integrative Nutrition community as an IIN Coaching Circle Coach.

"As a coach for IIN students, I'm in awe of the confidence students have acquired to become rock star Integrative Nutrition Health Coaches and go out to make a difference in the world. And, personally, I am grateful and blessed to be doing work that I'm passionate about. There have been so many lessons learned since graduating from IIN. But, the most important one to me is that I have accepted who I am."

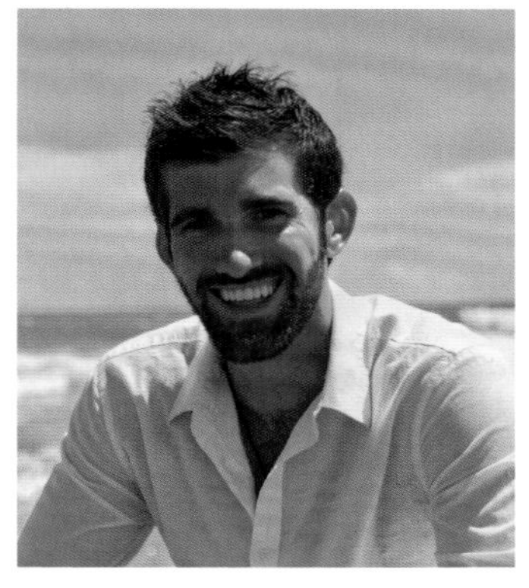

After losing his grandfather to cancer, **Devin Burke** *began to truly gain an understanding of how profoundly the lifestyle choices we make can impact our health and happiness as a result of his family striving to make healthier choices. This realization inspired his study of exercise science and health promotion in college and continuing education through the Institute for Integrative Nutrition.*

"IIN greatly impacted not just my physical health, but really accelerated and expanded my mental, emotional, and spiritual evolution. The program gave me perspective on how to make a massive positive impact on others while making a living at the same time."

Inspired by these changes in his family and within himself, Devin has founded and branded a "high-performance health" coaching practice which helps individuals who have roles that demand high performance—such as CEOs and community leaders. This optimizes not only their health and happiness, but ultimately their performance. Devin has been featured in top online publications, health and wellness podcasts, radio, and has authored *Healthy Eating in the 21st Century*. Currently, Devin is dedicated toward launching his own podcast on high-performance health, publishing his second book, and is also active as a Integrative Nutrition Health Coach and public speaker.

Devin has taken some big risks to communicate his important message of health and to really get it out there. But, he also feels a deep, ongoing sense of satisfaction from the lasting changes he has seen in his clients. He is hopeful about the future of health and what it may hold for individuals due to the positive impact Health Coaches have.

"I see the health and wellness industry moving more toward providing personalized health solutions rather than providing cookie-cutter, one-size-fits-all approaches to prevention and optimal health.

The future is in personalizing health and empowering individuals to take full responsibility for their health. It's really the simple consistent actions that create the largest impact on health for both individuals and communities."

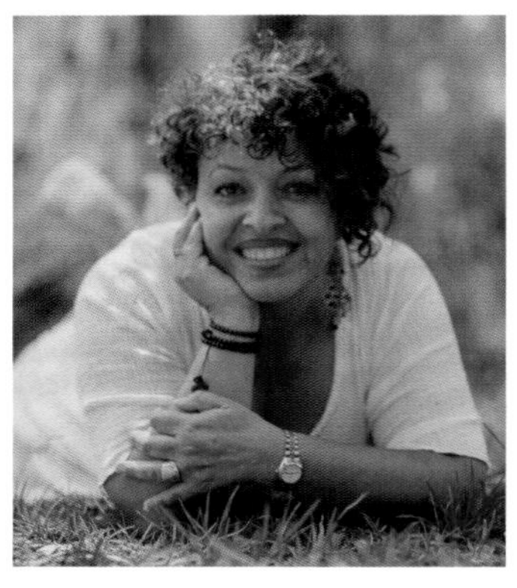

Irma Mejia *was born in Mexico City and dreamed of helping people from a young age. Having battled frequent physical illnesses and depression throughout her life, Irma had always been seeking information about nutrition, but she seemed to continually encounter barriers or controversy in her search. Finding IIN finally brought an end to her formerly fruitless searching and gave her a vision for her future.*

Irma lives in Mexico, where today she works as a full-time Integrative Nutrition Health Coach while also running an organic, vegan health store that hosts workshops in nutrition and healthy cooking. She also presents a weekly radio show on both primary and secondary nutrition, frequently hosting guest Health Coaches. She also gives back to the IIN community as a Spanish IIN Coaching Circles Coach. Irma is looking forward to working on her first book and opening a vegan bistro.

"At the beginning, I felt too old to start studying. But now, I say, 'It's never too late.' I'm finally helping people as I always dreamed about, and I'm so pleased to see my students living a better, more fulfilling life and starting their own healthy businesses."

Irma is presently working in tandem with the International Health Coach Association toward achieving recognition for Health Coaches by the Mexican government. She also has the joy of working toward her dreams of a healthier population alongside her daughter, who's also an Integrative Nutrition Health Coach. Together, they have created a coaching resource that offers a number of different programs to the people of Mexico.

"I really have a gorgeous life now and am even expecting my second grandchild. I'm so blessed to be surrounded by great people who are working to create a better world. And, I can say this is all possible because of IIN. I'm so thankful!"

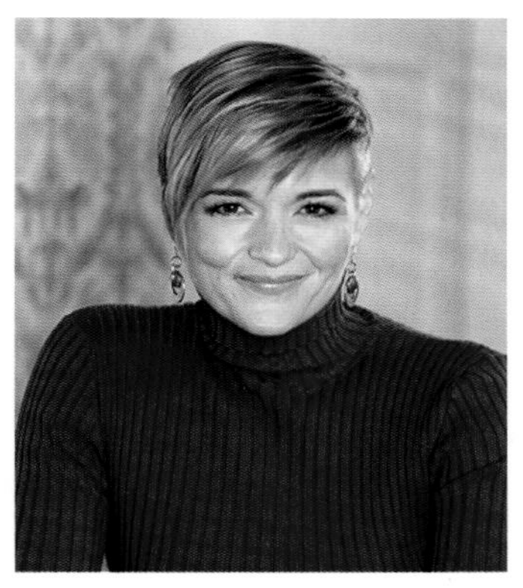

Despite her successful career as a medical doctor, **Shaunna Menard** *still found herself looking for a better way to help people live longer, happier, and healthier lives. She had begun her own journey, discovering the power of nutrition and the role of emotional wellbeing in overall health. But, still, she wanted more. When she discovered the Institute for Integrative Nutrition, the mission and the message resonated with her instantly.*

Since graduating from IIN, Shaunna has seen dramatic positive changes in both her own life and the lives of her patients and clients. Today, in addition to her coaching practice, she does multiple TV and public speaking appearances, serves as the Chair of Public Health for doctors in Manitoba, and has expanded her reach with her book, *Doctor Up the Recipe*. Shaunna also founded an online superfood meal planning service called "Meal Cure," which she developed to help busy clients reach their goals of eating healthier amidst a hectic schedule.

"As a traditional MD for over 25 years, as well as a holistic Health Coach, I have a unique perspective. I'm able to highlight the best of both worlds to optimize the best results for my clients, moving forward and helping people to break through plateaus of all kinds. I know that their body truly is a miracle, and we work together to allow their natural wellbeing to rise, focusing more on EASE than dis-ease."

Shaunna's time with the IIN guided her transformation into a holistic entrepreneur, which gives her the opportunity to spend plenty of time with her family and to practice health and wellness from her dream location in Canada. As this region has coincidentally been labeled as having the healthiest people in Canada, she has gained the added bonus of reaping the benefits of a healthy lifestyle on a daily basis.

Clients often come to Shaunna initially looking to resolve a physical issue, but they end up embodying a deep transformation of the mind, body, and spirit.

"I love the connection with people. I love and live for the transformation and being a witness to the process of them becoming their best self. I am fascinated by the power of mind/body medicine. It really is quite spectacular!"

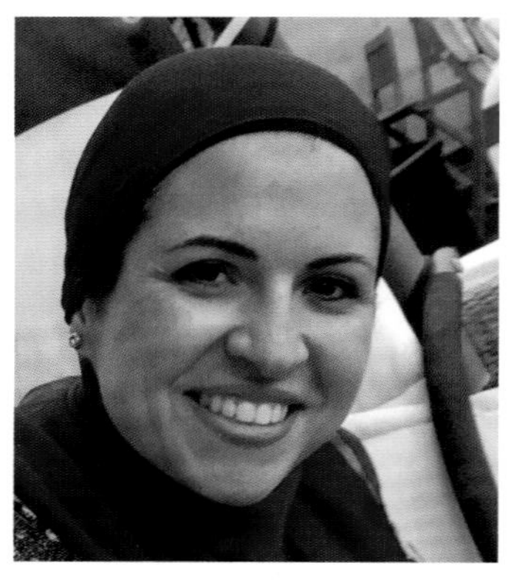

Wafaa Abdel-Hadi *had been leading a proud career in oncology for 13 years when her entire world was shaken with the loss of a precious family member to cancer. She decided she needed to move beyond silencing the symptoms of the disease and instead dive deeper into truly understanding the roots of the disease itself. So, she founded the AWARE Clinic to introduce "The Anti-Cancer Lifestyle Concept." Still struggling with grasping the overall picture, her naturopath recommended Integrative Nutrition to her as the best path to understanding the power of the body to heal. IIN helped Wafaa to begin looking differently at the connection between health and food, as well as at the positive effects of mental and spiritual wellbeing. She immediately started implementing her new approach into her clinic with amazing results. Her success has been such that her clinic now also supports education and prevention for those battling autoimmune and chronic disorders.*

In her thirst for more knowledge, Wafaa began to discover a large community of functional medicine doctors who, like her, spoke the language of natural medicine. She was inspired to begin additional studies and, as of publication of this book, became the first and only functional medicine doctor in Egypt through The Institute for Functional Medicine. Wafaa now includes the application of functional medicine in her practice and is experiencing wonderful results.

"Applying functional medicine in my practice has not only made my patients feel better and heal faster, but has given me hope and faith in a brighter, healthier future for our next generations."

Wafaa is always continuing to build and expand her practice with the concepts she learned through Integrative Nutrition, such as educational seminars, group therapy sessions, and maintaining an individualized approach to each of her patients. She also still subscribes faithfully to the #1 tool in an Integrative Nutrition Health Coach's toolbox—the Health History questionnaire, which she feels repeatedly delivers results beyond any expectations.

"For me, IIN is an eye opener to a world of infinite possibilities that I'm ready to explore and implement. I now look at my life differently and feel energetic from all of the work that I can do with IIN and functional medicine. My wish is to grow into an institute to guide and stimulate people to overcome their daily health challenges through finding the root cause of their imbalances and re-designing their life pattern."

Step by step, Health Coaches are creating a new future for healthcare and for humanity. Since coining the term Health Coach, it's been a goal of mine to continuously pioneer the field through diverse means, including advocacy, rights to practice, and continuing education.

Together, we have created a ripple effect that is bringing health and happiness to the world.

IIN Timeline

1992 Joshua Rosenthal, founder of IIN, begins teaching macrobiotics in a rented kitchen with 20 students.

1997 IIN enrolls its first international student.

2002 Integrative Nutrition celebrates continued growth, with 899 students and graduates.

2005 Joshua Rosenthal is teaching classes of more than 1,000 students with leading health experts LIVE in NYC.

2007 IIN establishes partnership with State University of New York, Purchase College.

2009 IIN is licensed by the New York State Department of Education.

2010 IIN works with Apple to figure out how to get the curriculum onto the iPod.

2012 IIN transfers curriculum to cutting-edge iPads and has 111 visiting teachers, 50,000 students and grads.

2015 Progress in Health Coach profession recognition: Health Coach Week 2015, Letter of Recognition from Tim Ryan, Health Coach Resolution submitted, IAHC Certification Exam.

2016 H.Res.552 (Health and Wellness Coach Recognition Resolution) introduced in U.S. House of Representatives, recognizing and supporting the work of Health Coaches.

2017 100,000 students and grads in 155 countries.

Health Coaches in Washington, D.C.

With leadership from Rep. Donald Payne, Jr. (D-N.J.) and Rep. Markwayne Mullin (R-Okla.), the bipartisan H.Res.552 (Health and Wellness Coach Recognition Resolution) was introduced in 2016 and recognizes and supports the work of Health Coaches in combatting the global health crisis. Currently, H.Res.552 has nine Congressional co-sponsors and is gaining more allies. Members of Congress from both parties understand and agree with the research and movement embracing a holistic approach to wellness, with food and lifestyle as the new prescription of choice and Health Coaches as the guides.

"We are in the midst of a global health crisis," said Rep. Tim Ryan, D-Ohio. "For the first time in history children will likely have a shorter life expectancy than their parents. Sadly, of the $4 trillion spent on healthcare in the U.S. this year, only 2% goes toward prevention. Preventive chronic diseases are costing us billions. It is imperative that we fight this epidemic with education and smarter lifestyle choices."

One of the ways I'm working to gain more allies is through Health and Wellness Coach Week. In 2016 we hosted a Capitol Hill briefing about the importance of Health Coaches with nearly 75 Congressional staffers. They learned from practicing area Health Coaches and speakers about the importance of health and wellness coaches. We also hosted a cooking demo that featured easy to prepare, delicious, and affordable food.

Other milestones include the addition of health coaching to the House and Senate Health Savings Acts of 2016 (H.R.4469 and S.2499). This provision was adopted, including health coaching as an allowable pre-tax expense. These bills allow more people control over their personal healthcare spending and improve their financial ability to hire Health Coaches.

IIN continues to host smoothie seminars, juicing classes, healthy cooking classes, and health coaching workshops on Capitol Hill for Congressional staff and members. In 2016 alone, we had more than 350 meetings.

We will continue to work with allies in Congress to get Health Coaches to play a larger role in preventative health care; highlight the essential role that Health Coaches can play to help reduce the onset of type 2 diabetes, during National Diabetes Awareness month; and keep promoting Health Coach Week for years to come.

I'm truly amazed at all the progress we have made, not just for Integrative Nutrition Health Coaches and the IIN community, but by all of those in the health and wellness world at large. I believe that everyone has a responsibility to do work that will make the world a better place. When health becomes the number one priority in this country and around the world, we will know that our community was part of that change and helped create a better world.

The IIN mission is to play a crucial role in improving health and happiness, and through that process, create a ripple effect that transforms the world.

Will you join the revolution?

Recipes

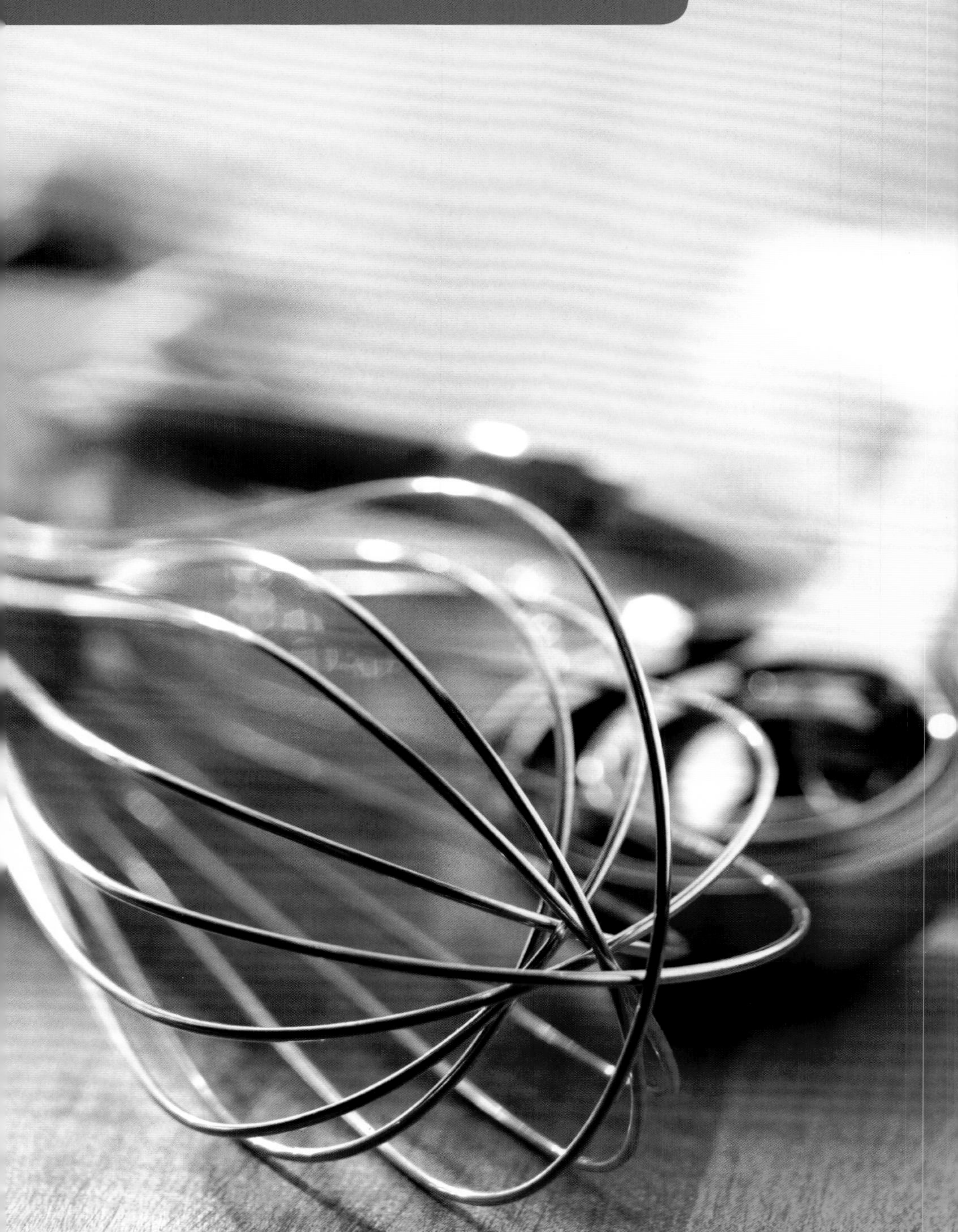

Recipes

Hunger is the best sauce in the world.
—Cervantes

For many more free recipes, please check out our website: www.integrativenutrition.com

breakfast

If you did the breakfast experiment in Chapter 2, you now have a better sense of the importance of breakfast. Starting your day with the fuel that works best in your body can set the tone for your whole day. Many people feel like they are too busy to eat breakfast, but once you get into the breakfast habit, you will see the benefits and a healthy morning meal will naturally become part of your day.

Try expanding your idea of what breakfast should look like. It doesn't have to be fruit and cereal or waffles and eggs. Vegetables, whole grains, fish, and other highly nutritious foods can be eaten at any time of day, including in the morning. These breakfast recipes are simple to prepare and will help broaden your breakfast palette.

Warm Gingery Oatmeal

Prep Time: 5 minutes
Cooking Time: 15 minutes
Serves 3

1 cup rolled oats
2 cups water
¼ cup raisins
¼ cup goji berries
¼ cup sunflower seeds
2 teaspoons grated ginger
1 tablespoon agave syrup

- Bring water to a boil.
- Add oats, raisins, goji berries, ginger, and a pinch of salt.
- Reduce heat to low.
- Continue cooking until water is absorbed and oats become nice and creamy, about 7 minutes.
- Add sunflower seeds and agave.

TIP: *Try using rice, soy, or nut milk instead of water to make it even creamier.*

Muesli

Prep Time: 5 minutes
Cooking Time: none!
Serves 3

1 cup rolled oats
2 cups almond or soy milk
5 to 6 dates, chopped
½ cup sunflower seeds

- Soak all ingredients overnight covered, and it will be done by the morning. Without cooking!

TIP: *Add shredded coconut, raisins, or a tablespoon of brown rice syrup before eating.*

Amaranth and Polenta Porridge

Prep Time: 5 minutes
Cooking Time: 40 minutes
Serves 4

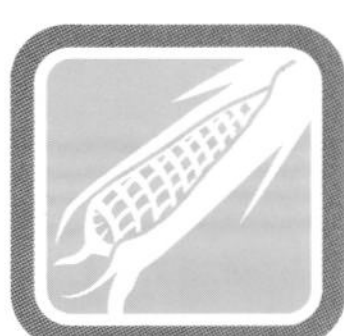

½ cup polenta
½. cup amaranth
3 cups water
½ teaspoon sea salt
½ cup dried cranberries
½ cup pine nuts
1-2 tablespoons honey
¼ cup milk (or non-dairy milk)

- Heat water with salt to boil.
- Add polenta and amaranth.
- Reduce heat and simmer, covered about 30 minutes, stirring occasionally.
- After 20 minutes, stir in cranberries.
- Taste to see if it's done. It should be soft and creamy.
- Add pine nuts, honey, and milk and enjoy!

Rice Porridge with Apples

***Prep Time:* 5 minutes**
***Cooking Time:* 15 minutes**
***Serves* 3**

2 cups leftover brown rice
1 apple
¼ cup water, rice milk, or coconut water
1 tablespoon brown rice syrup
1 teaspoon maple syrup
1 teaspoon ground cinnamon
pinch of sea salt

- Add rice, liquid, sweeteners, cinnamon, and salt to a pan and begin cooking over medium low heat.
- Peel and dice the apple, and add to the pot.
- Stir to mix everything well.
- Bring to a boil, then reduce heat to low and simmer.
- Continue cooking about 10 minutes, until the apple has become a little soft
- Enjoy hot!

Tofu Scramble

***Prep Time:* 5 minutes**
***Cooking Time:* 20 minutes**
***Serves* 2**

1 block firm tofu
2 to 3 tablespoons olive oil
½ teaspoon tamari soy sauce
⅛ teaspoon turmeric
1 red onion
½ red bell pepper
⅛ teaspoon paprika
1 tablespoon umeboshi vinegar
dash of black pepper

- Press tofu to remove excess water and then crumble into small pieces.
- Chop onion and pepper.
- Heat oil.

- Add tofu, tamari, and turmeric.
- Sauté for a few minutes.
- Add vegetables, paprika, umeboshi vinegar, and black pepper to tofu.
- Cook for 5 minutes or until mixture thoroughly heats and flavors blend.

TIP: *Use alfalfa sprouts or fresh parsley to garnish.*

Japanese Style Breakfast

Prep Time: 5 minutes
Cooking Time: 10 minutes
Serves 1

4 big bok choy leaves
1 teaspoon toasted sesame oil
1 tablespoon brown rice vinegar
1 tablespoon tamari
½ cup cooked brown rice

- Wash bok choy and chop into bite-sized pieces.
- Heat sesame oil in a sauté pan.
- Add bok choy and stir fry for one minute.
- Add vinegar, tamari, and rice.
- Stir gently and continue cooking about 3 minutes, until everything is warm.
- Transfer to a bowl to eat.

TIP: *Garnish with sesame seeds.*

TIP: *If you want some extra protein with your breakfast, add 4 ounces cooked salmon or other fish.*

Morning Sausage and Kale

Prep Time: 5 minutes
Cooking Time: 10 minutes
Serves 2

1 teaspoon olive oil
½ small yellow onion
1 precooked chicken apple sausage
½ bunch kale
1 tablespoon balsamic vinegar

- Slice onion into half moons (long, thin slivers)
- Heat oil in a frying pan and sauté onion for 5 minutes
- Meanwhile, slice sausage into ½-inch rounds and chop the kale into 1-inch pieces.
- Add sausage and kale to the frying pan and cook for 5 minutes, or until sausage is hot and kale has become soft.
- Remove from heat and sprinkle with balsamic vinegar before eating.

TIP: *If you are a vegetarian, try substituting marinated tempeh for the sausage.*

Scrambled Eggs and Greens

Prep Time: 10 minutes
Cooking Time: 12 minutes
Serves 1-2

1 tablespoon olive oil
1 leek, chopped into small pieces
1 clove garlic, minced
2 eggs
1 carrot, diced
1 cup chopped spinach, dandelion, watercress, or chard

- Beat the eggs in a small bowl.
- Heat the oil in a frying pan.
- Sauté leek for 3 minutes. Add garlic and sauté another minute.
- Add carrots, cover, and cook 5 minutes on low heat, until carrots are softened.
- Remove veggies and put on a plate.
- Add a little oil to the pan if it's dry, add the eggs, and cook over medium heat for 3 minutes until eggs are mostly cooked.
- Add greens and other veggies and stir everything together, scrambling the eggs.
- Add salt and pepper to taste and serve.

vegetables

Basic Cooking Methods for Vegetables

Steaming

Steaming is a simple way to cook vegetables, allowing you to experience their simple flavors in a pure form. Steaming takes 5 to 10 minutes for leafy green vegetables and 10 to 25 minutes for root vegetables. All you need is a steaming basket, a pot with about 2 inches of water at the bottom, and a lid.

Stir-Frying

Stir-frying is another quick and nutritious way to prepare vegetables. This method highlights their natural flavors. It takes just 5 to 10 minutes. You can stir-fry in oil or water. All you need is a skillet with a lid. If you choose to use oil, heat a skillet and add 3 to 5 tablespoons. Add vegetables and sprinkle them with a pinch of sea salt to enhance their flavor. To reduce fat but keep the flavor, you can use 2 to 3 tablespoons of water and 1 tablespoon of oil. This is called a wet sauté. After stir-frying the veggies for a few minutes in the oil, add the water and cover to give the vegetables extra steam and heat. Another option is a pure water sauté. Place 1 inch of water in your skillet and add garlic, ginger, or spices if desired. Bring to boil, add thinly sliced vegetables, cover, and simmer for 5 to 10 minutes.

Baking

Many vegetables taste best baked. Baking brings out the very essence of the vegetables, especially squashes and roots. You need a baking pan or sheet, vegetables, an oven heated between 375 and 450 degrees, and 50 to 60 minutes of cooking time. Be sure to use a nonstick pan or oil the vegetables so they don't stick.

Quick Boiling

When quick boiling vegetables, put them in boiling water and leave for 3 to 5 minutes. This method removes their raw flavor, makes them more digestible, and brightens their color. When you're done boiling, rinse vegetables with cold water to stop additional cooking and to preserve the color. You can save the boiled water and use it for drinking, cooking grains, watering your plants, or adding to soups.

How to Make Plain Steamed Vegetables More Exciting

- After cooking, add 1 tablespoon olive oil or toasted sesame oil to every 2 cups of veggies.
- Add 2 bay leaves or 1 teaspoon cumin seeds to the cooking water.
- Sprinkle cooked veggies with toasted pumpkin, sesame, flax, or sunflower seeds. Or sprinkle with almonds, walnuts, or dried shredded coconut.
- Sprinkle greens with fresh herbs: mint, dill, basil, parsley, cilantro, or scallion.
- Use tamari soy sauce or umeboshi vinegar to add extra flavor to cooked veggies.
- Squeeze fresh lemon or lime juice over steamed vegetables.
- After steaming, quickly stir-fry with a pinch of sea salt, olive oil, and garlic.

Steamed Kale

Prep Time: 5 minutes
Cooking Time: 15 minutes
Serves 4

1 bunch of kale
2 cups water
pinch sea salt

- Put water, salt, and a steamer basket in a medium-size pot and heat on high.
- Wash kale.
- Remove leaves from stems and cut or tear leaves in any size you like.
- Chop the stems into ½-inch pieces, discarding the bottom as it tends to be tough.
- When the water is boiling, add the stems to the pot, cover, and cook for one minute.
- Now add the leaves, cover, lower the heat, and steam for another 2-4 minutes. Leaves should be wilted, yet bright green.
- Carefully remove the steamer basket and transfer kale to a serving dish.

TIP: *Enjoy the kale plain, or add a little tamari or lemon juice.*

TIP: *Try this same technique with collard greens, bok choy, and mustard greens.*

Basic Blanched Greens

Prep Time: 5 minutes
Cooking Time: 15 minutes
Serves 4

1 bunch any leafy green (kale, collards, bok choy, chard, etc.)
½ inch water in a pot
umeboshi vinegar
tamari
flax oil

- Heat water in a large pot.
- Chop or tear greens into bite-size pieces, removing stems.
- Chop stems into small pieces.
- When water boils, add stems and cook 1 minute.
- Add leaves and cook another 3 minutes.
- Strain through a colander and transfer to serving dish.
- Add a bit of umeboshi, tamari, and flax to taste.

Brazilian Style Collards

Prep Time: 5 minutes
Cooking Time: 5 minutes
Serves 6

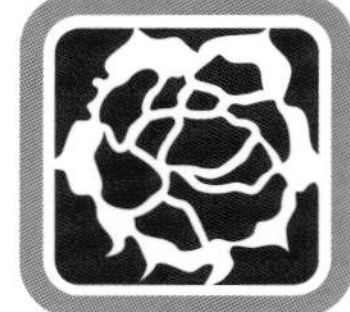

2 tablespoons olive oil
3 cloves garlic
2 bunches collard greens
salt and pepper to taste

- Wash collards.
- Remove leaves from stems, tear leaves in half, and stack into piles 4 leaves thick.
- Roll the stack tightly, turn to the side, and cut carefully into very thin strips. Repeat with all of the collards. The effect is that the leaves will be shredded.
- Mince the garlic.
- Heat oil in a frying pan and sauté garlic until golden brown, about 30 seconds.
- Add collards, salt, and pepper and toss quickly for about 3 minutes with tongs or a fork, making sure all greens get cooked.
- Remove from heat and transfer to a serving dish.

Sautéed Greens with Pine Nuts and Raisins

Prep Time: 10 minutes
Cooking Time: 10 minutes
Serves 6

½ bunch mustard greens
½ bunch kale
½ bunch dandelion greens
1 tablespoon olive oil
½ teaspoons sea salt
¼ cup pine nuts
⅓ cup raisins

- Toast pine nuts on a cookie sheet in a 325-degree oven for 5 minutes. Set aside.
- Wash and chop greens.
- Heat olive oil.
- Add greens, sea salt, and raisins. Stir and cook 5 minutes.
- Turn off heat. Add in pine nuts, and transfer to serving dish.

TIP: *Sprinkle with lemon juice before serving.*

Baby Bok Choy and Shiitakes

Prep Time: 8 minutes
Cooking Time: 8 minutes
Serves 6

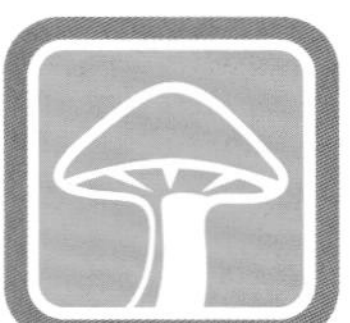

1 small yellow onion
4 heads baby bok choy
6 fresh shiitake mushrooms
1 tablespoon toasted sesame oil
3 tablespoons mirin
1 tablespoon tamari

- Peel onion and slice into long, thin strips.
- Heat oil in a frying pan.
- Add onions, turn heat down, and cook 5 minutes, stirring occasionally.
- Meanwhile, wash bok choy and slice each leaf in half.
- Thinly slice shiitakes.

- Add shiitakes, bok choy, mirin, and tamari to pan. Cover and cook 3 minutes.
- Spread on a flat surface to cool and stop greens from cooking.

TIP: *Garnish with toasted sesame seeds.*

Oh So Delicious Green Cleanser

This dish has got all of the five tastes: sweet, sour, bitter, salty, and pungent. It can be helpful in bringing balance to the system after a period of not-so-healthy eating.

Prep Time: 8 minutes
Cooking Time: 5 minutes
Serves 4

1 bunch lacinato kale
½ medium daikon radish
1 tablespoon tamari
1 teaspoon toasted sesame oil
1 tablespoon brown rice vinegar
1 tablespoon agave syrup
1 tablespoon nutritional yeast flakes

- Heat a medium sized pot with 2 inches of water.
- Chop the kale into 2-inch pieces (stems can stay on).
- Chop the daikon into 1-inch chunks.
- When the water boils, add veggies and blanch 2 minutes.
- Remove to a colander to drain and transfer to a large mixing bowl.
- Add all other ingredients and mix well, tasting to adjust amounts to your desire.

TIP: *It is even more amazing if you add some dulse flakes and sesame seeds.*

TIP: *Also try adding other vegetables as you like, such as cauliflower, broccoli, string beans, asparagus, etc.*

Gayatri Greens

These Indian-style greens bear the name of a powerful Hindu Goddess, and also a beautiful mantra (prayer) that is said to represent the divine awakening of the mind and soul.

***Prep Time:* 8 minutes**
***Cooking Time:* 10 minutes**
Serves 4

2 tablespoons coconut oil
1 teaspoon black mustard seeds
1 teaspoon ground cumin
1 teaspoon ground coriander
1 bunch swiss chard
½ cup organic plain yogurt
½ teaspoon sea salt

- Wash chard, cut out stems, and chop leaves into 1-inch pieces.
- Prepare spices and place them next to the stove.
- Heat oil in a frying pan on medium high.
- When the oil is hot, add mustard seeds and cook, stirring for 1 minute.
- Add cumin and coriander and cook for another 30 seconds, stirring.
- Add chard and salt, mix well, and cook 3-5 minutes, until chard is wilted.
- Turn off heat, stir in yogurt, and enjoy.

Lemon Broccoli with Avocado

***Prep Time:* 5 minutes**
***Cooking Time:* 15 minutes**
Serves 8

2 bunches broccoli
1 avocado
1 lemon
1 tablespoon olive oil
¼ teaspoon sea salt

- Chop broccoli into bite-size pieces, keeping stems separate from crowns.
- Fill a pot with 1 inch of water, place a steamer basket inside, cover, and heat to boiling.

- Add stem pieces, and steam for 2 minutes.
- Add crown pieces, cover, and steam for 5 minutes while you prepare the other ingredients.
- In a mixing bowl, combine the juice of the lemon, the olive oil, and salt.
- Chop the avocado into chunks and add to the bowl.
- Add the warm broccoli to the bowl, mix gently, and serve.

Bitter Greens with Walnuts

Prep Time: 10 minutes
Cooking Time: 15 minutes
Serves 8

1 bunch dandelion greens
1 bunch mustard greens
1 bunch collard greens
1 tablespoon olive oil
4 cloves garlic
½ cup walnut pieces
sea salt to taste

- Toast the walnuts in a 350-degree oven for 5-10 minutes, until they release a fragrant odor.
- Wash the greens and remove any coarse stems (especially from collards and mustard greens).
- Bring 3 inches of salted water to boil, add the greens, and boil for 5 minutes uncovered.
- Drain the greens, lay on a flat surface to cool, and then chop roughly.
- Heat the oil in a large sauté pan, add the garlic, and cook for 1 minute, stirring so the garlic doesn't burn.
- Add the greens, walnuts, and salt to taste and sauté for another minute.
- Enjoy!

Quick Daikon Pickles

Prep Time: 8 minutes
Cooking Time: none!
Serves 15

1 large daikon radish
¼ cup mirin
⅛ cup umeboshi vinegar
water

- Wash and peel daikon and slice into half circles that are ½-inch thick.
- Place daikon in a container.
- Add mirin, umeboshi, and just enough water to cover the daikon.
- Cover, shake, and store in the fridge.
- The pickles will be ready in 30 minutes and will stay good in the fridge for weeks.

TIP: *Use a few pieces as a condiment to go along with any other vegetable, grain, salad, or protein dish.*

Beet-Carrot-Parsnip-Fennel Extravaganza

Prep Time: 10 minutes
Cooking Time: 45 minutes
Serves 6

5 small beets
3 big carrots
2 parsnips
1 fennel bulb
2 tablespoons olive oil
½ teaspoon sea salt

- Preheat oven to 425 degrees.
- Scrub all your vegetables.
- Chop vegetables into 2-inch pieces and finely chop fennel bulb.
- Mix vegetables with oil and sea salt. Transfer them to a baking dish.
- Bake covered for 30 minutes.
- Uncover and bake for 15 minutes.

Roasted Rutabaga with Celery Root

Prep Time: 8 minutes
Cooking Time: 40 minutes
Serves 6

1 rutabaga
1 celery root
2 tablespoons olive oil
½ teaspoon sea salt
1 teaspoon fresh rosemary

- Preheat oven to 400 degrees.
- Wash and scrub vegetables. Cut them into 1-inch-thick rounds.
- Mix with oil, salt, and rosemary.
- Cover and bake for 30 minutes. Turn vegetables over and bake uncovered for 10 more minutes.

Carrot Burdock Strengthener

Prep Time: 10 minutes
Cooking Time: 20 minutes
Serves 6

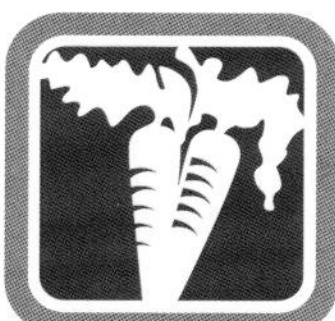

1 onion
1 large burdock root
1 large carrot
1 teaspoon olive oil
pinch of sea salt

- Wash and chop the vegetables into odd shapes.
- Heat oil in a skillet.
- Sauté veggies together with a pinch of salt on medium heat for 5 minutes.
- Add ½ inch of water to the skillet, cover, and simmer for 10-15 minutes on low heat.

TIP: *Try serving with a sprinkle of toasted sesame seeds or fresh parsley for variety.*

Baked Caraway Sweet Potato with Rosemary

Prep Time: 10 minutes
Cooking Time: 50 minutes
Serves 6

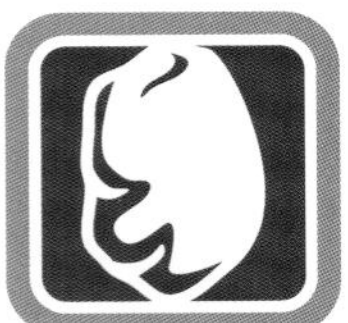

3 medium sweet potatoes
2 tablespoons olive oil
½ cup fresh rosemary
½ tablespoon caraway seeds

- Preheat oven to 400 degrees.
- Scrub sweet potatoes under running water and cut them into big chunks.
- Sprinkle baking dish with oil, place the sweet potatoes into the dish, and add rosemary and caraway seeds.
- Mix all ingredients together.
- Cover and bake for 50 minutes.

TIP: *Rosemary and caraway seeds can be substituted with cinnamon and 2 tablespoons of maple syrup or 1 tablespoon of ground cumin and a couple of dashes of cayenne.*

Veggie Bake

Prep Time: 20 minutes
Cooking Time: 50 minutes
Serves 4 or more

all the leftover veggies in your fridge that need to be used up
1 large can chopped tomatoes
1 can chickpeas
1-2 large yams, sliced into ⅛-inch-thick sheets
extra virgin olive oil

- Preheat the oven to 350 degrees.
- Chop veggies (not yams) and sauté in a bit of oil until soft, 5-10 minutes.
- Add can of tomatoes and drained can of chickpeas. Mix well and remove from heat.
- Slice yams into thin sheets.
- Spread a little olive oil on the bottom of a casserole dish and cover with a layer of yam sheets (as you would with lasagna noodles).
- Spoon out veggie-tomato-chickpea mixture and spread evenly on top of yams.

- Finish with a layer of yams.
- Lightly drizzle olive oil on top.
- Bake, covered, for 30 minutes.
- Take off the cover and turn up temperature to 450 degrees for 10 minutes to crisp up the top later.

TIP: *Add your favorite spices, like basil, oregano, fennel, cumin, chili pepper, or sea salt, when adding tomatoes and chickpeas.*

Spaghetti Squash Marinara

Prep Time: 10 minutes
Cooking Time: 45 minutes
Serves 4

1 spaghetti squash
olive oil
1 small onion
1 carrot
5 button mushrooms
2 fresh tomatoes
2 tablespoons minced fresh herbs (basil, oregano, or thyme)

- Preheat the oven to 425 degrees.
- Carefully cut the squash in half lengthwise and remove the seeds.
- Rub the inside with olive oil, and place open side down in a baking dish with ½ inch of water.
- Bake 45 minutes, or until a fork pierces easily through the squash.
- While squash is baking, prepare the sauce.
- Dice the onion, carrot, and tomatoes. Slice the mushrooms. Mince the herbs.
- Sauté the onions for 5 minutes in 1 tablespoon olive oil.
- Add the carrot and tomatoes and cook another 5 minutes.
- Add the mushrooms, herbs, and salt and continue cooking another 5-10 minutes.
- When the squash is cooked and cooled a little, use a fork to scrape the meat into spaghetti-like strands.
- Mix sauce and squash together in a bowl and serve.

TIP: *Add garlic, other veggies, or cooked chicken pieces to the sauce.*

Satisfying Sesame Burdock

Prep Time: 5 minutes
Cooking Time: 10 minutes
Serves 3

1 large burdock root
2 teaspoons toasted sesame oil
1 teaspoon Bragg liquid aminos
1 teaspoon tahini
a few squirts of umeboshi vinegar

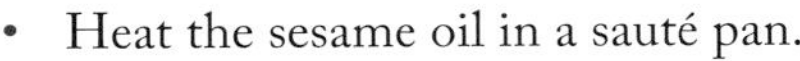

- Heat the sesame oil in a sauté pan.
- Slice the burdock in ½-inch rounds and add to the hot oil.
- Sauté for 5 minutes, stirring frequently.
- Add a little water, cover, and steam for 5 minutes.
- Meanwhile, add the other ingredients to a bowl and mix well.
- Add the burdock to the bowl and mix to coat with the sauce.

TIP: *Chop fresh spinach or dandelion greens and add during the last 2 minutes of cooking.*

meat & fish

When choosing meat and fish for cooking, always look for the best quality available. With meats, try organic, grass-fed meats that are leaner and full of more nutrients than meats from large factory farms. With fish, try wild varieties with vibrant colors and pick fish that smells fresh, like the ocean. If you are unsure about the quality of meat and fish available at your local store, ask the butcher or fishmonger for assistance in making the best choice.

Salmon Cakes

Prep Time: 10 minutes
Cooking Time: 10 minutes
Serves 4

4 ounces cooked salmon
6 rice crackers
½ onion, minced
2 cloves minced garlic
1 tablespoon fresh lemon juice
dash of black pepper
dash of coriander
1 tablespoon olive oil

- Break salmon and rice crackers into small pieces.
- Mix all ingredients together.
- Create several small patties.
- Refrigerate for 1 hour.
- In a skillet, heat oil on high.
- Quickly fry both sides of each patty for 3-4 minutes.

TIP: *Serve with brown rice and lemon slices.*

Ideal Dill Fish

Prep Time: 5 minutes
Cooking Time: 10 minutes
Serves 4

1 pound cod fish fillet
dash of sea salt
dash of black pepper
½ cup fresh dill
1 tablespoon fresh lemon juice

- Rinse fish.
- Season with salt and pepper.
- Finely chop dill.
- Fill skillet with about ½ inch of water and heat till steaming.
- Drop in fish, cover top with dill, and cook until it is soft, about 5 to 7 minutes.
- Serve immediately.

Honey-Macadamia Halibut

Prep Time: 10 minutes
Cooking Time: 10 minutes
Serves 4

4 4-ounce halibut fillets (1 inch thick)
¼ cup macadamia nuts
3 tablespoons honey
1 tablespoons coconut oil

- Chop nuts, spread on a cookie sheet, and toast in the oven or in a toaster on 350 degrees until golden brown, about 5-7 minutes. Check every minute or two and stir or spin tray around to toast evenly.
- Heat oil in a skillet.
- Sprinkle salt and pepper on both sides of each fish fillet, and cook first side over medium heat for 4 minutes.
- Flip each fillet and cook for 3 minutes on the other side.
- While fish is in the pan, spread a layer of honey on each fillet and add a layer of nuts on top.
- Flip over and cook for 2 minutes, while you add honey and nuts to the other side.
- Flip again and cook 2 minutes.

- Halibut is cooked when the meat is no longer translucent.
- Remove from heat and serve.

Moroccan Chicken Tagine with Prunes

Prep Time: 15 minutes
Cooking Time: 45 minutes
Serves 4

2 chicken breasts cut into 2-inch chunks
1 yellow onion, sliced into strips
½ teaspoons turmeric
2 cloves minced garlic
½ teaspoon powdered ginger
½ teaspoon powdered cinnamon
10 pitted prunes

- Heat 1 tablespoon of olive oil in a deep pan and sauté onions on low heat until translucent, 10 minutes or so.
- Add everything else except prunes and mix well.
- Add ½ cup water, cover, and cook over medium heat 30 minutes. Chicken should be cooked all the way through but should not be dried out. (Cut a piece open to check.)
- Add prunes and cook another 5 minutes, until they get soft and saturated with juice.

TIP: *Top with toasted sesame seeds and chopped parsley.*

Chai Chicken

Chai is the Indian way of drinking tea. You can buy chai tea bags, or make it yourself by putting shredded ginger, cinnamon powder, and ground cardamom seeds in a pot with 2 cups of water and bringing it to a boil. Cook for 2 to 3 minutes to bring flavor out of the spices, then add tea and stir.

Prep Time: 10 minutes
Cooking Time: 45 minutes
Serves 4

4 chicken legs
4 to 5 sliced carrots
1 cup coconut milk
2 cups chai tea

- Preheat oven to 350 degrees.
- Place chicken and carrots in a casserole dish. Sprinkle with a pinch of salt and pepper.
- In a pot, combine coconut milk and tea and bring to a boil.
- Pour over the chicken in the casserole dish.
- Cover with lid and bake in the oven at 350 degrees for 45 minutes, or until chicken is cooked through.
- Serve with brown basmati rice and greens. Use coconut milk mixture as a sauce.

Smoked Turkey with Kale

Prep Time: 10 minutes
Cooking Time: 20 minutes
Serves 4

2 teaspoons olive oil
1 red onion, sliced into thin strips
1 bunch curly kale, sliced into thin ribbons
½ pound smoked turkey breast, sliced into bite-size chunks
1 tablespoon balsamic vinegar
salt and pepper to taste

- Slowly sauté the onions over medium low heat for 15 minutes, until they start to turn a little brown.
- Add kale and stir until wilted, about 3 minutes.
- Add turkey and cook another 2 minutes until it is warm.
- Transfer to a serving dish and add balsamic vinegar, salt and pepper to taste.

Beef and Arugula Stir-Fry

Prep Time: 15 minutes
Cooking Time: 15 minutes
Serves 3

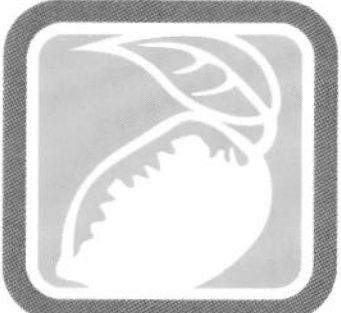

½ pound sirloin, cut into thin strips
2 teaspoons olive oil
1 tablespoon minced fresh ginger
1 clove minced garlic
2 red bell peppers, cut into very thin strips
1 to 2 bunches well-washed arugula
2 teaspoons kuzu
2 teaspoons tamari
2 teaspoons brown rice or apple cider vinegar
¼ cup water

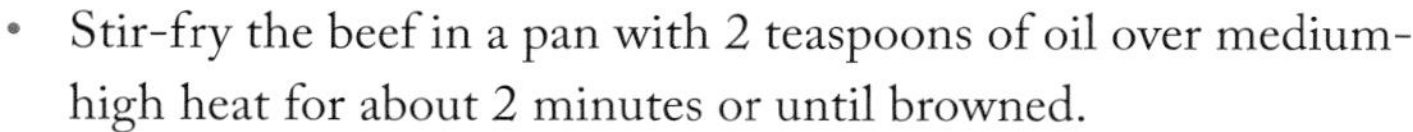

- Stir-fry the beef in a pan with 2 teaspoons of oil over medium-high heat for about 2 minutes or until browned.
- Remove beef with tongs or fork, allowing excess oil to drip off, and set aside.
- In same pan in remaining oil, stir-fry ginger and garlic for 2 to 3 minutes, and then add the bell pepper. Cook for another 2 to 3 minutes.
- Mix together fresh arugula and bell pepper mixture in a serving bowl.
- In a small bowl, combine kuzu, tamari, vinegar, and water.
- Place kuzu mixture into skillet and cook over medium heat until sauce starts to thicken.
- Return the beef to the skillet and cook for 1 minute, just enough to warm up the beef.
- Add the beef to the serving bowl with arugula and bell peppers.
- Mix and serve warm.

soup

Everyone craves comfort food. When we are busy and stressed, we tend to reach for our favorite convenience foods to get a soothing effect. Soup is the ultimate comfort food and a healthier choice. Remember eating soup as a child when you were sick? As adults, eating soup can still give us that cozy, nurtured feeling.

Soups are highly nutritious. Almost any vegetable can go into a soup; it is a great way to use leftover vegetables in your fridge. Cooking soup from scratch may sound like a big project, but in fact soups are incredibly quick and easy to make. The active prep time for all these soups is 10 minutes. You can prepare other components of your meal while you wait, or kick back with a magazine until your soup is done and ready to be enjoyed.

Roasted Vegetable Stock

Prep Time: 10 minutes
Cooking Time: 1 hour and 45 minutes

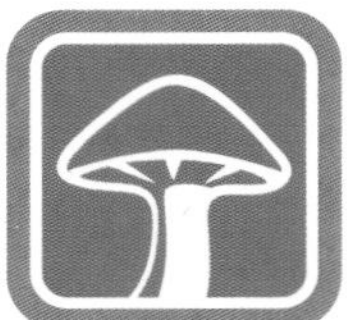

1 onion
1 parsnip
1 carrot
5 cloves garlic
4 mushrooms
1 bunch parsley
olive oil
sea salt and black pepper

- Preheat oven to 400 degrees.
- Peel and wash veggies, cut into chunks (you can leave garlic cloves whole), and spread on a cookie sheet.
- Drizzle a little olive oil over veggies and sprinkle with salt and pepper.
- Roast in the oven for 45 minutes, turning veggies occasionally until everything gets a little brown.
- Remove veggies from oven and place in a large soup pot with 10 cups of water.

- Bring to a boil, reduce heat to low, and simmer for at least one hour.
- Strain stock and it's ready to go!

TIP: *After you strain the stock, put it back on the stove on low heat for another hour or more. It will reduce to become more of a concentrate. To store it, pour it into an ice cube tray and freeze it. Then the next time you need some stock, just pop out a cube or two to flavor your rice or soup.*

Mighty Miso Soup

Prep Time: 10 minutes
Cooking Time: 15 minutes
Serves 4

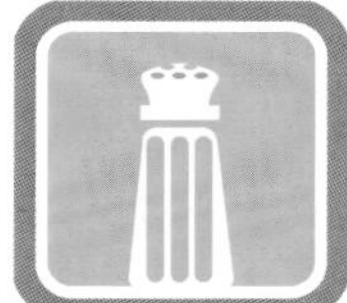

8-inch piece wakame
1 medium onion
1 medium daikon radish
½ block tofu
5 cups water
1 to 2 tablespoons miso paste
2 green onions

- Wash wakame, soak for 5 minutes or until softened, and cut into 1-inch pieces.
- Cut onion into long, thin strips.
- Cut daikon into half moons.
- Cut tofu into ½-inch cubes.
- Add veggies, wakame, and tofu to water and bring to boil.
- Reduce heat to low, and simmer for 10 minutes.
- Meanwhile, remove ½ cup of liquid from the pot and stir in the miso to dissolve.
- Return miso mixture to pot, reduce heat to very low, and cook for 2 to 3 more minutes. Do not boil.
- Garnish with chopped scallion.

Easy Breezy Soup

***Prep Time:* 10 minutes**
***Cooking Time:* 20-30 minutes**
Serves 4

Try any of these vegetable combinations to create a simply delicious soup: carrot, parsnip, celery, winter squash, yam ginger, broccoli, onion, cauliflower, daikon radish, leek, carrot, mustard greens, shiitakes, onion, kale, cabbage, rutabaga.

- Use one of each vegetable.
- Cut all veggies to roughly the same size, around 2-inch chunks.
- Place cut veggies in a pot with water just covering them.
- Bring to a boil, then lower to simmer.
- Cook until a fork inserts smoothly into each vegetable, probably about 20 minutes.
- Add your favorite condiments.
- Eat like this, or puree in a food processor, in a blender, or with a hand mixer.

TIP: *Garnish with parsley and scallion.*

TIP: *To add richness to soup, sauté one medium onion and add to water before cooking.*

Carrot Ginger Soup

***Prep Time:* 10 minutes**
***Cooking Time:* 30 minutes**
Serves 4

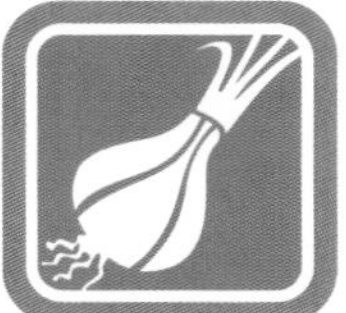

6 carrots
1 medium onion
1 teaspoon sea salt
4 cups water
6-inch piece fresh ginger
Fresh parsley to garnish

- Wash, peel, and cut carrots and onion into chunks.
- Place vegetables and salt in a pot.
- Add water. Bring to a boil. Cover with a lid.
- Simmer on low heat for 25 minutes.

- Transfer soup into blender, adding water if necessary to achieve desired consistency.
- When blending is done, squeeze juice from grated ginger and add to soup.
- Garnish with parsley.

TIP: *For extra flavor, sauté vegetables before cooking.*

TIP: *Substitute carrots with squash, parsnip, or beets. Squash and beets need 35 to 40 minutes to cook.*

Creamy Broccoli Soup

Prep Time: 10 minutes
Cooking Time: 30 minutes
Serves 4

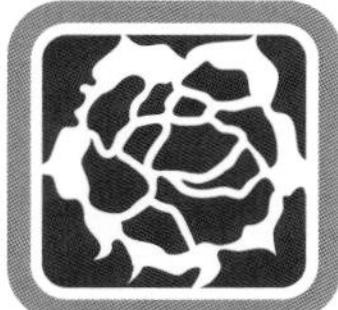

1 bunch broccoli
5 cups water
1 small onion
2 cloves garlic
2 tablespoons barley miso
1 cup cooked brown rice

- Wash broccoli and separate stems from florets.
- Chop onion.
- In a pot, bring water to a boil.
- Add broccoli stems and onion.
- Mince the garlic and add to the pot.
- Reduce heat and simmer for 15 minutes.
- Meanwhile, remove 2 cups of liquid from the pot, dissolve miso paste in the liquid, add brown rice, and return to the pot.
- Put soup in the blender and blend. When it is smooth, return to the pot.
- Add broccoli florets and cook 10 more minutes.

Garlic Lover's Soup

They say that garlic is as good as ten mothers due to its incredible healing properties. Try this soup when you are feeling a cold coming on.

Prep Time: 10 minutes
Cooking Time: 1 hour
Serves 4

2 heads garlic
2 teaspoons olive oil
5 cups vegetable stock
2 bunches spinach, chopped

- Preheat oven to 425 degrees.
- Slice off the top of each head of garlic, exposing the top of each clove.
- Pour a teaspoon of oil on each head.
- Place in a casserole dish with a lid or wrap in foil.
- Roast for 45 minutes or until cloves are completely soft.
- Let the garlic cool for a few minutes and squeeze cloves into a pot.
- Add stock and stir to break up the garlic and combine.
- Bring to boil, reduce heat, and simmer for 10 minutes.
- Just at the end, add in the spinach to wilt, stir well, and serve right away.

Cool Cucumber and Avocado Soup

Prep Time: 10 minutes
Cooking Time: none!
Serves 4

1 cucumber, peeled
1 avocado
2 green onions
juice of 1 lime
1 cup plain yogurt or soy yogurt
1 cup water
salt and pepper to taste

- Roughly chop the cucumber, avocado, and green onions and toss in the blender.
- Add other ingredients and process until smooth.

TIP: *Garnish with chopped fresh cilantro and a dash of cayenne pepper.*

salads

Ideas for Green Salads

Sometimes it's nice to get your greens from a good ol' salad of mixed greens. Here are some ways to put a new twist on an old favorite.

For the greens themselves, try a mixture using any of these:

- Romaine, red leaf, green leaf, butter lettuce, mesclun mix, spinach, blanched dark leafy greens, any cabbage, endive, radicchio, arugula, frisee, or whatever organic greens look fabulous at your market today.
- Add some veggies: use any that look and sound good to you. Try green beans, radishes, roasted winter squash, sugar snaps, corn from the cob, or root veggies.
- Add some fruits: fresh or dried berries, apples, tangerines, avocados, melons, figs, goji berries, or cucumbers.
- And don't leave out the nuts, seeds, and beans: sunflower seeds, pumpkin seeds, sprouts of all kinds, toasted nuts, sesame seeds, or coconut flakes.
- Be experimental! Add anything else you can imagine—dulse flakes, leftover grains, tofu, fish, toasted nori—just go for it!
- Then top it off with a delicious dressing (see Sauces & Dressings section) and enjoy!

Quinoa Salad

Prep Time: 15 minutes
Cooking Time: none!
Serves 8

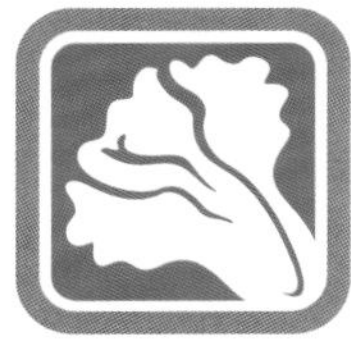

2 cups cooked quinoa
½ cup chopped radishes
½ cup chopped cucumber
½ cup chopped celery
½ cup chopped red onion
½ cup chopped fresh parsley
½ cup chopped red bell pepper
1 tablespoon olive oil
2 teaspoons balsamic vinegar

- Combine all ingredients together in a big bowl.
- Mix well.

TIP: *Garnish with cherry tomatoes and shredded garlic cloves and chill before serving.*

Carrot Raisin Salad

Prep Time: 10 minutes
Cooking Time: none!
Serves 6

2 carrots
handful of raisins
umeboshi vinegar
tamari
flax oil

- Grate carrots by hand or in a food processor.
- Place carrots and raisins in a mixing bowl.
- Dress with the other ingredients, to taste.

TIP: *This is a quick and easy salad to make when you get home from work, starving, and you want to devour everything in your fridge. Make this salad, sit down and relax for few minutes, and then move on to making dinner or whatever your evening entails.*

Barley Sun Salad

Prep Time: 20 minutes
Cooking Time: 1 hour
Serves 8

1 cup hulled barley
2 ¼ cups water
2 bunches arugula
½ cup sunflower seeds
1 carrot
½ bunch scallions
2 tablespoons olive oil
juice of 1 or 2 lemons

- Place barley water and ¼ teaspoon sea salt in a pot.
- Bring to a boil, reduce heat to low, and simmer, covered for 45 minutes.
- Meanwhile, wash arugula and chop into small pieces.
- Place sunflower seeds on a cookie sheet and toast for 5 minutes in a 350-degree oven, being careful not to burn them.
- Wash and chop the carrot into a small dice.
- Wash and finely chop the scallions.
- When the barley is cooked, transfer to a large mixing bowl, add all ingredients, and mix well.
- Add salt, pepper, oil, or lemon juice to meet your taste preference.

Cold Soba Noodle Salad

Prep Time: 20 minutes
Cooking Time: 15 minutes
Serves 4

8 ounces soba noodles
6 cups water
1 bunch chopped sunflower sprouts or pea shoots
½ cup chopped red radishes
½ cup chopped celery
½ cup chopped cucumber

- Put soba noodles into a pot of 6 cups boiling water.
- Cook until tender, no more than 8 minutes.
- Rinse with cold water when finished cooking.
- Mix all vegetables and noodles.

Dressing:
½ cup finely chopped fresh basil
1 tablespoon toasted sesame oil
¼ cup tahini
2 tablespoons tamari soy sauce
2-inch piece grated fresh ginger
juice of ½ lemon

- Mix all these ingredients and pour over noodles.

Beet Salad with Fennel and Mint

This salad is famous for converting non-beet eaters into beet lovers!

Prep Time: 20 minutes
Cooking Time: 30 minutes
Serves 6

2 beets
1 small fennel bulb
1 bunch mint leaves
2 oranges
¼ cup balsamic vinegar

- Place beets in a pot, cover with 1 inch with water, and boil for 20-30 minutes, until a fork pierces easily through the middle of each beet.
- While beets are cooking, wash fennel and slice very thin.
- Chop mint into thin ribbons.
- Zest oranges and juice them into a bowl.
- When beets are cooked, drain them in the sink.
- Cool them by rinsing under cold water, and peel the skin off with your hands. (It should slide right off.)
- Chop the beets into ¼-inch-thick quarter rounds.
- Add all ingredients into a large bowl and mix well.

Late Summer Corn Salad

Prep Time: 20 minutes
Cooking Time: 10 minutes
Serves 6

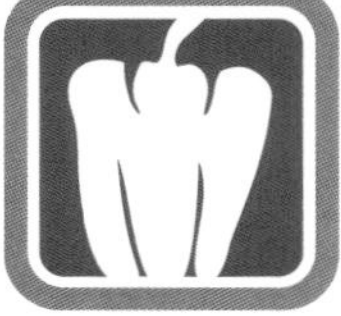

4 ears corn
½ small red onion
½ small green bell pepper
½ small red bell pepper
½ bunch cilantro
1 tablespoon olive oil
juice of 1 lemon
sea salt and pepper to taste

- Boil corn in a large pot for 5-10 minutes.

- Remove from pot and cool by running under cold water.
- Cut kernels from the cobs and place in a large mixing bowl.
- Finely dice the onion and peppers, mince the cilantro, and add them all to the corn.
- Add oil, lemon, salt, and pepper and mix well.
- Taste and adjust seasonings.

Raw, Nutty, Not Tuna Salad

Soaking Time: 8 hours or more
Prep Time: 15 minutes
Cooking Time: none!
Serves 4

1 cup almonds
1 cup sunflower seeds
1-2 stalks celery, finely chopped
1 tablespoon minced dill
½ small red onion, finely chopped
1 teaspoon kelp granules
juice of 1 lemon
½ teaspoon sea salt

- Place almonds in a bowl, cover with water, and let soak overnight.
- Do the same with the sunflower seeds.
- Discard most of the soaking water and combine nuts and seeds in a food processor or blender.
- Process until almost smooth.
- Combine with other ingredients in a bowl and mix well.

TIP: *Serve on a bed of mixed greens with a vinaigrette or as a sandwich filling, or roll in a sheet of nori.*

sauces & dressings

Tahini Lemon Dressing

Prep Time: 5 minutes
Serves 6

2 tablespoons tahini
juice of 1 lemon
½ cup water
¼ tablespoon tamari soy sauce

- Mix with a fork in small bowl.
- Adjust the amounts of each ingredient to meet your taste preference.

TIP: *Try adding a little miso paste too!*

Ginger Parsley Garlic Dressing

Prep Time: 8 minutes
Serves 8

4-inch piece fresh ginger
1 bunch fresh parsley
2 cloves garlic
juice of ½ lemon
½ tablespoon sesame oil
¼ tablespoon tamari soy sauce

- Dice ginger root. Put all ingredients in blender and blend until smooth.

Pumpkin Seed Dressing

Prep Time: 5 minutes
Serves 8

1 cup toasted pumpkin seeds
2 tablespoons brown rice vinegar
1 tablespoon umeboshi vinegar
1 teaspoon tamari soy sauce
1 cup water

- Mix in a bowl. Great on cooked greens!

Green Goddess Dressing

Prep Time: 5 minutes

½ pound silken tofu
1 bunch scallions
juice of 2 lemons
½ bunch flat leaf parsley
1 clove garlic
salt to taste

- Add all ingredients to blender and blend until creamy.
- Taste and adjust to your preference.

Maple Dijon Vinaigrette

Prep Time: 5 minutes

1 tablespoon Dijon mustard
½ cup balsamic vinegar
½ cup maple syrup
a couple pinches of sea salt and pepper
1 cup olive oil

- Blend first 4 ingredients in a food processor or with a whisk.
- Slowly add oil while mixing to emulsify.

Vegan Caesar Dressing

Prep Time: 15 minutes
Serves 8

¼ cup almonds
3 cloves garlic
3 tablespoons nutritional yeast flakes
2 tablespoons tamari
juice of 1 lemon
3 tablespoons Dijon mustard
1 tablespoon olive oil or flax oil

- Blanch the almonds by putting them in a bowl, pouring boiling water to cover them, and letting them sit for 1 minute.
- Drain and pat dry.
- Slip the skins off between your finger and thumb.
- Add all ingredients to a blender or food processor and blend until smooth.

TIP: *Serve with the classic combo of chopped romaine hearts and tempeh croutons.*

Simple Pesto

Prep Time: 5 minutes
Serves 8

¼ cup olive oil
1 cup basil leaves
1 cup pine nuts or walnuts
2 cloves garlic
2 tablespoons white miso
2 teaspoons umeboshi vinegar
1 teaspoon brown rice syrup
water

- Warm the oil over very low heat for 3 minutes.
- Combine all ingredients in a blender, except water.
- Blend together, adding as much water as necessary to get the consistency you desire.

Soothing Shiitake Gravy

Prep Time: 5 minutes
Cooking Time: 15 minutes
Serves 15

10 fresh shiitake mushrooms
1 heaping tablespoon kuzu root
1 teaspoon tamari
water

- Remove stems from shiitakes and slice caps thinly.
- Add to a pot with 2 quarts water.
- Bring to a boil, reduce heat, and simmer for 10 minutes.
- Add tamari.
- Dissolve kuzu root in ¼ cup cool water. It's nice to mash it up with your hand.
- Slowly add kuzu mixture to the pot, stirring as you pour it in.
- Stir for another minute, until the gravy thickens.
- Taste to see if you need to add more tamari, and serve.

Russian Dressing

Prep Time: 15 minutes
Serves 10

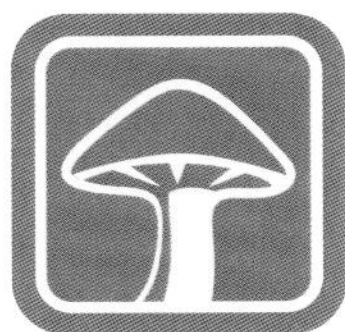

½ pound soft tofu
1 tablespoon lemon juice
3 tablespoons brown rice syrup
1 tablespoon olive oil
1 teaspoon mustard
1 tablespoon minced red onion
⅔ cup sun-dried tomatoes, soft and finely chopped
⅓ cup minced dill pickles
½ teaspoons sea salt

- Place sun-dried tomatoes in a bowl and cover with boiling water.
- Combine tofu, lemon juice, rice syrup, oil, and mustard in a food processor and puree until creamy.
- Chop and add tomatoes.
- Add pickles, onion, and salt.
- Pulse a few times to combine.

TIP: *Serve as part of a Reuben sandwich with baked tempeh, sauerkraut, and cheese on sprouted bread.*

savory snacks

We are a snack foods culture. Grab them on the go. Dip into a treat at that 3 p.m. to 4 p.m. energy slump. Many health-supportive alternatives can help you avoid processed, quick snack foods. They are tasty, simple, and easy to throw in your bag for those days on the go.

Snack Ideas

- **baked yam chips:** slice the yam and place on a baking sheet, bake for 20 to 25 minutes at 350 degrees.
- **carrot sticks with hummus:** a perfect blend of crunchiness and smoothness; make your own hummus or find spiced varieties made without preservatives at your natural food market.
- **edamame in a pod:** edible soybean found in frozen food section; defrost and sprinkle with sea salt.
- **fresh fruit:** an apple a day . . . so many different kinds, one day a granny smith the next a gala; or pick from what is in season: pears, plums, peaches, cherries, berries, or bananas.
- **granola:** a baked, crunchy mixture of rolled oats, nuts, dried fruit, and honey or maple syrup; eat on its own or with yogurt or nut milk.
- **mochi:** a traditional Japanese treat like puff pastry without wheat or flour, made from cooked, pureed rice and can be found in the refrigerator section of your health food store in savory and sweet flavors.
- **nori sheets:** found in the seaweed section of your health food store or Asian market; try nori with leftover brown rice or use it as a wrap for veggies.
- **rice cakes with nut butter:** spread any nut butter (try almond, peanut, or cashew) on these light crispy cakes.
- **trail mix:** a custom blend of nuts, seeds, and dried fruit, which offers a great protein boost.

- **various nuts and seeds:** cashews, peanuts, walnuts, tamari almonds, dry-roasted pumpkin or sunflower seeds.
- **yogurt:** try cow, goat, sheep, or soy; buy plain and add your own topping like jam, fresh fruit, granola, or maple syrup.

Afternoon Pick-Me-Up

Prep Time: 5 minutes
Cooking Time: none!
Serves 1

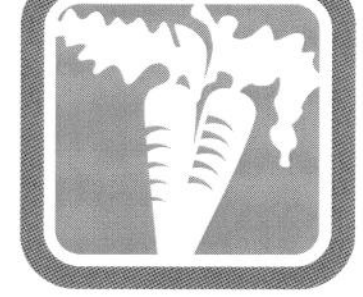

3 carrots or 12 ounces carrot juice
1 tablespoon spirulina or chlorella powder

- If you have a juicer, juice 3 carrots.
- If you don't have a juicer, buy some fresh or bottled organic carrot juice.
- Put green powder into the juice and shake well.
- Drink slowly, and enjoy your energy.

TIP: *Try different types of green superfoods to see how they affect you differently. I find this combination helps when I'm crashing in the afternoon.*

Ball-o-Nuts

Soaking Time: a few hours
Prep Time: 10 minutes
Serves 10

6 dates
½ cup rolled oats
¾ cup almonds
½ cup sesame seeds
½ cup apple juice
½ cup brown rice syrup
¾ cup poppy seeds

- Soak dates with oats in water for a few hours, then drain excess water.
- Add all remaining ingredients except poppy seeds into a blender and blend until chunks become very small but are still apparent.
- Form little balls with the mixture, then roll in poppy seeds.

TIP: *You can also squeeze lemon or ginger juice into the mixture.*

Kale Chips

Prep Time: 10 minutes
Cooking Time: 10 minutes
Serves 10 or more

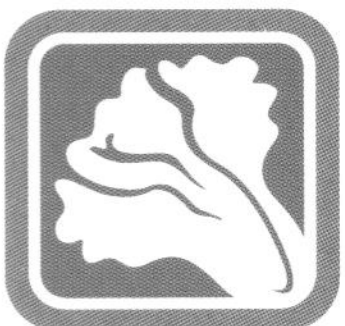

1 to 2 bunches kale
olive oil

- Preheat oven to 425 degrees.
- Remove kale from stalk, leaving the greens in large pieces.
- Place a little olive oil in a bowl, dip your fingers, and rub a very light coat of oil over the kale.
- Put kale on a baking sheet and bake for 5 minutes or until it starts to turn a bit brown. Keep an eye on it, as it can burn quickly.
- Turn the kale over and bake with the other side up. Remove and serve.

TIP: *For added flavor, sprinkle with a little salt or spice, such as curry or cumin, after rubbing on olive oil.*

Plantain Chips

Prep Time: 20 minutes
Cooking Time: 10 minutes
Serves 12

6 green plantains
juice of 6 limes
2 tablespoons coconut oil

- Peel and slice the plantains diagonally and very thin.
- Soak the slices in lime juice for 10 to 15 minutes.
- Dry thoroughly.
- Heat broiler.
- Toss plantains with coconut oil in a bowl. Make sure oil covers slices. (You may have to heat the oil just a bit so that it is not in solid form.)
- Place on a baking sheet and put under broiler for 3 to 5 minutes or until golden brown.
- Flip to the other side, and repeat.
- Store refrigerated in an airtight container once cooled down.
- They will keep for 1 week.

Veggie Muffins

Prep Time: 15 minutes
Cooking Time: 15 minutes
Serves 8

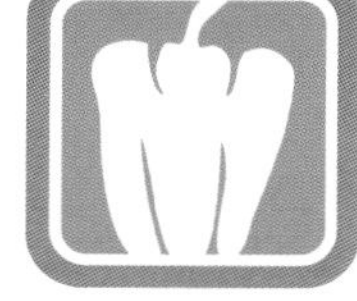

2 cups spelt flour
½ cup finely chopped fresh parsley
pinch of sea salt
2 beaten eggs
1 cup grated or finely chopped veggies
1 cup soy or rice milk

- Preheat oven to 325 degrees.
- Mix flour, parsley, and salt in a bowl.
- Make a well, add eggs and veggies.
- Mix lightly, gradually adding milk. This is supposed to be lumpy, so don't work too hard!
- Scrape into muffin tray that is lightly oiled.
- Bake for 12 to 15 minutes.
- Remove and allow to sit for 10 minutes, then serve.

Ants on a Log

Prep Time: 10 minutes
Serves 1

2 tablespoons almond butter
2 stalks celery
handful dried blueberries

- Wash celery.
- Spread nut butter inside each stalk.
- Dot with blueberries, or "ants."

TIP: *Try with any nut butter and any dried fruit that you like.*

Mixed Spicy Nuts

Prep Time: 5 minutes
Cooking Time: 15 minutes
Serves 8

2 cups mixed raw nuts—almonds, cashews, pecans
1 teaspoon coconut oil
1 tablespoon garam masala
1 teaspoon maple syrup
1 teaspoon sea salt

- Preheat oven to 300 degrees.
- In a bowl mix together nuts, oil, and maple syrup.
- Lay nuts on a cookie sheet and roast in the oven until lightly browned all over, about 15 minutes.
- Remove from heat and toss with garam masala and salt.

Guacamole with Jicama Sticks

Prep Time: 20 minutes
Serves 4

2 avocados
½ small red onion
1 small tomato
1 jalapeño pepper
¼ bunch cilantro
juice of one lime
½ teaspoon sea salt
1 large jicama

- Carefully cut open each avocado, remove the seed, and scoop out the meat into a mixing bowl.
- Finely dice the onion and tomato.
- Mince the jalapeño. Be careful, the seeds are hot!
- Mince the cilantro.
- Combine all ingredients by mashing and mixing with a fork in a mixing bowl.
- Peel the jicama and slice into sticks.
- Dip one into the guacamole to taste, and adjust seasonings as necessary.
- Enjoy!

Sautéed Edamame

Prep Time: 5 minutes
Cooking Time: 30 minutes
Serves 4

2 cups shelled edamame beans (get them pre-shelled in the frozen section)
1 tablespoon olive oil
½ teaspoons sea salt
juice of 1 lemon
2 tablespoons chopped cilantro
black pepper to taste

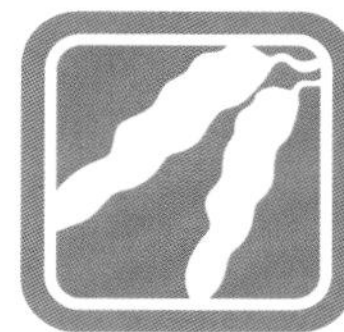

- Cook edamame in boiling water for 10 minutes.
- Drain beans and chill in the fridge for 10 minutes.
- Heat oil in a large sauté pan and sauté beans with salt for 5 minutes.
- Add lemon juice, cilantro and salt to taste.
- Mix well and serve hot.

Honey Sesame Treats

Prep Time: 5 minutes
Cooking Time: 10 minutes
Serves 8

¾ cup sesame seeds
1 ½ tablespoons raw honey

- Grind ½ cup sesame seeds in a coffee grinder or suribachi. Grind them well, but not so much that they become nut butter.
- Place in a bowl, add honey, and combine with a fork until it becomes a unified paste.
- Toast the rest of the seeds in a sauté pan for 5 minutes, stirring constantly until they turn golden brown.
- Transfer to a bowl.
- Make ½-inch balls out of the sesame paste and roll each ball in the toasted sesame seeds to coat.
- Eat warm or refrigerate.

desserts

Rice Pudding

Prep Time: 5 minutes
Cooking Time: 25 minutes
Serves 6

2 cups leftover cooked rice
1-2 cups coconut water,* rice milk, or water
1 cinnamon stick or 1 teaspoon ground cinnamon
10 cardamom pods or ½ teaspoon ground cardamom
½ cup raisins
½ cup shredded coconut
2 tablespoons raw honey or maple syrup

- Place all ingredients in a pot and bring to a boil.
- Reduce heat and simmer, stirring occasionally.
- Continue cooking until raisins are plump, coconut is soft, and most of the liquid has evaporated.
- Taste, and add more sweetener if necessary.

* Coconut water is simply the liquid inside a coconut. You can find it in the refrigerated drink section of the health food store. Also, you can often find fresh young coconuts in the health food store or in Asian markets.

Baked Bananas

Prep Time: 5 minutes
Cooking Time: 15 minutes
Serves 4

4 firm bananas
1 teaspoon olive oil
1-inch piece grated fresh ginger
1 tablespoon cinnamon
½ tablespoon nutmeg
½ cup raisins

- Preheat oven to 375 degrees.
- Peel and cut bananas in half lengthwise.
- Oil a baking pan and arrange bananas.
- Sprinkle with spices and raisins, cover, and bake for 10 to 15 minutes.

Mango Blueberry Sorbet

***Prep Time:* 5 minutes**
Serves 6

1 bag frozen mango
1 bag frozen cherries
1 tablespoon agave syrup or honey
¼ cup apple juice

- Put all ingredients into a blender or Vitamix.
- Blend until creamy, about one minute. You may have to scrape the sides of the machine down a few times if using a regular blender.
- Serve immediately.
- Put the rest in a freezer bowl and freeze to enjoy later.

TIP: *You can use any frozen fruits you like, or freeze fresh fruits such as bananas and strawberries.*

Melon, Avocados, and Figs

***Prep Time:* 15 minutes**
Serves 4

½ your favorite summer melon (cantaloupe, galia, ambrosia)
½ avocado
4 fresh ripe figs of your choice
2 tablespoons flax oil
1 tablespoon rice vinegar
1 teaspoon agave syrup
pinch of salt
1 tablespoon fresh mint, sliced into thin ribbons

- Slice fruit and arrange on a platter any way you like.
- Whisk together other ingredients.
- Pour sauce evenly over fruit.

TIP: *So delicious at the end of the summer, when melons and figs are both available!*

Tropical Breeze

Prep Time: 10 minutes
Serves 4

½ pineapple
1 cup plain yogurt
¼ cup dried coconut flakes

- Cut pineapple into bite-size chunks.
- Mix all ingredients together in a bowl and enjoy!

TIP: *This is the most simple and refreshing dessert to enjoy in warm weather. Depending on the sweetness of the pineapple, you may want to add a little honey.*

Kuzu: The Magic Sauce Thickener

Kuzu is a plant, originally from Japan. The white root is made into a powder that dissolves in cold water and becomes thick in hot water. It is all natural, with no bitter or sweet aftertaste. It has tremendous healing benefits in that it is alkalinizing and soothing, relieves stomach aches, controls diarrhea, helps relieve colds and flu, and restores overall strength.

Raisin Pudding

Prep Time: 5 minutes
Cooking Time: 25 minutes
Serves 4

1 cup raisins
2 cups water
1 teaspoon cinnamon
2 tablespoons kuzu

- In a saucepan, cook raisins in ½ cup water for 15 minutes.
- Add cinnamon.
- When finished cooking, blend in blender.
- Meanwhile, dissolve kuzu in 1 ½ cups water and mix in with blended raisins.
- Bring mixture back to saucepan and cook over medium heat for 5 more minutes.
- Dash with additional cinnamon and serve.

Almond Cherry Chocolate Pudding

Prep Time: 5 minutes
Cooking Time: 5 minutes
Serves 4

1 pint chocolate amazake
1 teaspoon almond extract
¼ cup chopped almonds, toasted
16 cherries, seeded and chopped
1 tablespoon kuzu root mixed with ¼ cup water

- Heat the amazake to just under boiling.
- Lower the heat, add vanilla, and stir in kuzu root. The amazake should thicken to the consistency of pudding.
- Pour the amazake into 4 pudding cups or small bowls.
- Sprinkle chopped nuts and cherries on top of each cup.
- Chill in the refrigerator for at least 30 minutes before serving.

Footnotes

CHAPTER 1

[1] Centers for Disease Control and Prevention. Death and Mortality. NCHS FastStats Web site. http://www.cdc.gov/nchs/fastats/deaths.htm

[2] Council on Foreign Relations, 2014. http://www.cfr.org/diseases-noncommunicable/NCDs-interactive/p33802?cid=otr-marketing_use-NCDs_interactive/#!/.

[3] Council on Foreign Relations, 2014. http://www.cfr.org/diseases-noncommunicable/NCDs-interactive/p33802?cid=otr-marketing_use-NCDs_interactive/#!/.

[4] Dr. Margaret Chan. "Adult Obesity Facts," Centers for Disease Control and Prevention, August 2012.

[5] World Health Organization. European Health Report 2015. http://www.euro.who.int/en/data-and-evidence/european-health-report/european-health-report-2015/ehr2015.

[6] National Center for Health Statistics. Health, United States, 2015: With Special Feature on Racial and Ethnic Health Disparities. Hyattsville, MD. 2016.

[7] Ying-xiu Zhang et al. "Trends in overweight and obesity among rural children and adolescents from 1985 to 2014 in Shandong, China" European Journal of Preventive Cardiology, Vol 23, Issue 12, 2016.

[8] World Disasters Report 2011, International Federation of Red Cross and Red Crescent Societies.

[9] World Health Organization. Diabetes fact sheet. http://www.who.int/mediacentre/factsheets/fs312/en/

[10] Ferlay J, Soerjomataram I, Ervik M, Dikshit R, Eser S, Mathers C, Rebelo M, Parkin DM, Forman D, Bray, F. GLOBOCAN 2012 v1.1, Cancer Incidence and Mortality Worldwide: IARC CancerBase No. 11. Lyon, France: International Agency for Research on Cancer; 2014.

[11] Mozaffarian D, et al. on behalf of the American Heart Association Statistics Committee and Stroke Statistics Subcommittee. Heart disease and stroke statistics – 2016 update: a report from the American Heart Association, December 16, 2015.

[12] Ibid.

[13] *Confronting Costs*, The Commonwealth Fund, January 10, 2013.

[14] World Health Organization. "*Health Systems Financing: The Path to Universal Coverage*," World Health Report 2010. http://www.who.int/whr/2010/en/

[15] Organisation for Economic Co-operation and Development (OECD), "OECD Reviews of Health Care Quality: Australia 2015. Raising Standards." http://www.oecd.org/australia/oecd-reviews-of-health-care-quality-australia-2015-9789264233836-en.htm

[16] Briefing Note USA, The Organization for Economic Co-operation and Development, 2012.

[17] *Dying for Coverage: The Deadly Consequences of Being Uninsured*, Families USA, June 2012.11 2012 Employer Health Benefits Survey, The Henry J. Kaiser Family Foundation.

[18] Makary, Martin A. Medical error—the third leading cause of death in the US, BMJ, 2016.

[19] *National Scorecard on U.S. Health System Performance*, The Commonwealth Fund, 2011.

[20] Marion Nestle, *Food Politics: How the Food Industry Influences Nutrition and Health* (University of California Press, 2003).

[21] *Food and Drink Weekly*, April 25, 2005.

[22] Fortune 500, 2012, Industry: Food Consumer Products.

[23] McDonald's Corporation, 2012 Annual Report, February 2013.

[24] Opensecrets.org, the website for The Center for Responsive Politics.

[25] D. M. Finkelstein, E. L. Hill, and R. C. Whitaker, "School Food Environments and Policies in US Public Schools." Pediatrics, vol. 122, no. 1, July 1, 2008, e251–e259.

[26] Mary Story, Karen M. Kaphingst, and Simone French, "The Role of Schools in Obesity Prevention," *The Future of Children*, vol. 16, no. 1, Spring 2006.

[27] Alexander Besant, "Pepsi Launches High-Fiber, Fat-Burning Soda in Japan," *GlobalPost*, November 12, 2012.

[28] Bruce L. Gardner, *American Agriculture in the Twentieth Century: How It Flourished and What It Cost* (Cambridge: Harvard University Press, 2002).

[29] United States Senate Committee on Agriculture, Nutrition & Forestry, Agriculture Reform, Food and Jobs Act of 2013.

[30] Patrick Leahy, S. 3240 (2012).

[31] Frank Lucas, www.opensecrets.org.

[32] *The Use of Medicines in the United States: Review of 2010*, IMS Institute for Healthcare Informatics, April 2011.

[33] Centers for Disease Control and Prevention. NCHS Data Brief No. 81, December 2011. https://www.cdc.gov/nchs/products/databriefs/db81.htm

[34] Youyoung Lee, "Celebrity Overdoses: Deaths Highlight Prescription Drug Epidemic," *Huffington Post*, August 28, 2012.

CHAPTER 2

[1] World Health Organization. Depression fact sheet. http://www.who.int/mediacentre/factsheets/fs369/en/

[2] Centers for Disease Control and Prevention. NCHS Data Brief No. 76, October 2011. https://www.cdc.gov/nchs/products/databriefs/db76.htm

[3] "U.S. Weight Loss Market Forecast to Hit $66 Billion in 2013," PRweb, December 2012.

[4] Adapted from *The Self-Healing Cookbook* by Kristen Turner.

CHAPTER 3

[1] "Phytochemicals: The Cancer Fighters in the Foods We Eat," American Institute for Cancer Research, 2013.

[2] "Industry Statistics and Projected Growth," Organic Trade Association, June 2011. UPDATE: "U.S. organic sales post new record of $43.3 billion in 2015," Organic Trade Association, May 2016.

[3] *Journal of Agricultural and Food Chemistry*, February 26, 2003, originally published on American Chemical Society's website on January 25, 2003.

[4] "Prop 37 Cheat Sheet: Labeling Genetically Engineered Foods," KCET.

[5] "Genetically Engineered Foods," Whole Foods Market.

[6] "Amazon Destruction: Why Is the Rainforest Being Destroyed in Brazil?" www.mongabay.com

[7] "Zero Net Deforestation by 2020," WWF Global Climate Policy.

CHAPTER 4

[1] Rupert Wheldon, *No Animal Food* (The Health Culture Company, 1910), 11–12.

[2] Claire Suddath, "A Brief History of Veganism," *Time*, October 30, 2008.

CHAPTER 5

[1] Dan Buettner, "The Island Where People Forget to Die," *New York Times*, October 24, 2012.

[2] Dan Buettner, "Power 9: Reverse Engineering Longevity," https://bluezones.com/2016/11/power-9/

[3] Daphne Miller, *The Jungle Effect* (HarperCollins, 2009).

[4] Fernando Martínez, *Why Did McDonald's Bolivia Go Bankrupt?*, 2011.

[5] "Bolivia—McDonald's Is Melted by Public Disinterest and Closes All Its Premises," *El Polvorin*, December 19, 2011.

[6] "Global and Regional Food Consumption Patterns and Trends," World Health Organization, 2013.

[7] Ewen Callaway, "Pottery Shards Put a Date on Africa's Dairying," *Nature*, June 22, 2012.

[8] Singhal Arvind, "India's Growing Appetite for Meat Challenges Traditional Values," AFP.

[9] Eliza Barclay, "Nordic Diet Could Be Local Alternative to Mediterranean Diet," NPR, *The Salt* (blog), May 31, 2013.

[10] Steve Inskeep and Maria Godoy, "Za'atar: A Spice Mix with Biblical Roots and Brain Food Reputation," NPR, *The Salt* (blog), June 11, 2013.

[11] Candido Astrologo Jr., "Statistical Indicators on Philippine Development," National Statistics Coordination Board (NSCB), 2008 Survey.

[12] "Health Benefits of Thai Soup Under Study," January 3, 2001.

[13] "10 Reasons to Add Bee Pollen to Your Diet," *The Fresh Network Blog*, January 17, 2013.

[14] Sophie D. Coe and Michael D. Coe, *The True History of Chocolate* (Thames & Hudson, 2013).

[15] Teya Skae, "Examining the Properties of Chocolate and Cacao for Health," *Natural News*, February 7, 2008.

[16] Lindsey Duncan, "Chia: Ancient Super-Seed Secret." www.droz.com

[17] David Wolfe, *Superfoods: The Food and Medicine of the Future* (North Atlantic Books, 2009).

[18] Ibid.

[19] Gero Leson and Walter Russell, "The Amazing Benefits of Hemp Seeds: Too Bad the DEA Is Curtailing the Industry," alternet.org, October 26, 2012.

[20] "Quinoa," The World's Healthiest Foods. www.whfoods.com

[21] "Manuka Honey," WebMD. www.webmd.com

[22] "Superfoods for 2012." www.drlindsey.com

CHAPTER 6

[1] Stephen D. Anton, Jacqueline Gallagher, Vincent J. Carey, Nancy Laranjo, Jing Cheng, Catherine M. Champagne, Donna H. Ryan, Kathy McManus, Catherine M. Loria, George A. Bray, Frank M. Sacks, and Donald A. Williamson, "Diet Type and Changes in Food Cravings following Weight Loss: Findings from the POUNDS LOST Trial," Eat Weight Disord. 2012.

[2] "Katie Fesler, The Craving Brain," *TuftsNow*, 2014.

[3] Sanjay Basu, Paula Yoffe, Nancy Hills, and Robert H. Lustig, "The Relationship of Sugar to Population-Level Diabetes Prevalence: An Econometric Analysis of Repeated Cross-Sectional Data," *PLOS ONE*, vol. 8, no. 2, 2013.

CHAPTER 7

[1] The Study of Adult Development. http://www.adultdevelopmentstudy.org

[2] Shen, Helen, "Neuroscience: The hard science of oxytocin," *Nature*, June 24, 2015.

[3] James Vlahos, "Is Sitting a Lethal Activity?" *New York Times*, April 14, 2011.

[4] Global Entrepreneurship Monitor 2015/2016 Global Report.

[5] "Women Entrepreneurs Thriving Worldwide," GEM News, Nov 18, 2015. http://www.gemconsortium.org/about/news

[6] Kerry Hannon, "Are Senior Start-Ups The Answer?" Forbes.com, September 9, 2012.

[7] Koenig, Harold G. "Religion, Spirituality, and Health: The Research and Clinical Implications," IRSN Psychiatry, Volume 2012.

CHAPTER 8

[1] Alyssa Oursler, "The Best-Selling Candy Brands of 2012," InvestorPlace.com, September 18, 2012.

[2] "Childhood Obesity Facts," Centers for Disease Control and Prevention, 2013.

[3] "BLS American Time Use Survey," A.C. Nielsen Co.

[4] Amanda Bruce, Rebecca Lepping, Jared Bruce, Bradley Cherry, Laura Martin, Ann Davis, et al., "Brain Responses to Food Logos in Obese and Healthy Weight Children," *Journal of Pediatrics*, vol. 162, issue 4, 2013.

[5] Dawn C. Chmielewski, "Disney Bans Junk-Food Advertising on Programs for Children," *Los Angeles Times*, June 6, 2012.

[6] South Carolina Department of Mental Health, "Eating Disorder Statistics," 2011.

[7] Galia Slayen, "The Scary Reality of a Real-Life Barbie Doll," *Huffington Post*, April 8, 2011.

CHAPTER 9

[1] John G. Rodwan Jr., "Bottled Water 2011: The Recovery Continues." www.bottledwater.org

[2] Jared Blumenfeld and Susan Leal, "The High Costs of Bottled Water," *San Francisco Chronicle*, February 18, 2007.

[3] Eurídice Martínez Steele, et al. "Ultra-processed foods and added sugars in the US diet: evidence from a nationally representative cross-sectional study," BMJ Open. http://bmjopen.bmj.com/content/6/3/e009892

[4] Vinícius Pedrazzi, et al. "Tongue-cleaning methods: a comparative clinical trial employing a toothbrush and a tongue scraper," National Center for Biotechnology Information. https://www.ncbi.nlm.nih.gov/pubmed/15341360?_ga=1.134415671.756900894.1483547473

[5] "10 facts on physical activity," World Health Organization. http://www.who.int/features/factfiles/physical_activity/en/

[6] The Peninsula College of Medicine and Dentistry. "Benefits of outdoor exercise confirmed" ScienceDaily, February 5, 2011. https://www.sciencedaily.com/releases/2011/02/110204130607.htm

[7] Do We Need a Daily Practice? https://www.ramdass.org/need-daily-practice

CHAPTER 10

[1] Alice G. Walton. "How Much Sugar Are Americans Eating?" Forbes.com, August 30, 2012.

[2] "Broccoli profile," USDA Economic Research Service, 2011.

[3] Walton, "How Much Sugar Are Americans Eating?"

[4] "The Global Burden," International Diabetes Federation, *Diabetes Atlas*, fifth edition.

[5] Basu, et al., "Relationship of Sugar to Population-Level Diabetes Prevalence." Notes 369

[6] Magalie Lenoir, Fuschia Serre, Lauriane Cantin, and Serge H. Ahmed, "Intense Sweetness Surpasses Cocaine Reward," *PLOS ONE*, vol. 2, no. 8, 2007.

[7] Qing Yang, "Gain Weight by 'Going Diet'? Artificial Sweeteners and the Neurobiology of Sugar Cravings," *Yale Journal of Biology and Medicine*, vol. 82, no. 2, 2010.

[8] David Barbano, "BST Fact Sheet," FDA Connection.

[9] "Quality Low Impact Food," Danish Institute of Agricultural Sciences and University of Newcastle.

[10] B. J. Abelow, T. R. Holford, and K. L. Insogna, "Cross-Cultural Association Between Dietary Animal Protein and Hip Fractures: A Hypothesis," *Calcified Tissue International* (Yale, 1992).

[11] "WHO Issues New Guidance on Dietary Salt and Potassium," World Health Organization. http://www.who.int/mediacentre/news/notes/2013/salt_potassium_20130131/en/

[12] "Raised Blood Pressure," World Health Organization, Global Health Observatory, 2013.

[13] "Who Consumes the Most Chocolate?" CNN Freedom Project, January 17, 2012.

CHAPTER 11

[1] FairShare CSA Coalition. www.csacoalition.org

[2] Ibid.

Index

B

C

E

F

G

H

I

J

K

N

O

P

Q

R

S

T

U

V

W

Y

Z

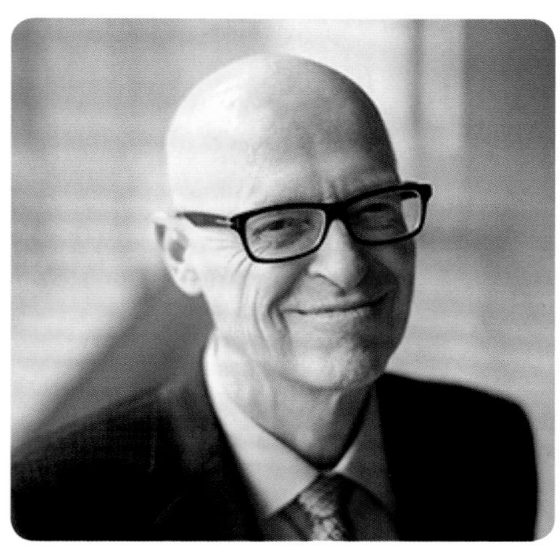

About the Author

Joshua Rosenthal is the founder, director, and primary teacher of the Institute for Integrative Nutrition (IIN)®, the world's largest nutrition school, based in New York City. His innovative whole-body approach to holistic nutrition has made him a highly respected thought leader in the health and wellness space. Joshua's revolutionary concepts and teaching methods allow people to quickly and successfully reach new levels of health and happiness. Joshua holds a Master of Science degree in Education, specializing in counseling, and has over 30 years of experience in the fields of whole foods, personal coaching, curriculum development, teaching, and nutritional counseling.

About the Institute for Integrative Nutrition

Founded in 1992, the Institute for Integrative Nutrition (IIN) has led the field of holistic nutrition education for more than 25 years and pioneered the concept of a Health Coach as a career. The mission of IIN is to play a crucial role in improving health and happiness, and, through that process, create a ripple effect that transforms the world. Its Health Coach Training Program allows students from all over the world to earn a Health Coach certificate. Today, 100,000 students in 155 countries have gone through the program.

A primary concept of the curriculum is "bio-individuality," which means that no one diet works for everyone. Each and every person has unique needs.

As a result, IIN is the only school in the world integrating multiple dietary theories—combining the knowledge of traditional philosophies like Ayurveda, macrobiotics, and Chinese medicine with modern concepts like the USDA food guides, raw foods, anti-inflammatory and gluten-free diets, and diets supporting gut and brain health. In total, the curriculum covers more than 100 different dietary theories and addresses fundamental concepts, issues, and ethics of eating in a modern world. In addition, the curriculum bridges the gap between nutrition and personal growth and development through a concept called "primary food." Healthy relationships, regular physical activity, fulfilling careers, and a spiritual practice feed your soul and satisfy your hunger for living. When primary food is balanced, the fun, excitement, love, and passion of your daily life nourish you on a deeper level than the food you eat.

The Health Coach Training Program also features course material on coaching techniques and running a successful business. The goal of the program is to not only provide the critical knowledge necessary to counsel others on nutrition, but to be an effective coach and business owner as well. The school is a place of profound learning, with guest teachers who are the world's greatest nutrition and personal development experts, including Dr. Barry Sears, Dr. Joan Borysenko, Dr. Deepak Chopra, Dr. Andrew Weil, Dr. Lissa Rankin, and Geneen Roth.

IIN graduates partner with physicians, chiropractors, fitness facilities, spas, schools, restaurants, retail stores, publishers, and corporations and work in private practice. For more information about IIN, visit www.integrativenutrition.com.